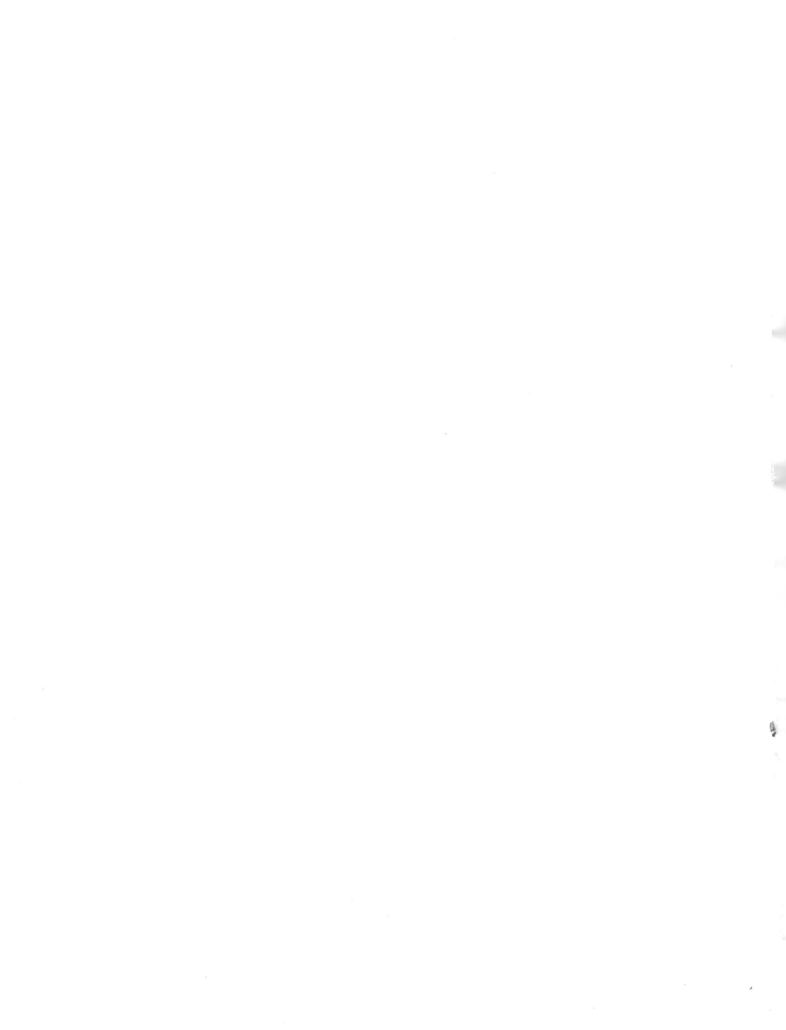

BUILDING MUSCLE AND PERFORMANCE

A Program for Size, Strength & Speed

Nick Tumminello

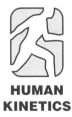

**HUMAN
KINETICS**

Library of Congress Cataloging-in-Publication Data

Tumminello, Nick.
Building muscle and performance : a program for size, strength & speed /
  Nick Tumminello.
Building muscle & performance
Champaign, IL : Human Kinetics, [2016] | Includes
  bibliographical references and index.
LCCN 2015042714 | ISBN 9781492512707 (print)
LCSH: Weight training. | Muscle strength. | Speed. | Physical
  fitness--Physiological aspects.
LCC GV546 .T86 2016 | DDC 613.7/13--dc23 LC record available at http://lccn.loc.gov/2015042714

ISBN: 978-1-4925-1270-7 (print)

Acquisitions Editor: Justin Klug; **Developmental Editor:** Laura Pulliam; **Managing Editor:** Nicole Moore; **Copyeditor:** Tom Tiller; **Senior Graphic Designer:** Fred Starbird; **Graphic Designer:** Tara Welsch; **Cover Designer:** Keith Blomberg; **Photograph (cover):** © MR.BIG-PHOTOGRAPHY/iStock.com; **Photographs (interior):** Neil Bernstein; **Visual Production Assistant:** Joyce Brumfield; **Photo Production Manager:** Jason Allen; **Art Manager:** Kelly Hendren; **Associate Art Manager:** Alan L. Wilborn; **Printer:** Sheridan Books

We thank BB3 Fitness & Nutrition Center at Bonaventure Resort & Spa in Weston, Florida, for assistance in providing the location for the photo shoot for this book. We also thank Varisport, Inc., for providing the Ultraslide Slideboard for the photo shoot for this book.

Human Kinetics books are available at special discounts for bulk purchase. Special editions or book excerpts can also be created to specification. For details, contact the Special Sales Manager at Human Kinetics.

Printed in the United States of America   10 9 8 7 6 5 4 3 2 1

The paper in this book is certified under a sustainable forestry program.

Human Kinetics
Website: www.HumanKinetics.com

United States: Human Kinetics
P.O. Box 5076
Champaign, IL 61825-5076
800-747-4457
e-mail: info@hkusa.com

Canada: Human Kinetics
475 Devonshire Road Unit 100
Windsor, ON N8Y 2L5
800-465-7301 (in Canada only)
e-mail: info@hkcanada.com

Europe: Human Kinetics
107 Bradford Road
Stanningley
Leeds LS28 6AT, United Kingdom
+44 (0) 113 255 5665
e-mail: hk@hkeurope.com

Australia: Human Kinetics
57A Price Avenue
Lower Mitcham, South Australia 5062
08 8372 0999
e-mail: info@hkaustralia.com

New Zealand: Human Kinetics
P.O. Box 80
Mitcham Shopping Centre, South Australia 5062
0800 222 062
e-mail: info@hknewzealand.com

E6585

This book is dedicated to my mother, Faith Bevan, and my father, Dominic Tumminello. Although you both have very different outlooks on life and on raising me, you both have done one thing the same: being not just a wonderful and loving parent but also a best friend to me.

I'd also like to dedicate this book to my late grandmothers, Rita Whitehouse and Mary Jane Tumminello. From the day I was born until the day each of them passed on, they spoiled me and always made me feel as if their world revolved around me. And that's the kind of love that every kid should grow up with.

CONTENTS

PART III Workout Programs

PREFACE

You want more muscle. That's what most people are in the gym for. This book will help you get the muscle—and far more. The hybrid training concepts and workout programs will improve your athletic performance and boost your conditioning while you pack on muscle.

You most likely don't want to be all show and no go. You're looking to get stronger and build a better-looking body that can also get things done. Achieving that requires a comprehensive mixture of both muscle- and performance-based training. That's what separates this book from the rest: It gives you the best of both worlds, whereas most books on building muscle are essentially bodybuilding books that neglect the performance and conditioning components. The training strategies and workouts will challenge you on multiple levels so you will build the physique you're after while improving your overall athleticism. So, not only will you look better, but you can also be better at every athletic pursuit in your sight. It won't be easy. Hard work and consistency are what you need for growth and improvement.

Put simply, improving your physique and performance, along with your overall health, requires several training components because no single type of training will address all demands. With that reality in mind, it makes sense that taking a mixed approach to exercise programming—an approach that uses the entire functional spectrum of training—will give you better results than you'd get by using only one training method.

The concept of functional training has long been an area of great confusion, at times even heated debate. As hot button a topic as it is, functional training is a subject worthy of intelligent discussion, which is exactly what chapter 1, Functional-Spectrum Training, provides. Chapter 1 defines what functional training truly is, and especially what it isn't. From there, you'll learn about the sources of the confusion and separate the sense from the nonsense. You'll discover the four types of foundational exercises in the functional-spectrum training system and the benefits and limitations of each type of exercise. Every workout program in this book uses all four types of exercises.

Chapter 2, Building Muscle, Increasing Strength, presents the three Ss of the functional-spectrum training system—speed, strength, and size—that the resistance training portion of all the workout programs in this book will help you improve. It describes the scientific principles behind the practical applications used in the functional-spectrum training system and workout programs to enhance each quality.

In chapter 3, Cardio Conditioning, you'll learn how to incorporate polarized training to improve your endurance to complement the speed-, strength-, and size-oriented training. Supramaximal interval training (SMIT), steady-state cardio, metabolic conditioning protocols, and a variety of exercise applications for each protocol are presented.

Chapters 4 through 7 detail training for the upper and lower body, including the core. These chapters contain a variety of total-body exercise applications, cross-body exercise applications, compound exercise applications, and isolation exercise applications using all the training tools—medicine balls, barbells, dumbbells, kettlebells, cables, machines and body weight. You'll also learn about the "Core 4" and some common myths in core training.

In chapter 8, Warm-Up and Cool-Down, you'll get a variety of warm-up sequences and self-massage drills that will bookend your workouts and make your training well rounded.

The workout programs in chapter 9, Foundational Programming, will help you build a solid training foundation to ensure your body is ready to safely perform the more intense workouts using the three Ss of the functional-spectrum training system. Four phases of workout programs ensure you begin with the appropriate workout phase for your current training level.

When you've developed your training base or if you're an advanced exerciser, chapters 10, 11, and 12 present five training programs, each consisting of three workouts that you can do three, four, or five times per week. Because some people train only twice per week, these chapters include three program variations consisting of two workouts.

The programs in chapter 10, Performance Programming, emphasize improvements in performance while still having a concern for muscle. The programs in chapter 11, Muscle Programming, emphasize improvements in muscle while still having a concern for performance. The programs in chapter 12, Performance and Muscle Programming, address both without emphasizing one over the other.

Keep in mind the titles of chapters 10 and 11 refer to the main focus of the workout programs in each chapter, but overall, the functional-spectrum training system is a mixed-training (i.e., hybrid) approach. In all workout programs in chapters 10, 11, and 12, you'll get a mixture of exercise applications that enhance each of the three Ss along with some cardio work. What separates the workout programs in each of these chapters is the order in which each S is addressed and the amount of time you spend on each, which can be manipulated based on which physical qualities the program emphasizes.

Finally, in chapter 13, Customizing Programs for Personal Results, you'll review the five principles and guidelines of safety and exercise selection you should apply, regardless of training goal, in order to tailor workouts to suit your needs and to ensure that you continue to achieve the best training results—whether you're using the workout programs provided or designing your own workouts based on the training concepts and techniques you've learned in this book.

Each chapter can be used as a stand-alone resource for scientifically founded programming concepts and training techniques. If you're an inexperienced exerciser, you will appreciate the step-by-step presentation on muscle and performance training. If you're an advanced exerciser, fitness professional, or sport coach, you will certainly recognize the effectiveness of the training methods and will gain exciting new ideas, insights, and organizational strategies for hybrid training. If you want the muscle and the hustle while also learning what will help you get the most out of your training time and enjoy every workout, read on.

ACKNOWLEDGMENTS

This book would not be possible if it weren't for my exercise models: Korin Sutton, Megan Supko, Jay Bozios, and Jaclyn Gough (who is also my beautiful girlfriend who gives me unwavering support). Or if it weren't for my great friend and one of the best trainers I know, Billy Beck, who allowed us to do the photo shoot at his facility, the BB3 Training Center in Weston, Florida. And the Human Kinetics family—with special thanks to Justin Klug, Laura Pulliam, Neil Bernstein, Nicole Moore, and Sue Outlaw—for giving me the opportunity to share a piece of myself and the Performance University training concepts and techniques with the fitness world. It's truly an honor to work with these professionals in bringing this project to life.

And to all the people in the fitness and performance training field or related fields, I owe them a debt of gratitude for their friendship, continued support of my work, and help in my professional growth, I'm reminded that there's no such thing as a self-made person: Marc Spataro, Kate Grevey Blankenship, John Rallo, John Cavaliere, Gary Stasny, Mark Simon, James "Binky" Jones, Ryan Mackin, Rick Desper, Nick Clayton, Brad Schoenfeld, Jim Kielbaso, Bert Sorin, Richard Sorin, Peter Bognanno, Andrew Connor, Matt Paulson, Mike T. Nelson, Mike Bates, Ryan Ketchum, Nick Bromberg, Lindsay Vastola, Eric Cressey, Jonathan Ross, Bret Contreras, Alan Aragon, Lou Schuler, Luke Johnson, Chris Burgess, Mark Comerford, Bob and Ron Rossetti, Greg Presto, Sean Hyson, Vince McConnell, Billy Beck, Jason Silvernail, Lars Avemarie, Bill Sonnemaker, Cassandra Forsythe, David Barr, Justin Kompf, Spencer Nadolsky, Jose Antonio, Gunnhildur Vilbergsdóttir, Helgi Gudfinnsson, James Fell, Tony Gentilcore, Dan Blewett, Jennifer Widerstrom, Amy Rushlow, Aleisha Fetters, Dave Parise, Stephen Holt, Marie Spano, David Jack, Charles Staley, Quinn Sypniewski, Luka Hocevar, Jonathan Goodman, Claudia Micco, Espen Arntzen, Sally Tamarkin, Steve Weatherford, Juma Iraki, Andrew Heffernan, Jose Seminario, John Spencer Ellis, Bryan Krahn, Stacey Veronica Schaedler, Sibilla Abukhaled, Adam Bornstein, Ann Gilbert, Ethan and Liz Benda, Lee Boyce, John Meadows, Nick Ng, Jonathan Mike, Kara Silva, Robert Linkul, Per Gronnas, Micheal Easter, Ray Klerck, Sean Huddleston, Lavanya Krishnan, Ryan Huether, Jen Sinkler, James Krieger, Kimberly Mills, Louie Guarino, Brandon Poe, Nick Collias, Lisa Steuer, Ann-Marie Saccurato, Chad Landers, Jennifer Cavallero, Ben Brewster, Susan Singer, Leah Lyons, David Crump, Rob Simonelli, Deanna Avery, Paul Christopher, and Joe Drake. I'm sure there are people that I'm leaving out whose names deserve to be on this list. And, I owe those people a big handshake and a hug.

Taking existing ideas and building something new with it or putting your own spin on it is just how art works. And training is the art of applying the science. So, if you build a chair you certainly don't owe the first chair builder money, but you do owe those that came before you and influenced you your gratitude and recognition for paving the way. That said, there have been several people that have influenced my training approach and philosophies: Bruce Lee, Mel Siff, Juan Carlos Santana, Paul Chek, Mark Comerford, Gary Gray, Vern Gambetta, Mike Boyle, Alwyn Cosgrove, Gray Cook, and Michael Clark. There's plenty that I disagree with from each of these individuals—some more than others—but that doesn't change the fact that the information each of these people has worked hard to provide has influenced me in some way, shape, or form.

I also owe a big debt of gratitude to everyone at Reebok, Hylete, Sorinex Exercise Equipment, and VersaClimber for supporting my work over the years and for providing me with the best fitness apparel and training equipment on the planet.

Finally, I thank all of my clients—past, present, and future—for allowing me to continue to do what I love.

PART I

Principles and Rationale

1
Functional-Spectrum Training

Resistance training is a multifactorial endeavor that helps athletes achieve multiple goals. If done right, it not only improves the athlete's overall health, but also builds both muscle and general athletic capability. When pursuing these multiple goals, one can achieve better training results by taking a mixed approach than by using only one type of exercise; in fact, the best results are achieved by using the entire functional spectrum of resistance exercise.

For this purpose, I have developed the functional-spectrum training system, which forms the foundation of this book. The system uses four primary types of resistance-training exercise: total-body power, cross-body, compound, and isolation. Each of these types, much like each unique style of martial arts training, benefits the athlete in areas where the other types fall short. In order to talk about the system in greater depth, we must first define the word *functional* in terms of exercise and performance.

What Is Functional Training?

The word *functional* is commonly used in the fitness and performance-training community. The problem is—does anyone really know what it means in relation to strength and conditioning? Despite the uncertainty, however, let's not fall for the nonsense (put forth by many trainers and coaches) that *functional* is meaningless just because "it means different things to different people." The word *strength* also means different things to different people, but no one says it's meaningless. The different treatment given to these two words creates logical inconsistency. To clear the air, let's avoid blindly repeating what others are saying and start thinking with consistent logic.

In school, we were taught to understand a word's meaning by looking it up in the dictionary—not by making up our own definition. That would cause chaos and confusion, which is the case with the often-contradictory ways in which *functional* is used in the fitness and performance training community. To resolve that confusion, *functional* is used in this book not as a buzzword but in a manner consistent with its accepted, dictionary definition. When the word is used in that way, the term *functional training* refers to a meaningful, legitimate, and fundamental training concept.

Let's start by defining exactly what functional training is—and what it is not. The word *functional* applies to something that has a special task or purpose; therefore, the term has nothing to do with what an exercise *looks* like or with the type of equipment used to perform it. Rather, functional training for improved human performance involves applying the principle of specificity to improve in special (i.e., specific) athletic actions (i.e., tasks).

The principle of specificity holds that adaptations to training are specific to imposed training demands. For instance, in order to maximize improvement in pushing performance while standing, you've got to use standing exercises for pushing. This is the case because the common bench-press and the standing-press actions in sport involve very different patterns of force production and neuromuscular coordination (more on this a bit later). In short, it is legitimate to gear training toward improving specific, targeted sport movements by working to improve specific force-generation and neuromuscular coordination patterns that transfer into the targeted movement actions. In fact, this approach is as legitimate a training concept as you can get.

Transfer for Improved Performance

The goal of exercise programming for enhanced human performance is to maximize training transfer. Some exercises provide obvious and direct transfer to improved performance in sporting actions and overall functional capacity, whereas others provide less obvious transfer—that is, indirect transfer.

Functional capacity is one's range of ability; in other words, higher functional capacity means that a person can perform a broader range of specific tasks. Within this framework, the four primary types of exercise addressed in the functional-spectrum training system (again, total-body power, cross-body, compound, and isolation) are each classified as either *specific* or *general* based on how they transfer functionally. These two categories of exercise—specific and general—offer different benefits; more specifically, each type benefits certain interdependent components of fitness and performance that the other category may miss.

Specific Exercises

Specific exercises provide obvious and direct transfer to improved performance and functional capacity because they are based on the principle of specificity. That principle has been defined as follows by Dr. Everett Harman in the National Strength and Conditioning Association's *Essentials of Strength Training and Conditioning* (2000, 25-55)

> "The concept of specificity, widely recognized in the field of resistance training, holds that training is most effective when resistance exercises are similar to the sport activity in which improvement is sought (the target activity). Although all athletes should use well-rounded, whole-body exercise routines, supplementary exercises specific to the sport can provide a training advantage. The simplest and most straightforward way to implement the principle of specificity is to select exercises similar to the target activity with regard to the joints about which movement occur and the direction of the movements. In addition, joint ranges of motion in the training should be at least as great as those in the target activity." [1]

Specific exercises create a more ideal environment than general exercises for enhancing the specific force-generation and neuromuscular-coordination patterns of the targeted athletic movements.

General Exercises

General exercises are essentially conventional strength-training exercises and may consist of either compound or isolation movements using free weights, cables, or machines. In most cases, general exercises create a more ideal environment than specific exercises for stimulating increases in overall muscle strength and size. Therefore, these applications offer general transfer into improvements in human performance by increasing muscle hypertrophy, motor-unit recruitment, bone density, and connective tissue strength, which can improve overall health and reduce injury risk.

On the other hand, because these exercises do not necessarily reflect the specific force-generation and neuromuscular coordination patterns of many common movements in athletics, their positive transfer into improved performance potential is less obvious. This fact has led some personal trainers and coaches into mistakenly labeling them as "nonfunctional" and therefore not valuable. That is a false belief.

Granted, the further an exercise gets away from replicating the specific force-generation patterns of a given movement, the less directly it carries over to improving the neuromuscular coordination of that movement. However, this fact doesn't make an exercise bad, and it certainly doesn't make it nonfunctional. It simply means that the less specific an exercise is, the more general it is.

For this reason, instead of referring to some exercises as "functional"—which implies that others are "nonfunctional"—it is more accurate (and less confusing) to refer to exercises as either general or specific. Each of these types offers a unique set of benefits that transfers into improvements in performance and overall functional capacity.

Common Confusion Associated With Specific Exercises

Working on sport skills with specific exercises is not the same thing as working to improve specific force-generation and neuromuscular coordination patterns, which transfer into targeted athletic movements. Unaware of this distinction, some strength and conditioning professionals advise athletes and clients to perform what they call "sport-specific exercises" or "functional exercises" by attaching a resistance band to the end of a golf club or hockey stick, for example, or shadow-boxing against bands strapped around the back. Loading specific sport skills in this manner misapplies the principle of specificity and rests on a misunderstanding of how to properly use specific exercises.

In reality, improving one's ability to perform certain sport skills is not about replicating what a specific movement *looks* like but about replicating the specific force-generation patterns involved in the movement pattern. In other words, when training focuses only on what an exercise looks like, one can easily make the mistake of loading sport-specific skills instead of working to improve the specific force-generation patterns used to perform sport movements.

The problem lies in the fact that sport movement skills involve accuracy components that are not just similar but exact. For example, consider studies of the use of weighted bats in baseball. Contrary to general public understanding, studies have found that the heavy bat not only alters the batter's perceptions of bat heaviness and swing speed, but also slows the batter's swing speed for as many as five swings after using the weighted bat (2,3)! Sure, some baseball players might prefer to "warm-up" by using a weighted bat, but the smart ones will also take several more swings with an unweighted bat to normalize themselves before stepping up to the plate.

You can test this effect for yourself: Shoot 10 free throws with a regular basketball, then take 10 more shots with a 2-to 4-pound (1 to 2 kg) medicine ball. You'll quickly find that the fine-motor pattern (i.e., skill) used to throw the heavier ball accurately is completely different, and your shots with that ball will likely come up short until you hone the pattern. After shooting with the medicine ball, go back to the normal basketball for 10 more shots. Your first few shots may go over the backboard because shooting the much lighter basketball involves a different fine-motor sequence than shooting the medicine ball.

The Four Types of Resistance Exercise

Improving both your physique and your overall athletic ability is a multifaceted goal that requires a multifaceted training approach. That is exactly what the functional-spectrum training system was developed to provide, and the programs presented in this book show you how to carry it out. The following sections detail the qualities of each of the four primary types of resistance exercise used in this training system, as well as their unique benefits, so that you know why the exercises are used as they are in the training programs provided later in the book.

Total-Body Power Exercises

Let's start with a simple equation: power = strength × speed. By definition, everything we do in life—in or out of the gym, on or off the field of competition—involves an expression of power. Whoever finished the marathon first produced the most power. Whoever does the most push-ups in a minute produces more power than anyone who does fewer. If your grandfather used to take two minutes to get up a flight of stairs but now, after working out, can do it in only one minute, then he's producing more power.

To prevent confusion, I want to be specific about this: Just about everything you do in your training can improve your ability to generate power. The goal of these total-body power exercises, however, is specifically to improve total-body *explosive* power. These exercises involve a coordinated effort by the entire body (the individual muscles added together) to summate force in an explosive manner. Athletic movements—whether throwing a punch; swinging a bat, club, or racket; or sprinting and jumping—are driven not by power generated in just one specific area of the body but by the combination of individual muscles producing power in a smooth, coordinated sequence.

Total-body power exercises use as many muscle as possible in a sequential and explosive (i.e., fast) manner to obtain maximal force in what I refer to as the three pillars of power:

- Vertical or diagonal power
- Horizontal power
- Rotational power

Though each sport involves its own unique set of skills, these three pillars of power provide the source for all explosive actions in athletics. That is, regardless of the skill being expressed, explosive sport movements involve a total-body expression of power that is primarily either vertical (or diagonal), horizontal, or rotational. Whether you're jumping up to catch a ball (the vertical or diagonal pillar), pushing an opponent backward (the horizontal pillar), or swinging a golf club (the rotational pillar), your power is initiated by the larger, stronger muscle groups in the central part of your body, whereas the smaller muscles of your extremities are used in fine movements and coordination (i.e., skills).

Total-body power exercises are categorized as *specific* exercises, not because they load the specific skills required in any given sport—you've already learned why loading sport skills is a mistake—but because they replicate the force-generation and neuromuscular coordination patterns that form the foundation of *all* explosive sport actions. For example, the rotation sequence (i.e., the rotational power pillar) is the same for swinging an implement (such as a racket, club, or bat) as for throwing a punch. Both actions involve producing force from the ground up, beginning with the legs and hips, followed by the trunk, and terminating with the arms, which handle the accuracy component (i.e., the individual sport skill).

For this reason, that same force-production sequence is used in all of the rotational-power exercise applications included in the functional-spectrum training system. Therefore, total-body power exercises enhance your body's ability to summate force using all of its levers—legs, hips, torso, and arms—in an explosive manner that transfers directly (functionally) into most explosive rotary actions, regardless of the individual sport skill being executed.

These total-body power exercises also closely match the force-production patterns of fast, ballistic, sport-type actions, which involve what is called a *triphasic* muscle-firing pattern. Whereas slow movements produce a single, continuous activation of the agonist muscles (i.e., the muscles creating the movement), research has shown that performing the same movements fast leads to a triphasic muscle-firing pattern of predominantly burst-like muscle activation (4,5,6). The triphasic muscle-firing pattern involves alternating bursts of muscle activation in agonist and antagonist muscles (i.e., the muscles that work counter to those muscles creating the movement). This sequence of activity begins with an agonist burst (AG1), which is followed 30 to 40 milliseconds later by an antagonist burst (ANT), which in turn is followed 30 to 40 milliseconds later by another agonist burst (AG2).

Research findings indicate that the triphasic muscle-activation pattern is always present during fast, ballistic movements. Therefore, the principle of specificity dictates that we incorporate fast, ballistic exercises into training in order to maximize our potential to safely and effectively perform a variety of fast, explosive athletic movements.

In short, the total-body power exercises used in the functional-spectrum training system enable you to train and potentially refine the triphasic muscle-firing pattern involved in high-speed actions, and to enhance your body's ability to summate force in an explosive manner, in all directions—vertically (or diagonally), horizontally, and rotationally. This is important because research also indicates that power and agility are direction-specific. As for both men and women, the single-leg vertical, horizontal, and lateral jump tests measure mostly *different* leg-power qualities. As a result, they should not be used interchangeably (7).

Cross-Body Exercises

The anatomical characteristics of the human body dictate that it commonly functions in a crisscross manner. More specifically, the arm-and-shoulder mechanism on one side links diagonally through the torso mechanism to the hip-and-leg mechanism on the opposite side. Consider, for example, the motions used in walking, running, punching, throwing, and batting. Such cross-body linkages are foundational to human functioning and thus are also a big part of athletic movement. For this reason, a variety of cross-body exercises are incorporated into the functional-spectrum training system, in which they are classified as *specific* exercises

Cross-body actions involve specific muscular relationships, which are often referred to by means of certain terms, such as the serape effect (8), and the posterior oblique sling (9). The serape effect was a term coined to describe the diagonal prestretch of four pairs of muscles (rhomboids, serratus anterior, external obliques, and internal obliques) that occurs when rotating the shoulders and hips in opposite directions. The pre-stretch of these four pairs of muscles creates a snap-back effect (like snapping a rubber-band), which increases force production and movement efficiency in rotational actions such as throwing or kicking.

Similarly, the posterior oblique sling is a term used to describe the interaction of the latissimus dorsi with the opposite gluteus maximus and biceps femoris through the thoracolumbar fascia and erector spinae during rotational actions and locomotion (i.e., walking, running, etc.)

On a broader scale, when we take into account the entirety of the muscular relationships responsible for the human body's various cross-body actions (which certainly involve more anatomical relationships than those identified within any such terms like the ones just described), we can refer to the collective interaction between these relationships as the body's *X factor*.

The unique benefit offered by the variety of cross-body exercises provided in this book lies in the consistency between these exercises and the patterns of force generation and neuromuscular coordination that commonly occur when movement involves the body's X-factor linkages. In that, these exercises use movements that involve single-arm loading or offset loading (e.g., two unevenly-loaded dumbbells) which either create rotation or force you to resist rotation from various stances. Although traditional compound exercises (e.g., barbell squat, barbell bench press) can help strengthen the entire body, they are not ideally suited for improving coordination of the X-factor linkages.

This reality is highlighted in research (10) comparing the single-arm standing cable press (a cross-body exercise) and the traditional bench press (a compound exercise). The study found that performance in the single-arm standing cable press is limited *not* by maximal muscle activation of the chest and shoulder muscles, but by the activation and neuromuscular coordination of the torso muscles. In other words, the limiting factor when pushing an offset load or with a single arm from a standing position—the position and manner from which field, court, and combat athletes commonly push during competition—is the stiffness of the torso muscles that maintain body position and enable coordination of the hips and shoulders while stabilizing the forces created by the extremities (arms and legs).

Granted, standing cross-body movements also rely on strength in the shoulder and chest musculature. This is true, for instance, of the standing single-arm cable press, which more closely resembles the standing push actions of athletics than does the bench press. However, in such cross-body movements, force generation is still limited *primarily* by whole-body stability, as well as joint stability (10).

In short, different load placement and body position during an exercise changes the force generation and neuromuscular coordination demands of the exercise. Cross-body exercises utilize a different type load placement and body position than compound exercises. The specific force generation and neuromuscular coordination demands of performing cross-body exercises more closely replicate those of athletic movements (e.g., running, punching, throwing, batting, golfing, etc.), therefore using cross-body exercises adds more specificity to one's training.

Compound Exercises

Simply put, compound exercises are multijoint movements that involve several muscle groups. These exercises consist primarily of traditional strength and bodybuilding lifts, such as squats, deadlifts, bench presses, chin-ups, and rows. Compound exercises can be classified as general exercises because they don't necessarily reflect any specific force-generation patterns. Rather, they indirectly benefit functional capacity by increasing muscle mass, motor-unit recruitment, bone density, and connective-tissue health.

Some coaches and trainers, usually those with a powerlifting bias, say something like the following: "Don't worry about replicating force-generation and neuromuscular patterns of specific athletic movements. Just get strong in the basic compound lifts and you'll be more athletic." Improving strength in general compound lifts absolutely does contribute to improved sport performance, which is why these lifts play an integral role in the functional-spectrum training system.

With that in mind, let's quickly discuss what some strength coaches would have you do to improve your strength in (for example) the bench press. In addition to improving your bench press technique, they'd have you do lots of bench-press variations (e.g., close-grip, wide-grip, two- or three-board) and perform the bench press using chains or bands at various speeds, with various loads, and in various rep ranges. These exercises are all commonly referred to as "assistance exercises" because they help you improve bench-press performance by replicating the specific force-generation and neuromuscular coordination patterns involved in the bench-press movement.

The same principle applies to assistance exercises used by powerlifters to maximize their strength in the squat or deadlift. That is, they all replicate the specific force-generation and neuromuscular coordination patterns of the movement they're supposed to be assisting. Surely, however, you don't think that using assistance exercises to improve performance in a specific movement pattern applies only to the bench press, squat, and deadlift?

Indeed, this very same wisdom used by powerlifters is also used in the *specific* exercise applications included in the functional-spectrum training system (i.e., the total-body power exercises and the cross-body exercises) to improve target movements in a variety of sports. In short, specific exercise movements are used essentially as assistance exercises for the specific movement patterns that form the foundation of athletics.

As you can see, using *general* exercises to get bigger and stronger does help you improve your overall athletic ability and functional capacity. But this approach has its limitations, which is why the functional-spectrum training system also incorporates specific exercises—to produce benefits in the areas where the general exercises fall short.

Still, many trainers and coaches who preach to athletes that they should "just get strong in the basic lifts"—and not worry about replicating force-generation and neuromuscular coordination patterns of specific, target movements of athletics— are often the same people who tell athletes to avoid using machines because they don't resemble the movement patterns involved in athletics. Now if that isn't the king of all training contradictions, I don't know what is!

Isolation Exercises

Isolation exercises are single-joint movements that focus on individual muscle groups. These exercise applications consist primarily of classic bodybuilding exercises, such as biceps curls, triceps extensions, shoulder raises, and machine-based exercises (e.g., leg extensions and hamstring curls).

Like compound exercises, isolation exercises are classified as general exercises in the functional-spectrum training system because they don't necessarily reflect specific force-generation patterns. Instead, they indirectly benefit functional capacity by increasing muscle mass, motor-unit recruitment, bone density, and connective-tissue health. In addition, both isolation and compound exercises can help you improve your overall health and physique.

Many trainers and coaches claim that they don't use bodybuilding concepts (e.g., isolation exercises focused on specific muscles to enhance muscle size) because they don't want their athletes to become overly muscle-bound and less athletic like many bodybuilders. This view, however, lacks a certain sense of reality. Doing some biceps curls and leg extensions doesn't automatically turn you into a professional bodybuilder any more than doing sprints on a track turns you into an Olympic sprinter. Nor is the central nervous system so fragile that performing a few sets of isolation exercises or a few sets on weight machines per week could somehow undercut the functional abilities and movement skills acquired from long hours of sport practice and competition.

You see, it's not that bodybuilding (i.e., size) training concepts make you less athletic; rather, it's that if *all* you do is bodybuilding, *then* you'll become less athletic simply because you're not also regularly requiring your body to do athletic actions. As the old saying goes, "If you don't use it, you lose it." However, you won't lose athletic ability if you regularly do athletic actions while integrating some general bodybuilding concepts.

This is precisely why the functional-spectrum training system uses a variety of specific exercises (e.g., total-body power exercises and cross-body exercises) in conjunction with general exercise applications (e.g., compound and isolation exercises). In addition, chapter 2 presents three reasons that using bodybuilding concepts to get *bigger* can help you improve your overall athletic performance.

The field of training and conditioning has gone from viewing muscles purely in isolation to recognizing more integrated movement patterns that show how muscles coordinate to create movement, both in athletics and in activities of daily living. As a result, some have advised us to "train movements, not muscles," in order to direct people away from the general, muscle-focused bodybuilding style of training and toward a specific, movement-focused performance-based training approach.

However, as you've now learned, these arguments about specific versus general (i.e., movement focused versus muscle focused) are ridiculous because they're like arguing about whether you should eat vegetables or fruits. Avoiding one or the other will leave your diet deficient. This is why nutrition experts always encourage eating a 'colorful diet' with a variety of both vegetables and fruits because they all have a different ratio of vitamins and minerals.

Similarly, a training plan that exclusively focuses on either general or specific exercises leaves some potential benefits untapped since each method offers unique training benefits the other lacks. In contrast, a training plan that combines both specific and general methods—one that utilizes all four types of resistance exercises—enables you to achieve superior results by helping you build a more athletic body that's got both the hustle and the muscle you seek.

You now understand the exercise components used in the functional-spectrum training system. You also recognize that improving your overall health, physique, and performance requires multiple exercises components. With this foundation in place, we can now discuss how to *use* the various exercise components to gain muscle and increase strength and speed.

2

Building Muscle, Increasing Strength

This chapter gives you the three Ss of the functional-spectrum training system: speed, strength, and size. Like the training system as a whole, the specific workout programs in this book will help you improve these three qualities. Both the overall system and the particular workout programs enable you to train through a spectrum of movement speeds and loads in order to enhance your explosiveness, improve your strength, and increase your muscle.

The Three Ss of the Functional-Spectrum Training System

This section explores each of the three Ss—speed, strength, and size—to help you understand exactly what each quality is. It also addresses the scientifically founded principles behind the practical exercise applications used to enhance each quality.

Movement-Speed Training

In the context of this book, movement-speed training focuses on improving your rate of force development—that is, how quickly you can use your strength. Remember: power = strength × speed. Therefore, the exercises used to improve your movement speed are the total-body power exercises. The heavier the load you're working against, the slower your movement becomes. For this reason, the principle of specificity dictates that, in order to do all you can to improve your explosive power, you don't just do exercises that involve moving against high loads (i.e., strength exercises). You also do exercises that require you to move at high *speeds*.

As you may recall from chapter 1, adaptations to training are specific to the demands that the training puts on the body. Therefore, regularly performing exercises that require you to move fast in certain directions makes your body more capable of moving fast in those or similar directions. With this principle in mind, the functional-spectrum training system includes exercises for each of the three pillars of power—vertical (or diagonal), horizontal, and rotational—in order to improve your functional capacity by enhancing your capability to move fast in multiple directions.

Since the goal is to move fast, the exercises provided in this book for improving total-body power (i.e., movement speed) use loads that are not heavy (relative to the loads used to improve strength). In fact, they involve very light loads (sometimes just body weight), but they demand that you move at high speed as fast as you can.

In addition to training movement speed, we also need (as addressed in chapter 1) to better adapt to and potentially refine the triphasic muscle-activation pattern used only during fast, ballistic athletic movements. One of the best workout methods to achieve both of these goals is to perform medicine-ball throwing exercises. When throwing the ball, unlike when lifting weights, you don't have to slow down at the end of the range of motion; you can just let the ball fly. Therefore, simply throwing the ball in different directions (remember, power is direction specific) trains your body to generate explosive power without putting on any brakes.

Also, whereas Olympic weightlifting can be difficult to learn and trains only in the vertical or diagonal power pillar, the explosive medicine-ball throwing exercises provided in this book are easy to learn and require you to move fast and explosively in all three pillars of power (as described in chapter 1). To do so, the functional-spectrum training system and the various specific workout programs use a variety of medicine-ball throwing exercises—throwing either against a wall or into open space (e.g., field or parking lot)—to help you become more explosive and therefore more powerful and athletic.

With this system, then, unless you are limited to outside workouts and the weather is horrible, you have no excuse not to get the most out of your training! All you have to do is find a place where you can throw a medicine ball against a wall, and both of these pieces of equipment are cost effective and easy to come by.

Movement-Strength Training

Training for improved strength means improving one's capability to produce force in various movements. Put simply, the more force you can produce in a given movement, the stronger you are in that movement.

Like power, strength is task specific; therefore, the further an exercise gets away from the specific force-generation and neuromuscular coordination patterns of a given movement, the less directly it carries over to that movement. A stated in chapter 1, this fact in no way makes the exercise bad, and it certainly doesn't make it nonfunctional. It simply means that the less specific an exercise is, the more general it is.

That said, the functional-spectrum training system incorporates a wide variety of cross-body and compound exercises to help you improve your functional capacity by developing strength in various movement patterns, directions, and body positions. Remember, if you can perform a broader range of specific tasks, you possess a higher functional capacity. This relationship is crucial because you don't want your body to be merely more *adapted* to a limited number of gym-based exercise movements (only Olympic lifters and powerlifters need to specialize in specific exercise movements). Instead, you want your body to be more *adaptable* so that you can successfully take on a variety of physical demands.

Although training for strength gains and training for size gains (i.e., hypertrophy) are certainly not mutually exclusive, the size–strength continuum is characterized by some important differences between the two. Although both involve creating mechanical tension on the muscles, *strength* training is geared toward increasing force production. *Size* training, on the other hand, is geared toward getting a muscle pump and creating microscopic damage in the muscle, which causes the muscle to repair itself and grow larger (more on this in the next section).

When training for strength, the rule of thumb calls for keeping reps low and the resistance load high; in practical terms, this rule means using a weight load that allows you to perform only 1 to 5 reps. In addition, strength work that is truly low-rep is highly neuromuscular. If you think of your body as a computer, then strength training is geared more to upgrading your software (your central nervous system, or CNS) than to upgrading your hardware (your muscles). In contrast, training for size is geared more to upgrading your body's hardware—bones, connective tissues, and, of course, muscles. In short, strength training involves teaching your CNS how to bring more muscle into the game by increasing motor-unit recruitment.

Muscle-Size Training

The rule of thumb in training for size calls for using more reps and lower loads than when training for strength. In practical terms, this approach means using a weight load that allows you to perform about 9 to 15 reps per set; performing 6 to 8 reps per set serves as a nice middle ground between the general strength range and the general size range.

Although all types of training can provide neurological benefits—especially early on—the goal of training for size is more physiological than neurological. In fact, contrary to popular belief, increasing muscle size depends not on the specific exercises you do but on the specific physiological *stimulus* you create. To build muscle, you need to create a training stimulus that elicits the three mechanisms for muscle growth (i.e., hypertrophy): mechanical tension, muscle damage, and metabolic stress (1).

- *Mechanical tension*: This tension is exerted on the muscles from movement and external loads to reduce, produce, or control force. Muscle tension can be created either by lifting heavy loads for lower volumes (i.e., lower numbers of reps) or by lifting medium loads for higher volumes (i.e., higher numbers of reps). Therefore, either can create a stimulus for muscle growth (2).

- *Muscle damage*: Muscle fibers generate tension during the action of actin and myosin cross-bridge cycling. The actin and myosin filaments are proteins that create cross bridges and are responsible for the contractions (i.e. shortening) of a muscle fiber. With this in mind, the term muscle damage refers to muscle-tissue microtears that occur when working muscles tire and struggle to resist the weight while the muscle fiber is lengthening eccentrically. This can cause the actin and myosin to be forcibly ripped apart, thereby causing damage. This damage often leads to delayed-onset muscle soreness (DOMS) after an intense exercise session. It's important to note that soreness is not needed for muscle development (3).

- *Metabolic stress*: Increasing time under tension (TUT) increases metabolic stress and gives you incredible pump, or muscle-cell swelling. This swelling can cause both an increase in muscle-protein synthesis and a decrease in protein breakdown, which are essential components of the process by which the body repairs and grows muscle tissue after exercise (4,5,6). Research shows that maximizing TUT by lifting a lower load to (or near) failure produces hypertrophy (i.e., gain in muscle size) similar to that produced by lifting a heavy load to failure (7).

Three Ways Bodybuilding Can Improve Athletic Performance

It's well established that getting stronger can help your overall athletic performance. Here are three specific ways in which using strength training and bodybuilding concepts to get bigger—that is, to increase muscle size—can indirectly transfer into improved performance.

1. Stronger From Your Feet

Unless you're a race-car driver, it is crucial for you as an athlete to be strong from a standing position. More specifically, the same study we discussed in the cross-body exercises section of Chapter 1, which compared the single-arm standing cable press and the traditional bench press, not only showed that the two actions involve very different force-production and neuromuscular-coordination patterns, but it also demonstrated that in a standing position, one's horizontal pushing force is limited to about 40 percent of body weight, rather than your bench press (8).

This tells us that it's mathematically and physically impossible for anyone to match, or even come close to replicating what they can bench press in a push from a standing position. It also tells us that the heavier you are, the more horizontal and diagonal pushing force you can produce from the standing position (regardless of your weightroom numbers) because you have more bodyweight from which to push.

Although it's clear the bench press is one of the most overemphasized and misunderstood exercises in the sports performance world, this isn't to deny that developing a stronger bench press can help your standing push performance. Rather, these results indicate that *also* getting bigger (gaining weight) can help you better use your strength by providing a greater platform from which to push against your opposition. It can also give you a better chance to avoid getting knocked over or knocked off balance. So, putting on 20 pounds of muscle mass—it is rarely good to gain weight in the form of extra body fat—through hypertrophy training (i.e., bodybuilding) can give you more push-force production ability (i.e., strength) from your feet.

To summarize, the functional-spectrum training system and its associated workout programs include exercise applications for each of the three Ss in order to help you update your body's software (neurological efficiency) and improve your body's hardware (muscle mass) to accommodate the enhanced software.

Programming Strategies for the Three Ss

Now that you have a clear understanding of the training principles behind each of the three Ss, we can talk about the practical programing strategies that put those principles into practice and help us to enhance speed, strength, and size.

Varying the Order and Volume of the Three Ss

It is generally considered appropriate to place the most neurologically demanding exercises (i.e., exercises in the movement-speed category) earliest in the training program because they require the most coordination and concentration and are therefore the most affected by mental and physical fatigue (9). For this reason, the exercises in the speed and power category are placed *first* in both the performance training programs and the

2. Harder Hitting

In a similar vein, another study, this one focused on baseball pitchers, found that increased body weight is highly associated with increased pitch velocity (10). In other words, pitchers who weighed more tended to throw the ball faster than those who weighed less.

Since throwing and striking are similar total-body actions—both summate force from the ground up—this finding about pitching correlates with what we see in combat sports. All other things (e.g., technical ability) being equal, bigger athletes simply tend to punch (and throw) harder than their smaller counterparts do because they have more bodyweight behind their punches (and throws). This gives them a greater platform (more weight into the ground) from which to generate force and use their power.

Now, if you're someone who worries about gaining too much muscle, here's something to think about: Although a gain of 10 pounds (4.5 kg) of muscle mass constitutes a significant increase, that additional muscle is not so noticeable if it is spread throughout the body.

3. Better Ability to Dissipate Impact Force (More Body Armor)

Physics tells us that a larger surface area dissipates impact force and vibration better than a smaller surface area of the same stiffness. In athletic terms, bigger muscle mass better dissipates the impact force and vibration caused by events such as falling, getting punched, and taking or delivering a football hit.

To go into a bit more detail, the way to better dissipate force is to spread it out over a greater area so that no single spot bears the brunt of concentrated force; one good example is an arch bridge. Accordingly, those who wish to improve functional capacity and participate in impact sports should consider bodybuilding exercises—both for the physique benefits and as a way to build the body's physiological armor. In fact, a larger muscle not only helps dissipate external impact forces but also sets the stage for increased force production (by upgrading your hardware), provided that your central nervous system (your software) can muster the neural charge to maximize it!

performance-and-muscle training programs provided in this book. However, these same exercises are placed *last* in the muscle-training programs, which focus on maximizing your ability to execute the exercises in the strength and size category because they are more directly related to creating a stimulus for improved muscle growth.

In other words, one of the biggest differences between the performance workout programs and the muscle workout programs lies in the choice of which exercise category you do first (when you're freshest) and which you do at the end of the workout (when you're more fatigued). Still, all three program types use strength exercises earlier in the workout than size exercises (see table 2.1). This approach reflects the fact that high-load, strength-oriented exercise applications are generally more neurologically demanding than size-oriented (i.e., bodybuilding) exercise applications, which involve medium loads.

In addition, as you can see in table 2.2, another difference between a functional-spectrum *muscle*-training program and a functional-spectrum *performance*-training program involves the number of exercises placed in the speed and power category and in the size category. Specifically, the performance programs use the most exercises in the speed and power category and the fewest in the size category, whereas the muscle programs reverse that pattern.

TABLE 2.1 Program Comparison: Pulling Exercises

Performance program 1: workout A—pulling	Muscle program 1: workout A—pulling	Performance and muscle program 1: workout A—pulling
SPEED	**STRENGTH**	**SPEED**
• Medicine-ball step-and-overhead throw • Medicine-ball front-scoop horizontal throw • 30-yard shuttle	• Barbell bent-over row	• Medicine-ball step-and-overhead throw • Medicine-ball front-scoop horizontal throw
STRENGTH	**SIZE**	**STRENGTH**
• One-arm cable row	• Leaning lat pull-down • Wide-grip seated row • Suspension biceps curl • Bent-over dumbbell shoulder fly • One-arm cable row	• One-arm cable row
SIZE	**SPEED**	**SIZE**
• Wide-grip seated row • Suspension biceps curl • Bent-over dumbbell shoulder fly	• Medicine-ball step-and-overhead throw	• Leaning lat pull-down • Wide-grip seated row • Dumbbell biceps curl • Bent-over dumbbell shoulder fly

TABLE 2.2 Program Comparison: Lower-Body Exercises

Performance program 1: workout B—lower body and core	Muscle program 1: workout B—lower body and core	Muscle and performance program 1: workout B—lower body and core
SPEED	**STRENGTH**	**SPEED**
• 25-yard-dash • 180-degree squat jump with cross-arm drive	• Trap-bar squat • Ab snail	• 25-yard dash
STRENGTH	**SIZE**	**STRENGTH**
• Trap-bar squat • Ab snail	• Machine leg press • Leg lowering with band • 45-degree hip extension • Dumbbell plank row • Barbell calf raise • One-leg one-arm dumbbell Romanian deadlift	• Trap-bar squat • Ab snail
SIZE	**SPEED**	**SIZE**
• One-leg one-arm dumbbell Romanian deadlift • Dumbbell plank row • Bench step-up • Leg lowering with band • 45-degree hip extension	• 180-degree squat jump with cross-arm drive	• One-leg one-arm dumbbell Romanian deadlift • Dumbbell plank row • Bench step-up • Leg lowering with band • 45-degree hip extension • Barbell calf raise

Varying Sets and Reps for Better Gains

Chapter 1 suggests that arguing about which type of resistance-training exercise is best for building muscle and performance is just as ridiculous as debating whether you should eat only fruits or only vegetables for nutrition. Similarly, the scientific evidence on sets and reps tells us that another debate we shouldn't be having is whether to use high-load or high-volume lifting. Rather, the smartest approach is to incorporate *both* heavy-load, low-volume work *and* lighter-load, higher-volume work in an undulating fashion. In short, it's best to think about the types of resistance training exercise—and the sets and reps you use—in the same way that you think about your nutrition: Make sure to get enough variety, because each type offers unique training or nutritional value that the other type doesn't.

The training system and workout programs provided in this book enable you to incorporate not only the full spectrum of exercise types but also a full spectrum of set and repetition ranges. This variety is the reason that they can be so effective at helping you improve your strength, your size, and your speed (i.e., explosiveness).

For instance, research has shown that daily variations in intensity and volume (sets and reps) are more effective than weekly volume variations for increases in maximal strength; they may also lead to greater gains in muscle size (11,12,13,14). Mixing your sets and reps in this manner throughout the week is commonly referred to as daily undulating periodization. The term *periodization* refers to a form of workout planning that systematically varies the acute variables of training (e.g., sets, reps, loads, rest) at regular intervals.

This book includes three chapters that present functional-spectrum workout programs (chapters 10, 11, and 12). Chapter 10 features workout programs emphasizing speed and strength gains, chapter 11 emphasizes gains in muscle size, and chapter 12 occupies a nice middle ground.

In this chapter, I've indicated very general rep ranges for focusing on strength or size training, and these ranges are emphasized in the corresponding workout programs presented later in the book. Recall, however, that muscle growth can result from using the lower rep ranges generally associated with strength building, and strength increases can result from using the higher rep ranges generally associated with size (i.e., hypertrophy). Again, the two types of training aren't mutually exclusive; in fact, increasing strength can help you better recruit your muscles when focusing on size, and increasing size along with connective-tissue strength can help you lift heavier loads.

Therefore, regardless of whether a given workout program emphasizes strength or size, all of the full-spectrum training programs incorporate some *daily* undulating variations in sets and reps along with some linear-based strength training where, each week, you perform more weight for the same amount of reps, or perform more reps using the same amount of weight you did in the workout previously.

In short, there are two ways to get stronger and build a great-looking body *that can get things done*: neurologically and physiologically. Both approaches are addressed by the functional-spectrum training system, which helps you reprogram your body's software *and* improve its hardware for more muscle and better performance capability.

You now understand the three Ss of the functional-spectrum training system. You also know the principles for improving each element, as well as the benefit of using daily undulating variations in sets and reps. With that foundation in place, it's time to examine the cardio-conditioning component of this training system.

PART II

Exercises

3

Cardio Conditioning

To complement the training geared to speed (power), strength, and size, the functional-spectrum training system also incorporates polarized training to improve your cardio conditioning. Polarized training, which originated in the arena of endurance training, involves training at either low intensity (aerobic work) or high intensity (anaerobic work) and minimizing the training time devoted to moderate-intensity work.

Research shows polarized training to be more effective than medium-intensity work at improving aerobic performance (1). For example, in one study, participants who used polarized training improved their 10K race times by an average of 41 seconds more than those who emphasized more moderate training (i.e., at a level between high intensity and low intensity). The groups spent about the same amount of time on high-intensity training; the only thing that differed was how much time they spent in the low- and moderate-intensity ranges (2).

Polarized training is now a battle-tested concept in the endurance training world. It is adapted in the functional-spectrum training system to help athletes and athletic-minded individuals increase their aerobic (i.e., cardio) capacity and improve their *conditioning*, which is their ability to resist fatigue during anaerobic activity. You see, the training methods used for strength and power in the functional-spectrum system (covered in chapters 1 and 2) are great for improving your strength and explosive power, but they're not designed to directly improve your *power endurance*. This capacity enables you to produce the same level of power for a longer time—ideally, for the length of competition.

In other words, the power-training and strength-training methods discussed in chapters 1 and 2 help you peak your power in short bursts, but they don't prepare you to go five rounds or beat your opponent to the ball at the end of the fourth quarter. To fill that gap, the functional-spectrum cardio-conditioning protocols provided in this chapter are just what the doctor ordered to help you outlast the competition.

Types of Cardio Conditioning

The functional-spectrum cardio-conditioning aspect of the workout programs provided later in this book incorporates three methods:

- Supramaximal interval training
- Steady-state cardio training
- Metabolic conditioning protocols

These methods are detailed in the following sections.

Supramaximal Interval Training

Even if you're familiar with high-intensity interval training (HIIT), you may not be familiar with supramaximal interval training (SMIT), which may be more effective at improving fitness and performance. One study found greater improvements in 3000-meter time-trial performance after SMIT than after continuous running; In short, the results demonstrated that SMIT worked better in improving shorter and longer distance performance than doing both HIIT and continuous running (3).

To better understand how to use SMIT—and HIIT, for that matter—you must understand the differences between the two. HIIT involves interspersing high-intensity work (exercise) intervals performed at 100 percent of your $\dot{V}O_2$max with either active-recovery (i.e., low-intensity) phases or passive-recovery phases (e.g., standing or sitting fairly still). SMIT, on the other hand, involves interspersing maximal-intensity (all-out) bursts of work (exercise) intervals performed at *more* than 100 percent of your $\dot{V}O_2$max with passive-recovery phases.

Now, if you're not familiar with $\dot{V}O_2$max, you may wonder how it is possible to work at more than 100 percent of it. The answer depends on understanding just what $\dot{V}O_2$max is—the highest rate of oxygen consumption attainable during maximal or exhaustive exercise. As exercise intensity increases, so does oxygen consumption; eventually, however, a point is reached where exercise intensity can continue to increase without an associated rise in oxygen consumption. What we're really talking about here is *aerobic* ("with oxygen") training versus *anaerobic* ("without oxygen") training, and the main thing that separates the two is intensity.

To understand these dynamics in more practical terms, here's a real-world example. Let's say that you and a friend are jogging together and carrying on a conversation. If you're able to speak in normal (full) sentences without huffing and puffing between words, then you're in an aerobic state (i.e., with oxygen). However, if you both increase the pace to a fast run or a sprint, you'll still be able to talk to one another, but you'll be unable to get out full sentences without huffing and puffing. In other words, you'll be in an anaerobic state (i.e., without oxygen).

The preceding example uses what is referred to as the "talk test"—an easy but legitimate method of telling whether you're in an aerobic or an anaerobic state. It's that simple: If you can speak a full sentence as you normally would in a conversation, then you're in an aerobic state. But if you have to take a breath (or a few breaths) during a single sentence, then you're in an anaerobic state.

Now you can see that $\dot{V}O_2$max is just the maximum volume of oxygen you can consume and use. In other words, it is the level at which you cannot increase your intake of oxygen. Crucially, however, it is *not* the maximal amount of work intensity you can achieve. You can work at a higher intensity—an *anaerobic* intensity—and that is what supramaximal training involves.

Steady-State Cardio Training

As HIIT has grown in popularity, there has been a decline in the popularity of the standard 30-minute bout of steady-state aerobic training (e.g., low- to medium-intensity exercise on a treadmill, elliptical trainer, or bicycle). However, if you're just starting (or restarting) an exercise program, beginning with HIIT may increase the chance for injury and muscle soreness. Therefore, it's probably a good idea to start with low-intensity aerobic exercise until you can run (or use the elliptical trainer or bike) for about 30 consecutive minutes at moderate intensity in order to increase your aerobic fitness, and thus giving you a better fitness platform (i.e., training base) for using high-intensity conditioning methods (4).

Steady-state cardio has also been demonized for interfering with, or even killing, muscle gains produced by strength training. However, scientific evidence indicates that in previously untrained men, adding low-impact aerobic exercise (e.g., cycling) does not jeopardize gains in strength or muscle size; in fact, it may even increase muscular gains (5). Other evidence indicates that aerobic exercise not only created improvements in muscle size and aerobic capacity, but that these improvements were similar between younger and older men (6). It's likely that these results also apply to women because research has demonstrated that aerobic exercise acutely and chronically alters protein metabolism and induces skeletal muscle hypertrophy, and it can also serve as an effective countermeasure for populations (both women and men) prone to muscle loss (7).

Now, we must keep these study results in perspective because they involved untrained individuals. So, the question is: What impact does doing some steady-state cardio training have on muscle for trained individuals? To get the answer, we have to look no further than what bodybuilders have been doing for years as they get closer to getting on stage. In that bodybuilders do bouts of steady-state cardio training while prepping for their shows and are able to maintain impressive amounts of muscle mass while doing so. This cannot be simply chalked up to the influence of drugs because there are plenty of natural bodybuilders out there.

So, with this reality in mind, it's unrealistic to think that doing some steady-state cardio training will automatically causes you to lose your hard-earned muscle, especially if you're using it to complement a workout program that emphasizes resistance training.

For intermediate and advanced athletes and exercisers who already possess a solid training base, it's unrealistic—not to mention unnecessary—to do high-intensity interval-style training (i.e., SMIT and HIIT) during each workout. This is especially true if you're using SMIT or HIIT in combination with intense strength training. This is because, as the name suggests, high-intensity interval training, along with supramaximal interval training and the metabolic conditioning protocols, can be intense and push your body hard. Therefore, you don't want to do too much in a given week, and it's important to allow plenty of recovery time between workouts. A great method to use on recovery days—between the more intense anaerobic (conditioning) interval-training days— is to perform light to moderate aerobic (i.e., cardio) exercises. This is exactly how such exercise is used in the functional-spectrum workouts.

Metabolic Conditioning Protocols

You want to be able to repeat your power throughout a contest, right? Sure you do, since most sports often require you to call upon every ounce of strength you have and explode—even when you're tired. If you want to be explosive at the end of a competition when you're fatigued, then you must train for that specific goal. To do so, you must mix conditioning and strength work, which is precisely what these metabolic conditioning protocols (MCPs) do.

In other words, as stated several times throughout this book, the principle of training specificity tells us that adaptations to training are specific to the demands that the training puts on the body. Given this fact, the MCPs and the SMIT exercises featured in this book can help you increase your power endurance because they require you to give strong effort for extended periods of time—which is exactly what power endurance is.

Even if you're not currently participating in a sport, just about everyone is looking to make the most of his or her time at the gym. When the rubber hits the road, metabolic complexes assure you that, regardless of whether or not you improve on your lifts in a given session, you leave knowing that you left it all on the gym floor and did what you could to ensure as effective a workout as possible. In addition, if you value mental toughness and the satisfaction of pushing yourself, then metabolic conditioning protocols, as well as SMIT and HIIT exercises, are tough to beat.

Combining Cardio Conditioning With Strength Training

Each form of cardio conditioning used in the functional-spectrum training system—supra-maximal interval training, steady-state cardio, and metabolic conditioning protocols—has its benefits and limitations. Therefore, as with the various forms of resistance training, any argument for favoring one of these methods over another is misplaced because the types are *not* mutually exclusive; rather, they are complementary training components. In other words, the question isn't about doing either this or that but about how it all goes together.

Let's now consider how these great training and conditioning concepts go together in the functional-spectrum workout programs. As covered in chapter 2, the resistance-training portion of your functional-spectrum workouts uses primarily undulating periodization. This approach means that some resistance-training sessions take longer than others; for example, it takes less time to perform 2 sets of 15 reps than it does to perform 4 sets of 6 reps. This is where the modified polarized training fits perfectly with your undulating strength training.

In the functional-spectrum workout programs, the type of cardio conditioning you do corresponds to the set-and-rep scheme used in the preceding strength-training portion of the workout. On days when you spend the most time on the strength-training portion—the workouts with the most sets (e.g., four per exercise)—you use SMIT, because it takes the least time of the cardio-conditioning methods. In contrast, on days when you do the fewest sets (e.g., two per exercise)—which is where you spend the least time on strength training—you perform steady-state cardio because it takes the longest of the cardio-conditioning methods. And on days when you do three sets per exercise, you use one of the metabolic conditioning protocols because they require a moderate amount of time.

In other words, the cardio-conditioning portion of the functional-spectrum workouts is undulated just like the strength training is (as covered in chapter 2). On days when the strength-training portion of your workout is the longest (i.e., where you're doing more sets), your cardio-conditioning activities are the shortest, and vice versa. This approach not only keeps your workouts consistent in terms of time but also makes them more comprehensive, effective, and interesting.

Cardio-Conditioning Exercises

You now understand the benefits of the three cardio-conditioning methods used in the functional-spectrum training workouts. With that foundation in place, the following sections of the chapter present recommended exercise applications for each method.

Supramaximal Interval Training

The following exercises for supramaximal interval training are used in the functional-spectrum training system to enhance power endurance.

Shuttle Run

The term *shuttle run* may give you flashbacks to high-school gym class. I, for one, advocate keeping the memory alive by adding some old-school shuttle sprints to your workouts as a way of applying your new-school knowledge of how this kind of training can benefit your fitness, physique, and performance. In fact, shuttle sprints offer one of the best ways to incorporate SMIT into your workouts because they don't require any special equipment, or even a gym. You just need the will to go through super-intense work, which—no secret here—is just plain tough. But with the right mind-set, you'll realize that it's *not* tougher than you are!

Setup
Place two cones 25 yards apart (see figure).

Action
Jog up to the start cone, then sprint as fast as you can back and forth between the cones. On each reversal of direction, touch the cone, alternating hands from one touch to the next.
Lengths are as follows:

- 200-yard shuttle run = four round-trips between the cones
- 250-yard shuttle run = five round-trips
- 300-yard shuttle run = six round-trips

Between rounds, use a work-to-rest ratio of 1:3 or 1:2, depending on your fitness level. For example, using a 1:3 ratio, if it takes you one minute to complete a 300-yard shuttle sprint, then rest for three minutes before starting the next round.

Coaching Tips
- You can start your shuttle runs from the starting line. However, I recommend jogging up to the starting point in order to reduce the potential risk of injury, such as a hamstring strain, that can come from quick starts.
- Drive with your arms while sprinting.
- If you're not comfortable with touching the cone each time you change direction, simply eliminate that aspect of the drill. Instead, stay upright as you turn around (in a controlled manner) and run back toward the other cone.

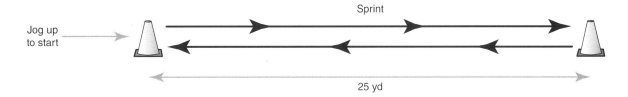

Gasser

Gassers have been used by American football coaches for years in order to get their players in great condition for the upcoming season. They were originally performed by running the width (sideline to sideline) of an American football field, which is about 53 yards (49 m), for four laps; half-gassers involved running two laps. In the context of the functional-spectrum workouts presented in this book, gassers involve running laps between two cones located 50 yards apart, since this distance makes for a nice round number and not everyone has access to an American football field.

Setup

Place two cones 50 yards apart (see figure).

Action

Jog up to the start cone, then run as fast as you can back and forth between the cones. Unlike in shuttle sprints, you don't touch the cones at the turns; therefore, you stay more upright.

Use a work-to-rest ratio of 1:3 or 1:2 between rounds, depending on your fitness level. For example, using a 1:3 ratio, if it takes you one minute to complete a full round of gassers, then rest for three minutes before starting the next round. How many rounds you do will depend on the workout plan chosen from the programming options presented later in this book.

Coaching Tips

- You can start your gasser runs from the starting line. However, I recommend jogging up to the starting point in order to reduce the risk of injury that can come from quick starts.
- Drive with your arms while running.
- If you're not comfortable with touching the cone each time you change direction, simply eliminate that aspect of the drill. Instead, stay upright as you turn around (in a controlled manner) and run back toward the other cone.

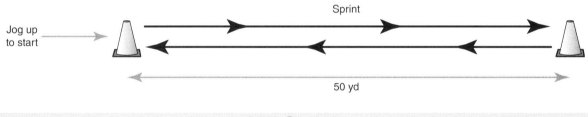

Hill Sprint

Hill sprints help you improve not only your cardio conditioning but also your stride length and leg drive. Both components help you build a great-looking and better-performing body.

Setup

Find a fairly steep hill at least 20 yards long. If you're lucky, you'll find one that is 40 yards or even longer.

Action

Run up the hill as fast as you can, then walk down slowly to set up your next run.

Use a work-to-rest ratio of 1:3 or 1:4 between rounds, depending on your fitness level. For example, using a 1:3 ratio, if it takes you 20 seconds to complete a hill sprint, then rest roughly 60 seconds before starting the next round.

Coaching Tips

- Do not take short, choppy steps; take a full stride on each step.
- Drive with your arms while running.
- To vary your leg movement, you can walk backward down the hill between sprints.

Airdyne Bike

The Airdyne bike (see figure) has been around for some time but is rarely found in larger gyms today. This bike provides a fantastic option for SMIT because it incorporates upper-body exercise with the pedaling action of the legs and allows you to speed up and slow down without manipulating settings. Although the Airdyne is low impact, supramaximal intervals performed on it create a very challenging conditioning workout.

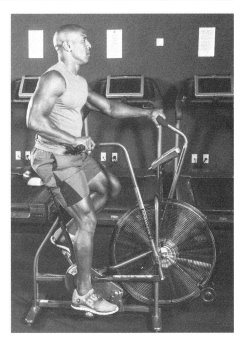

Setup

Find an Airdyne bike to use.

Action

Pedal your feet and drive your arms as hard and as fast and as you can for 15 to 45 seconds. Rest fully for 45 seconds to 3 minutes between intervals.

Coaching Tips

- It's okay to lean forward as you're performing the intense portions of each interval.
- During the rest position between each work interval, you can stay seated on the bike or get off the bike and stand or pace around a bit before beginning your next work interval.

VersaClimber

Like the Airdyne bike, the VersaClimber (see figure) has existed for a number of years but is rarely found in gyms these days. The VersaClimber offers a unique climbing action that incorporates the arms and legs, thus making it another great option for performing supramaximal interval training. In addition, because it puts you in an upright position, the VersaClimber is very back friendly, which makes it a good substitute for people who struggle with sitting on a bike due to back issues.

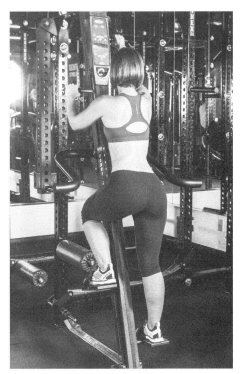

Action

Using short to medium strides, drive your feet and arms as hard and as fast and as you can for 30 to 90 seconds. Rest fully for 90 seconds to 3 minutes between intervals.

Coaching Tips

- Minimize shifting your body from side to side as you perform each work interval. Keep your body fairly centered on the machine.
- During the rest position between each work interval, get off the machine and either stand or pace around a bit before beginning your next work interval.

Rower

Supramaximal interval training can also be performed with a rowing machine (see figure), which is a fairly common feature in gyms. To avoid overusing your low back, perform the rowing motions primarily with your legs and arms.

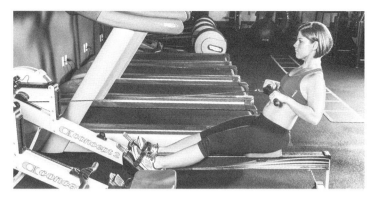

Action

Drive your legs and pull with your arms as hard and as fast and as you can for 30 to 90 seconds. Rest fully for 90 seconds to 3 minutes between intervals.

Coaching Tips

- Perform each rowing action by coordinating the action of your legs in a smooth and rhythmic fashion with the action of your arms.
- During the rest position between each work interval, get off the machine and either stand or pace around a bit before beginning your next work interval.

Treadmill

The treadmill allows you to walk or run no matter the weather. It's readily found in just about every gym.

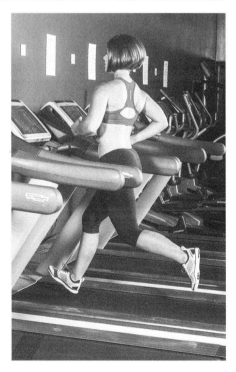

Setup

Set the treadmill to a combination of speed and incline that forces you to go as hard as you can for the time frame indicated in the chosen workout program.

Action

Drive your legs and arms to run as fast as you can for 8 to 15 seconds while staying centered on the treadmill track. Rest fully for 30 to 45 seconds between intervals. To transition from running to resting, or vice versa, keep the treadmill running and simply jump on and off. For rest periods, use the side handles to lift yourself off of the track and place your feet on the side rails.

Coaching Tips

- Do not take short, choppy steps; take a full stride on each step.
- Drive with your arms while running.

Steady-State Cardio Exercises

The functional-spectrum cardio-conditioning system allows for a variety of machines. Some of these machines are found in almost every gym, whereas others are less common. The following options are recommended for performing steady-state cardio exercise in the functional-spectrum workout programs.

Brisk Walking

Since you'll be doing sprint variations on SMIT training days, the functional-spectrum training programs presented in this book do not recommend light running as a steady-state cardio option. This isn't to say that doing some light roadwork is a bad thing; it's simply to focus on a lower-impact version of steady-state cardio that minimizes the risk of overuse injury and helps you improve your recovery from intense workouts.

Action
Walk at a brisk pace (approximately 2.5 to 3 miles per hour) outside or on a treadmill for 25 to 35 minutes.

Coaching Tips
- Do not take short, choppy steps; take a full stride on each step.
- Drive with your arms while walking.

Elliptical Trainer

The elliptical trainer (see figure) is another piece of equipment readily found in just about every gym. It can serve as a lower impact alternative to the treadmill.

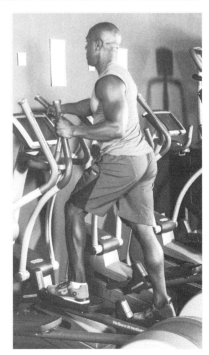

Action
On a scale of 1 to 10, with 10 being as fast as you can move, stay at a pace that puts you around a 4 for 25 to 35 minutes.

Coaching Tips
- Stay tall as you perform this exercise.
- Don't just use your legs. Also use your arms to push and pull the handles.

Upright Bike

The upright bike (see figure) is a great steady-state cardio option because it's very knee friendly, which makes it especially valuable for people whose knees may be irritated by steady-state running.

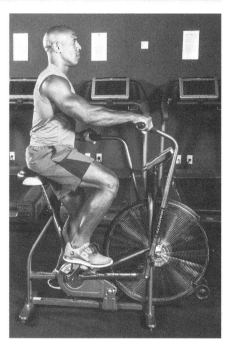

Action

Upright bikes are a staple piece of equipment at most gyms, and some facilities will also have the Airdyne bike (pictured) that also allows you to use your arms. On a scale of 1 to 10, with 10 being as fast as you can move, stay at a pace that puts you around a 4 for 25 to 30 minutes.

Coaching Tips

- Adjust the seat position so that when standing next to it, it aligns with your hip joint.
- Avoid slouching as you perform this exercise.

Metabolic Conditioning Protocols

This section presents a variety of metabolic conditioning protocols (MCPs) that are used (along with SMIT) in the functional-spectrum training system to help you develop the conditioning (i.e., work capacity) to outlast the competition. Some MCPs use only your body weight, whereas others use a variety of common exercise equipment, such as medicine balls, barbells, dumbbells, kettlebells, weight plates, and weight sleds.

Boxing and Kickboxing on a Heavy Bag

Used as training methods, boxing and kickboxing can help you improve both your athleticism and your conditioning. Because this program is geared toward usefulness for everyday gym users and home exercisers, it focuses on the use of a heavy bag (see figure), which can be found in most gyms and even some homes, rather than on hitting mitts and sparring for timing. If you'd like to take your boxing skills to the next level, seek out training from a boxing coach or join a boxing gym.

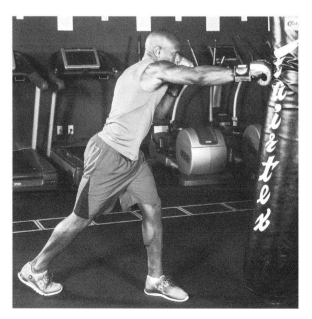

Setup

You'll need a set of boxing gloves and a heavy bag.

Action

From a fighting stance with your hands up, perform combinations of punches—jabs, crosses, and hooks (you can't really throw an uppercut on a regular heavy bag). Alternatively, perform combinations of punches, kicks, and knee strikes. Between combinations, circle the bag by side-stepping around it. Perform 2- or 3-minute rounds with 1 or 2 minutes of rest between rounds.

Coaching Tips

- Stay light on your feet when circling the bag.
- Focus on using your entire body when striking the bag—good punches involve the legs and hips.

Reaction Ball

The reaction ball is rubber and usually has six sides. Due to its shape, when the ball lands on the ground it makes an unpredictable bounce, forcing you to make quick decisions and multi-directional movements to catch the ball. This makes the reaction ball a great and cost-effective addition to one's training tool-box.

Setup

With at least 10-feet of open space around you, hold the reaction ball in one hand while standing in an athletic stance with knees slightly bent and feet roughly shoulder width apart.

Action

Drop the reaction ball onto the ground and allow it to bounce. Try to catch the reaction ball with one-hand after the first bounce (see figure a). If you're unable to catch it on the first bounce, chase the ball down and attempt to catch it in as few bounces as possible (see figure b). After you've caught the ball, return to the starting position and repeat. Try to perform as many catch and release reps as possible for 2 to 3 minute rounds. Rest 1 to 2 minutes between each round.

Coaching Tips

- Be sure to begin every rep from an athletic stance and stay light on your feet.
- Sometimes the reaction ball will bounce straight back to you. Other times it will take odd bounces and force you to constantly change direction in order to catch it. So, make sure you're ready to move fast each time you drop it.

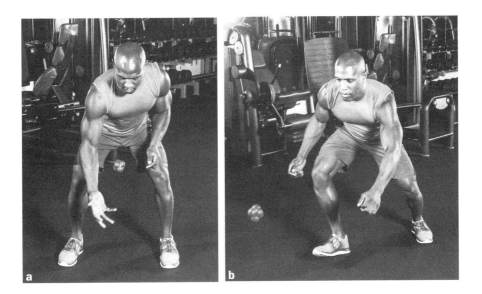

Six-Minute Body-Weight Complex

Perform the following four moves as a circuit. Do one move for 30 seconds, rest for 15 seconds, and then move on to the next move. Repeat the circuit twice for a total of 6 minutes.

1. Prisoner Speed Squat

Setup

Stand tall with your feet shoulder-width apart and your toes turned out slightly (about 10 degrees). Interlace your fingers behind your head and point your elbows out to the sides (see figure a).

Action

Perform a squat by bending your knees and sitting back at your hips (see figure b). Go down so your thighs reach just below parallel to the floor without allowing your lower back to round out. Move as fast as you can.

Coaching Tips

- As you squat, do not allow your heels to come off of the ground or your knees to come together toward the midline of your body.
- Your knees should track in the same direction as your toes.

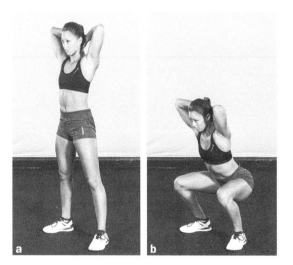

2. Burpee

Setup

With your feet slightly farther than shoulder-width apart, hold your arms straight in front of your body so that they hang between your feet (see figure a).

Action

Bend your knees and hinge forward at your hips so that your torso leans forward. Place your hands on the ground, with your wrists directly below your shoulders (see figure b), and jump your legs backward (see figure c) to move into a push-up position (see figure d). Jump your feet back up to the outside of your hands (see figures e and f), then return to a tall standing position to complete the rep (see figure g).

Coaching Tips

- Make sure that your body forms one straight line and that you do not allow your hips to sag toward the floor in the push-up position.
- Each time that you jump your feet up to the outside of your hands, drop your hips down into a squat-type position before you stand up tall.

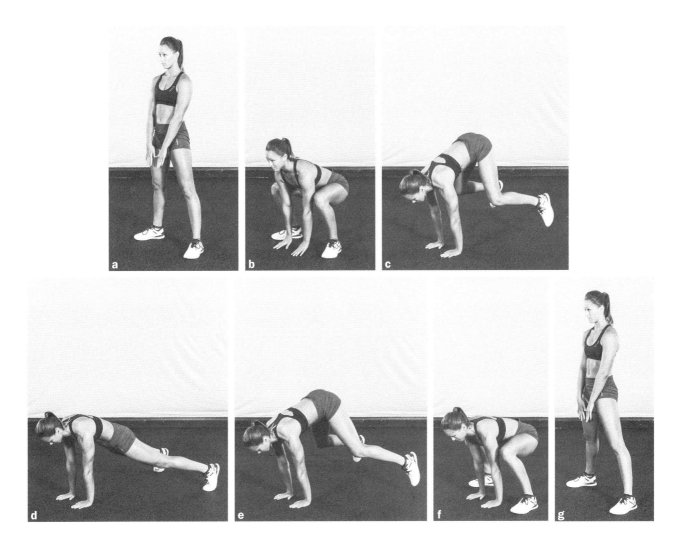

3. Mountain Climber

Setup

Start at the top of a push-up (see figure *a*).

Action

Pick up your right foot and bring your knee toward your left elbow (see figure *b*). Quickly switch your legs so that your right leg goes back to the start position and your left knee moves up to your right shoulder. Continue to alternate legs at a rapid pace.

Coaching Tips

- Keep your hips no higher than your shoulders.
- Do not allow the leg that's pulled toward your shoulder to touch the floor.
- Keep your wrists underneath your shoulders throughout.

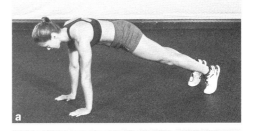

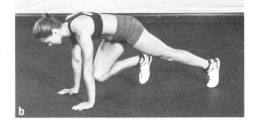

> *continued*

4. In-Place Speed Skip

Setup

Stand tall with your feet hip-width apart and your elbows bent roughly 90 degrees.

Action

Lift your left knee just above your hip while also lifting your right arm and moving your left arm back (see figure *a*). Quickly reverse your arm position and simultaneously drive your left leg down to the ground while elevating your right knee (see figure *b*). As in rope jumping, skipping requires a double-foot strike pattern, or right-right hops followed by left-left hops. Skip in place as fast as possible.

Coaching Tips

- This is not running in place. To skip in place, you must coordinate your arm pumping with the double-foot strikes.

- Keep your torso upright throughout.

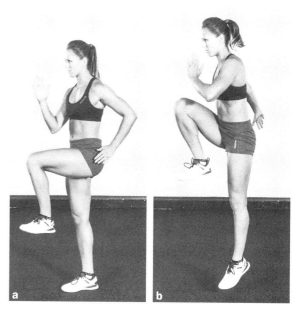

Unilateral Leg Complex

Leg complexes can help you build legs that don't quit; they can also make your wheels feel like you just squatted a ton without ever putting a heavy bar on your back. This makes leg complexes a nice option for giving your back an occasional break from the spinal compression brought on by high-load squats and deadlifts.

This complex involves all unilateral-dominant (i.e., single-leg-dominant) exercises, which can help you make your legs equally strong, improve symmetry, and increase carryover to your chosen sport. To perform these exercises, you'll need a weight bench. Perform them back to back.

1. Split Squat

Setup

Assume a split stance with your hands interlaced behind your head and your rear heel off the ground (see figure *a*).

Action

Lower your body toward the floor allowing your back knee to lightly touch the floor (see figure *b*). Drive your front heel into the ground to raise your body to the starting position, thus completing one rep. Perform 8 to 12 reps per leg. Perform all reps on one side before switching to the other leg.

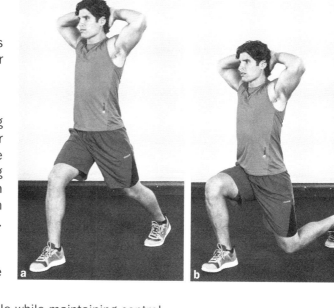

Coaching Tips

- Keep a slight bend in your front knee at the top of each rep.

- Perform each rep as fast as possible while maintaining control.

2. Reverse Lunge

Setup

Stand tall with your feet hip-width apart and your fingers interlaced behind your head (see figure *a*).

Action

Step your left leg backward, placing the ball of your foot on the floor while bending both knees, and lower your body into a lunge (see figure *b*). Once your back knee lightly touches the floor, reverse the motion by stepping back up into the starting position. Perform the same motion by stepping back with your other leg. Alternate legs on each rep. Perform 8 to 12 reps per leg.

Coaching Tips

- Perform each rep as fast as possible with control.
- Your knees should track in the same direction as your toes.

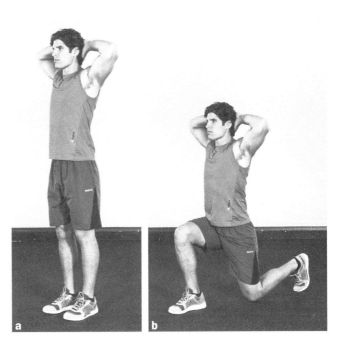

3. Single-Leg Step-Up With Knee Drive

Setup

Facing a weight bench, stand with your feet hip-width apart and your arms at your sides. Place your left foot on top of the bench (see figure *a*).

Action

Step up onto the bench by extending your left knee. As you step up, simultaneously drive your right knee up above your hip (see figure *b*). Reverse the motion by stepping down, with your right foot touching the ground first. Perform all reps on the same leg before switching legs. Perform 8 to 12 reps per leg.

Coaching Tips

- Perform each rep as fast as possible with control.
- On each step-up, drive your knee through powerfully.
- Perform each rep as fast as possible with control.

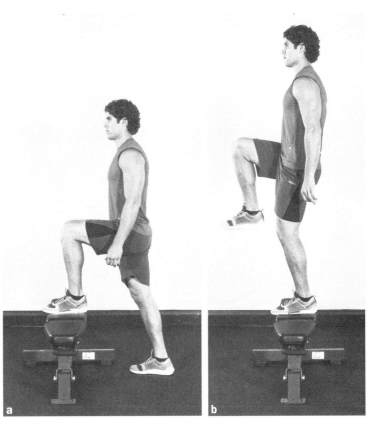

> continued

4. Anterior-Leaning Lunge Scissor Jump

Setup

Assume a split-stance position with your legs hip-width apart and your rear heel off the ground so that most of your weight is placed on your front leg. Lean your torso slightly forward by hinging at your hips. Reach your arms down toward the floor (see figure *a*).

Action

Jump into the air as high as possible while scissoring your legs (see figure *b*) so that you land in the same starting position but with the opposite leg forward (see figure *c*). Jump into the air again and repeat the action. Perform 8 to 12 reps per leg.

Coaching Tips

- Land as quietly and lightly as possible, using each landing to load the next jump.
- Each time you land, keep your knees in the same line as your toes; at no time should your knees come toward your body's midline.
- Each time you land, hinge forward at your hips while keeping your spine straight.
- Each time you explode back into the air, raise your torso.

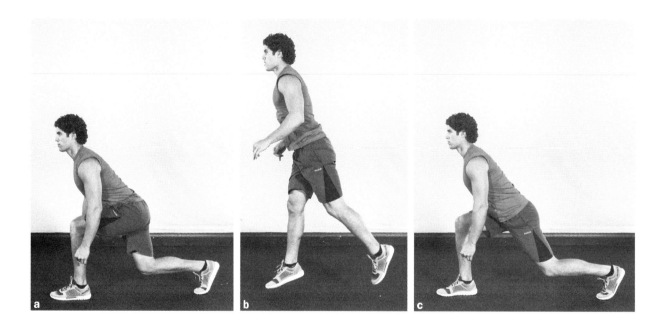

20-20-10-10 Leg Complex

This complex gets your legs burning and your heart pumping. Its name comes from the number of reps you perform for each of the four exercises. Perform the exercises back to back without rest—20 reps for the prisoner speed squat and the zombie squat hold. Then 10 reps for the burpee and 10 reps for the squat jump with arm drive.

1. Prisoner Speed Squat

Setup

Stand tall with your feet slightly more than shoulder-width apart and your toes turned out slightly (about 10 degrees). Interlace your fingers behind your head with your elbows pointed out to the sides (see figure *a*).

Action

Perform a squat by bending your knees and sitting back at your hips (see figure *b*). Go down so your thighs reach just below parallel to the floor without allowing your lower back to round out. Move as fast as you can.

Coaching Tips

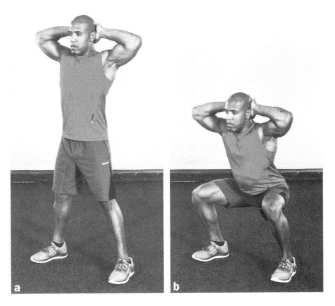

- As you squat, do not allow your heels to come off of the ground or your knees to come together toward the midline of your body.
- Your knees should track in the same direction as your toes.

2. Zombie Squat Hold

Setup

Stand tall with your feet shoulder-width apart and your toes turned out slightly (about 10 degrees). Extend your arms in front of you at shoulder height.

Action

Squat until your thighs are parallel to the ground (see figure). Hold this position for 20 seconds without allowing your lower back to round out.

Coaching Tips

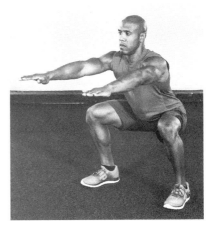

- As you squat, do not allow your heels to come off of the ground or your knees to come together toward the midline of your body.
- Your knees should track in the same direction as your toes.

> continued

3. Burpee

Setup

With your feet slightly wider than shoulder-width apart, hold your arms straight in front of your body so that they hang in front (see figure *a*).

Action

Bend your knees and hinge forward at your hips so that your torso leans forward. Place your hands on the ground, with your wrists directly underneath your shoulders (see figure *b*), and jump your legs backward (see figure *c*) so that you move into a push-up position (see figure *d*). Jump your feet up to the outside of your hands (see figure *e* and *f*) and return to the tall standing position, thus completing the rep (see figure *g*).

Coaching Tips

- Make sure that your body forms one straight line and that you do not allow your hips to sag toward the floor in the push-up position.
- Each time you jump your feet up to the outside of your hands, drop your hips into a squat-type position before you stand up tall.

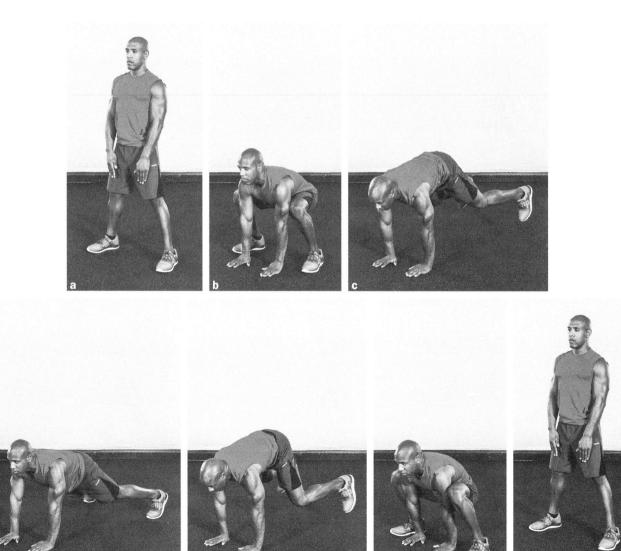

4. Squat Jump With Arm Drive

Setup

Stand with your feet roughly shoulder-width apart and your arms by your sides.

Action

Squat by bending at your knees and hips so that your thighs are just above parallel to the ground. Reach your arms slightly behind your hips, keeping your elbows slightly bent (see figure *a*). Jump straight up into the air, simultaneously extending your legs and swinging your arms above you (see figure *b*). Land as lightly and as quietly as possible, returning to the starting position for the next jump.

Coaching Tips

- Jump as high as you can on each repetition.
- Each time you squat, keep your knees in the same line as your toes; your knees should not come toward one another at any time.
- Do not allow your back to round out at the bottom of each repetition.

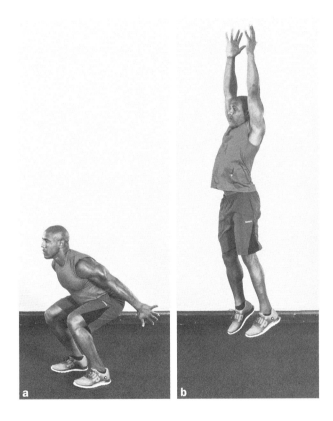

Weight-Sled Forward Pull

Using a sled to increase your cardio conditioning differs from using a sled to improve your strength only in the resistance and the distance that you use. For cardio conditioning, use a lighter load for 50 to 100 yards per set.

Setup

Attach a pair of handles to the rope or straps of the sled. Holding a handle in each hand, stand with the sled about two yards behind you. Position your body at roughly a 45-degree angle with one leg in front of the other and your arms in line with your torso (see figure *a*). If using handles, keep your arms by your sides, in line with your torso.

Action

Drive your legs into the ground and move forward by stepping one leg after the other (see figure *b*). Drag the sled for 40 to 100 yards per set, depending on the weight of the sled.

Coaching Tips

- Unlike using a shoulder harness, the handles add an additional grip challenge and force you to control two separate handles.
- Use a load that's heavy enough to force you to lean in and move in a deliberate manner.
- Avoid short strides, push hard from your legs, and drive your feet diagonally into the ground with each step.

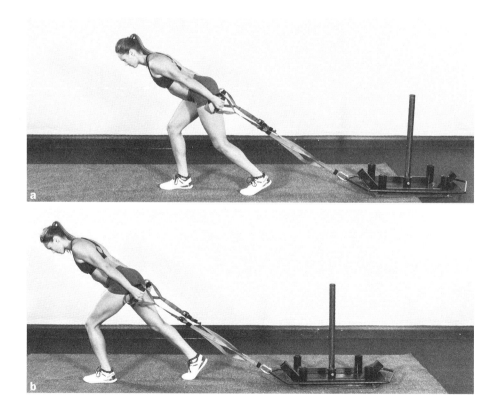

Weight-Sled Push

Setup

You'll need a weight sled with upright poles attached. With your arms extended in front of you, position your body at a forward-leaning angle with one leg in front of the other (see figure *a*).

Action

Keeping your arms straight, drive your legs into the ground and move forward by stepping one leg after the other (see figures *b* and *c*). Avoid short, choppy strides. Drag the sled 40 to 100 yards per set, depending on the weight.

Coaching Tips

- Avoid short, choppy strides.
- Use a load that's heavy enough to force you to lean in and move in a deliberate manner.

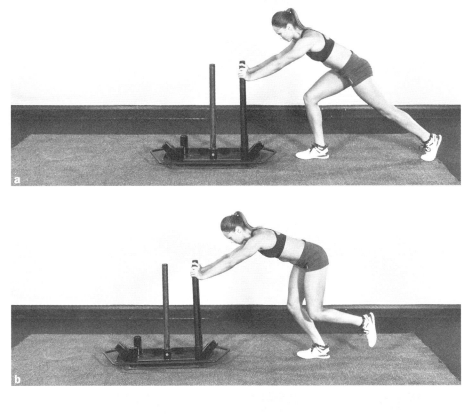

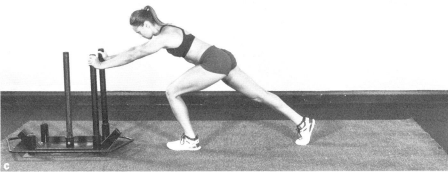

Medicine-Ball Diagonal Squat Push Throw Run Combination

Setup

In a large space (e.g., field or parking lot), stand with your feet roughly shoulder-width apart. Hold a medicine ball weighing 3 to 5 kilograms (about 6.5 to 11 lbs.) at your chest with your elbows underneath the ball.

Action

Lower your body in a motion similar to that of a deadlift by shifting your hips backward and bending your knees so that your thighs become roughly parallel to the ground and your torso leans slightly forward (see figure a). Explode out of the bottom position by simultaneously extending your arms and legs and launching the ball diagonally (at a 45-degree angle) as far as you can out in front of you (see figure b). After you've released the ball, sprint to it (see figure c). Allow the ball to bounce once or twice but grab it before it bounces a third time. Reset your feet to begin the next throw, which is followed by another run to grab the ball. Repeat this sequence, moving across the field or parking lot or throwing it back to where you started, for a total of 8 to 12 throws.

Coaching Tips

- As you throw the ball, your forward lean causes you to jump forward, which sets you up nicely to sprint forward.
- Do not try to throw the ball on the run. Stop after you've grabbed the ball to properly set up each throw so that you can throw the ball in the most powerful manner.
- If you're using a sand-filled, non-bounce medicine ball, throw the ball into open space as far as possible at a 45-degree angle, then sprint to where it lands and throw it back to where you started.

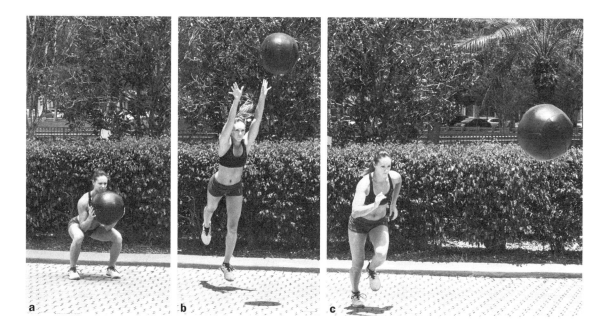

Medicine-Ball Side-Scoop Diagonal Throw Run Combination

Setup

In a large space (e.g., field or parking lot), stand with your feet shoulder-width apart and your knees slightly bent. Hold a medicine ball weighing 3 to 5 kilograms (about 6.5 to 11 lbs.) by your right hip.

Action

Shift your weight to your right leg while hinging forward slightly at your hips (see figure a). Explosively shift your hips to your left while turning your hips and shoulders to throw the ball at a 45-degree trajectory (see figure b). Throw with both hands in a scooplike motion as if throwing a hay bale into the back of a truck by explosively shifting your weight to the left. After you've released the ball, sprint to it (see figure c). Allow it to bounce once or twice but grab it before it bounces a third time. Reset your feet to begin the next throw, which is followed by another run to grab the ball. Repeat this sequence, moving across the field or parking lot and switching sides each time you throw or throwing it back to where you started, for a total of 8 to 12 throws (4 to 6 throws on each side).

Coaching Tips

- On each throw, simultaneously extend your legs and rotate your torso; keep your elbows slightly bent throughout.
- On every throw, your feet should leave the ground and your rotation should cause you to land facing the spot to which you threw the ball.
- Do not try to throw the ball on the run. Stop after you've grabbed the ball to properly set up each throw so that you can throw the ball in the most powerful manner.
- If you're using a sand-filled, non-bounce medicine ball, throw it into open space as far as possible at a 45-degree angle, then sprint to where it lands and throw it back to where you started.

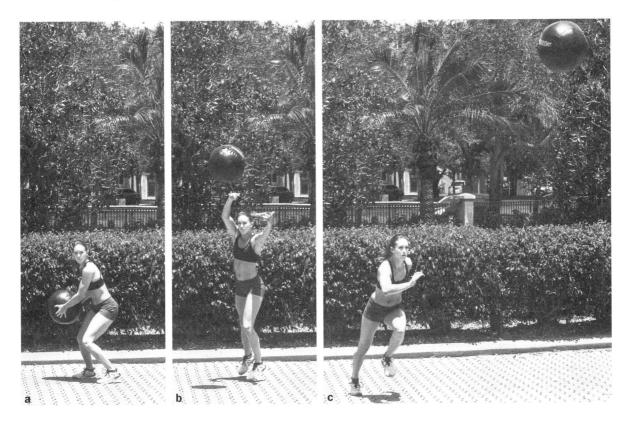

a   b   c

Medicine-Ball Throw Complex

Obtain a medicine ball weighing 3 to 5 kilograms (about 6.5 to 11 lbs.) and find a solid wall at which to hurl it. You can use either a rubber (bouncing) medicine ball or Dynamax-type (minimal-bounce) medicine ball. Perform the following exercises back to back and explosively.

1. Vertical Squat Push Throw

Setup

Stand with your feet roughly shoulder-width apart and hold the medicine ball at your chest with your elbows underneath the ball.

Action

Squat so that your thighs are roughly parallel to the floor with your torso fairly upright (see figure a). Explode out of the bottom position by simultaneously extending your arms and legs and launching the ball vertically into the air as high as possible (see figure b). Do not catch the medicine ball; allow it to land after each throw or catch it on the bounce before resetting for the next rep. Perform 6 to 10 reps.

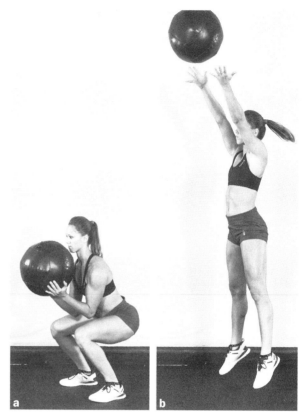

Coaching Tips

- When squatting to prepare for each repetition, do not allow your knees to drop in toward the midline of your body, your heels to lift off of the ground, or your lower back to lose its arch.
- On each throw, explode out of the starting position as fast as you can while throwing the ball as hard as you can.
- Your feet should leave the ground, and at the end of each throw your body should be fully extended with your arms overhead.

2. Step and Overhead Throw

Setup

Stand with your feet roughly hip-width apart and hold the medicine ball over your head (see figure a). Step back with one foot and lean backward, thus causing your abdominal region to stretch (see figure b).

Action

Lean forward on the front foot as you explosively throw the ball at the wall in a manner similar to that of soccer throw (see figure c). Aim for a target on the wall that's roughly at your torso height. Stand far enough back from the wall to allow the ball to bounce at least once before you catch it and reset for the next rep. Alternate the lead leg on each rep. Perform 6 to 10 reps total.

Coaching Tips

- At the start of each rep, do not lean back so far as to overextend your lower back. Lean back just enough to initiate a stretch in the front of your torso.
- On each throw, initiate with your legs and follow through with your arms.
- If you're using a Dynamax-type medicine ball, which has limited bounce, you can stand much closer to the wall than if using a rubber medicine ball. Stand at a distance from the wall that allows the ball to bounce back to you after each throw without forcing you to feel rushed.

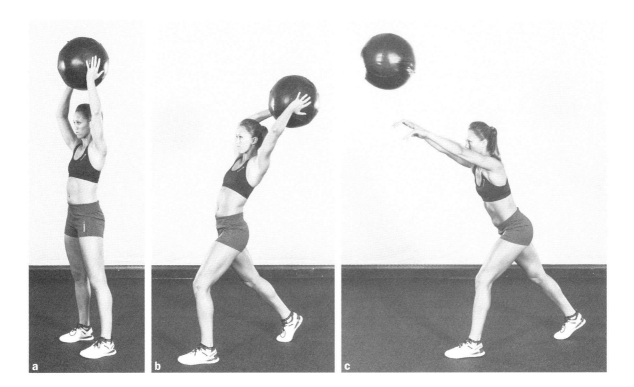

3. Side-Scoop Horizontal Throw

Setup

Stand perpendicular to a solid wall at your right side with your feet shoulder-width apart and your knees slightly bent. Hold the medicine ball by your left hip.

Action

Shift your weight to your left leg while hinging forward slightly at your hips (see figure a). Explosively shift your hips toward your right while turning your hips and shoulders to throw the ball horizontally with both hands in a scooplike motion (see figure b). Aim for a target on the wall that's roughly at your torso height. Alternate sides on each throw. Perform 8 to 10 reps (4 to 5 per side).

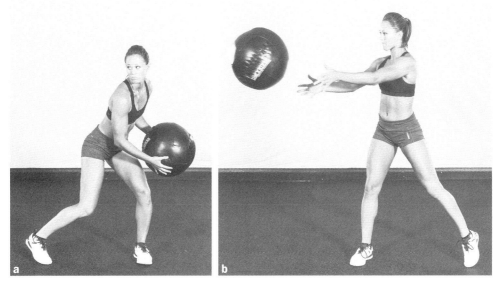

> continued

Coaching Tips

- Keep your back in good alignment when setting up each throw.
- Keep your elbows slightly bent throughout.
- As you throw, lift your back heel off of the ground and rotate in the same direction you're throwing by pivoting on the ball of your foot.
- If you're using a Dynamax-type medicine ball, which has limited bounce, you can stand much closer to the wall than if using a rubber medicine ball. Stand at a distance from the wall that allows the ball to bounce back to you after each throw without forcing you to feel rushed.

4. Rainbow Slam

Setup

Stand with your feet hip-width apart while holding the medicine ball above your head with your elbows slightly bent (see figure *a*).

Action

Slam the ball to the ground at roughly a 45-degree angle, just outside your opposite foot, while shifting your weight to the same side (see figure *b*). Allow the ball to take a very small bounce, catch it, and reverse the motion to perform the next repetition on the other side. Perform 10 to 12 total reps (5 to 6 per side).

Coaching Tips

- As you slam the ball, allow your shoulders and hips to rotate slightly.
- To avoid getting hit in the face when the ball bounces, do *not* keep your face directly above the spot where the ball is slammed.
- At the top of the range of motion, when your arms are overhead, reach as high as possible to create a stretch in your torso musculature.

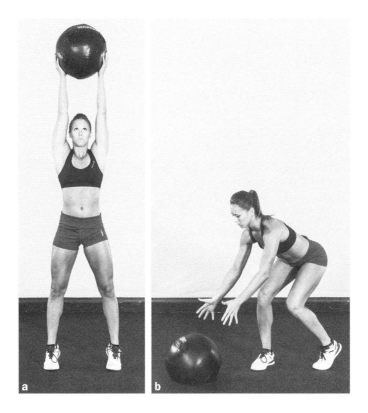

Four-Minute Rope Complex

Rope-conditioning protocols can greatly benefit your upper-body power endurance, especially since many of the conditioning protocols shared up to this point are lower-body dominant. Perform the following four rope exercises back to back. Perform each exercise twice in row—20 seconds on and 10 seconds off—for a total of one minute per exercise and four minutes for the entire complex.

1. Rope Tidal Wave

Setup

Anchor a heavy rope at its center, 15 to 20 feet (about 4.5 to 6 m) away from where you're standing and around a stable object. Stand facing the rope with your feet hip-width apart, your knees slightly bent, and one end of the rope in each hand with your arms extended in front of your body (see figure a).

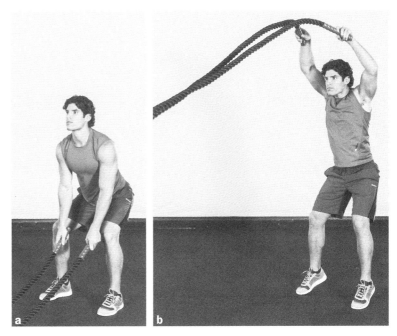

Action

Start swinging your arms up and down at the same time to create a parallel wavelike motion with the rope. Extend your legs each time you lift your arms slightly overhead (see figure b), and allow your knees to bend each time your arms come down.

Coaching Tips

- Do not allow your back to round out when you slam the ropes toward the floor.
- Do not just use your arms; allow your entire body to contribute to rapidly moving the ropes.
- Move as fast as possible without pausing at any point until the set is completed.

2. Rope Spiral

Setup

Anchor a heavy rope at its center, 15 to 20 feet (about 4.5 to 6 m) away from where you're standing and around a stable object. Stand facing the rope with your feet hip-width apart, your knees slightly bent, and one end of the rope in each hand with your arms in front of your body (see figure a).

Action

Keeping your elbows slightly bent, make outward circular motions with both hands, moving your arms from your knees to above your head to create a spiral pattern (see figures b and c). Repeat this motion as fast as you can.

> continued

Coaching Tips

- Move as fast as possible without pausing at any point until the set is completed.
- Don't just use your arms. Allow your entire body to contribute to the motion of rapidly moving the ropes.

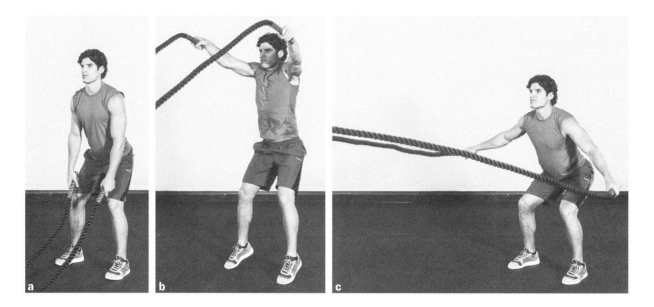

3. Rope Press Wave

Setup

Anchor a heavy rope at its center, 15 to 20 feet (about 4.5 to 6 m) away from where you're standing and around a stable object. Stand facing the rope with your feet hip-width apart, your knees slightly bent, and one end of the rope in each hand with your arms in front of you at roughly waist height (see figure *a*).

Action

Extend your legs and explosively drive your arms out in-front of your body at roughly a 45-degree angle (see figure *b*). Quickly reverse the motion, pulling your arms back down and return to the starting position. Continue this total-body action, whipping the ropes up and down as fast as you can.

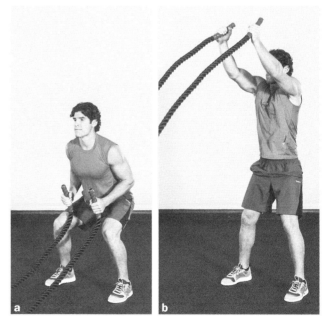

Coaching Tips

- Move as fast as possible without pausing at any point until the set is completed.
- Don't just use your arms. Allow your entire body to contribute to the motion of rapidly moving the ropes.
- Since this exercise uses the opposite grip than the rope tidal wave, the emphasis of this exercise is reversed. It emphasizes a pushing action—driving the rope away from you—instead of a pulling action—driving the rope down into the floor—to create the waves.

4. Rope Rainbow

Setup

Anchor a heavy rope at its center, 15 to 20 feet (about 4.5 to 6 m) away from where you're standing and around a stable object. Stand facing the rope with your feet hip-width apart while holding one end of the rope in each hand above your head with your elbows bent and your hands underneath the rope (see figure *a*).

Action

Explosively pivot your body while flipping the ropes over as if throwing them to the floor to one side and then the other (see figures *b* and *c*). Move your arms explosively in an arching, rainbow-like motion. This movement should create a rhythmic, wavelike motion in the ropes.

Coaching Tips

- Move the ropes back and forth in a manner that is fast but smooth and coordinated; do not use a jerking, stop-and-start motion.
- Use your legs a bit by allowing your knees to bend as your arms lower to each side and by extending your legs each time your arms are overhead when you go back to center.

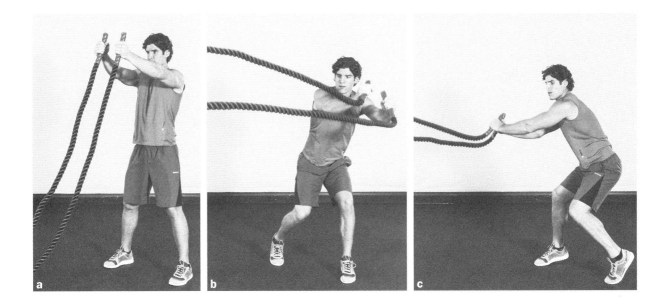

Weight-Plate Push

Setup

Place a heavy weight plate—try 35 to 45 pounds (about 15 to 20 kg)—on top of a towel so that it glides or on a turf surface. For an additional challenge, you can also place a set of dumbbells (25 to 35 lbs., or about 11 to 15 kg) inside of the weight plate. Get into push-up position with your hands on top of the weight plate or the dumbbells.

Action

Drive with your legs by bringing your knees up toward your chest in alternating fashion to push the plate quickly across the floor for 40 to 50 yards (see figures a-c).

Coaching Tips

- Maximize muscle tension by keeping your elbows straight and your arms at a 45-degree angle above your head.
- Take long strides and keep your hips no higher than your shoulders.
- As you improve, increase the load challenge by placing a pair of heavier dumbbells inside the weight plate.

Barbell Complex

Grab an Olympic-style barbell with no more than 25 pounds (11 kg) loaded onto each side and perform the following exercises back to back in a fast but controlled manner.

1. Barbell Bent-Over Row

Setup

Stand with your feet roughly hip-width apart. Hold the barbell with an overhand grip, keeping your hands just outside shoulder-width apart. Bend over at your hips, keeping your back straight so that your torso is parallel to the floor and your knees are bent 15 to 20 degrees (see figure a).

Action

Row the bar into the middle of your torso, between your chest and belly button (see figure b). Lower the bar to complete the rep. Perform 8 to 10 reps.

Coaching Tips

- At the top of each rep, pinch your shoulder blades together.
- Do not allow your back to round out at any time.
- Do not allow the fronts of your shoulders to round forward at the top of each repetition.

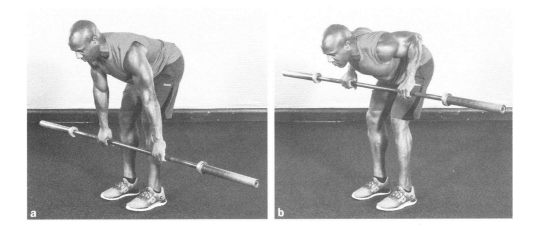

2. Barbell Romanian Deadlift

Setup

Standing tall with your feet hip-width apart, hold a barbell in front of your thighs with your arms straight; grip the bar just outside your hips (see figure *a*).

Action

Keeping your back straight, hinge at your hips and bend forward toward the floor with your knees bent at a 15- to 20-degree angle (see figure *b*). Once your torso is roughly parallel to the floor, drive your hips forward toward the barbell, then reverse the motion to stand tall again. Perform 12 to 15 reps.

Coaching Tips

- As you hinge forward, drive your hips backward; do not allow your back to round out.
- Lift the bar by extending your hips—not by overextending at your lower back.
- Keep the barbell close to you throughout; the barbell should touch your shins at the bottom and track against the front of your legs as you perform the repetitions.

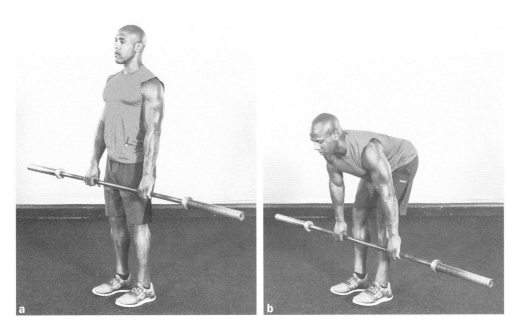

> *continued*

3. Barbell Jump Shrug

Setup

Standing tall with your feet hip-width apart, hold a barbell in front of your thighs with your arms straight; grip the bar just outside your hips.

Action

Keeping your back straight, hinge at your hips and bend forward toward the floor with your knees bent at a 15- to 20-degree angle (see figure *a*). Once the barbell is just above your knees, take a small jump into the air as you shrug the bar, driving your shoulders toward your ears (see figure *b*). Reverse the motion by lowering the barbell in a controlled manner. Perform 8 to 10 reps.

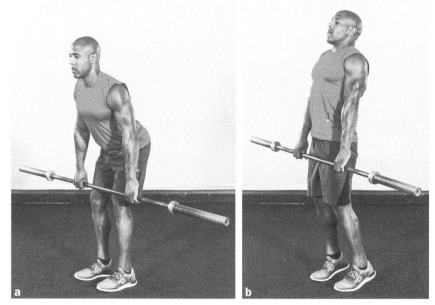

Coaching Tips

- As you hinge forward, drive your hips backward; do not allow your back to round out.
- Lift the bar by extending your hips—not by overextending at your lower back.
- Keep the barbell close to you throughout.
- Although the word *jump* appears in the name of this exercise, there's no air under your feet on each lift. Your heels explode off of the ground, but the balls of your feet remain in contact with the ground.

4. Barbell Hang Clean

Setup

Stand with your feet shoulder-width apart and hold a barbell with your hands just outside shoulder-width apart. Hinge slightly at your hips, keeping the bar against your thighs (see figure *a*).

Action

Explode your hips into the bar as you pull the bar upward (see figure *b*). Once the bar reaches shoulder level, quickly flip your elbows underneath the bar to catch it at the top of your chest (see figure *c*). Perform 6 to 8 reps. After performing your last hang-clean repetition, hold the barbell at the top of the position, thus setting up to begin the barbell overhead push press.

Coaching Tips

- Your heels leave the ground as your drive the bar upward, but do not allow your entire foot to leave the ground (doing so reduces your potential for power production).
- Perform this exercise fast but with deliberate control; your motion should be smooth and coordinated on each lift and on each lowering to set up for the next rep.

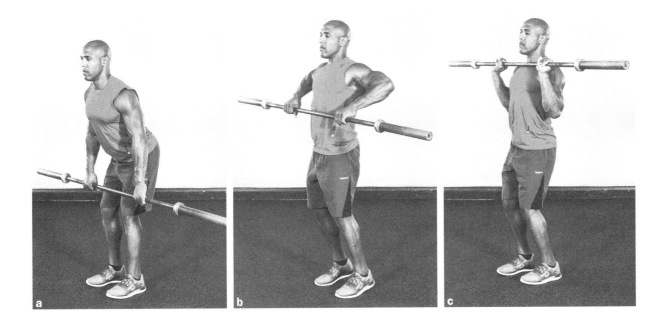

5. Barbell Overhead Push Press

Setup

Stand with your feet shoulder-width apart and hold the barbell with your hands just outside shoulder width.

Action

Slightly bend your knees (see figure a), then quickly reverse the motion, exploding into the bar and driving it overhead with your arms and legs in a coordinated fashion (see figure b). Once the bar is completely overhead, slowly reverse the previous motions, replacing the bar on the floor to complete a full repetition. Perform 6 to 8 reps. After performing the last repetition, lower the barbell behind your head and place it across your shoulders to set up for the barbell reverse lunge.

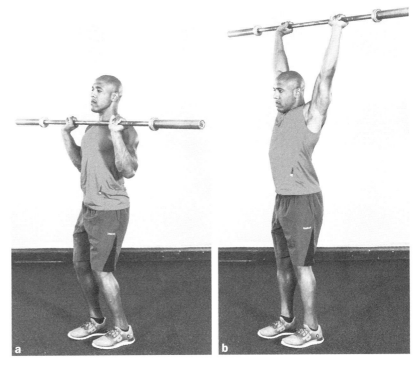

Coaching Tips

- Keep your wrists straight; do not allow them to bend backward at any time.
- Do not allow your lower back to overextend as you press the barbell overhead.

> continued

6. Barbell Reverse Lunge

Setup

Stand with your feet hip-width apart and a barbell across your shoulders behind your head; grip the barbell outside your shoulders (see figure a).

Action

Step your right leg backward, placing the ball of your foot on the floor while bending both knees and lowering your body into a lunge (see figure b). Once your back knee lightly touches the floor, reverse the motion by stepping back up so that your feet are once again parallel. Perform the same action with the other leg. Perform 5 to 6 reps per leg.

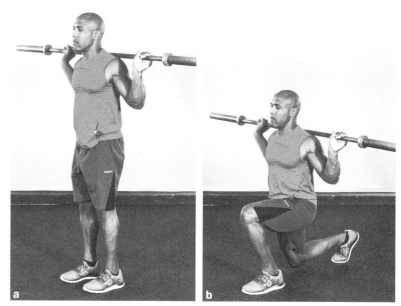

Coaching Tips

- It's ok to hinge at your hips and lean your torso slightly forward during each lunge, which better recruits the glute musculature and makes the exercise more knee friendly.
- Keep your knees in line with your toes on each rep.

Unilateral Kettlebell Complex

Perform these kettlebell exercises while holding the kettlebell in the same hand. Once you've finished the entire sequence, switch hands and repeat. Rest once you've completed all of the exercises with both arms.

1. One-Arm Kettlebell Swing

Setup

With your feet roughly hip-width apart, hold a kettlebell in one hand with your arm straight and in front of your body.

Action

Keeping your back and arm straight, drive the kettlebell between your legs as if hiking a football and hinge forward at your hips. Keep your knees bent at roughly a 15- to 20-degree angle (see figure a). Once your

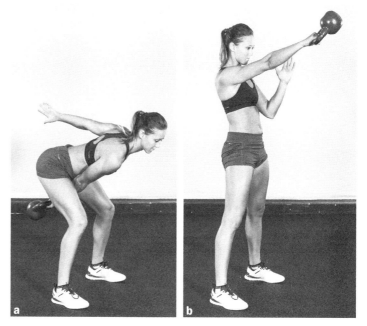

forearm comes into contact with your thigh, explosively reverse the motion by simultaneously driving your hips forward and swinging the kettlebell upward to eye level (see figure b). Perform all reps on the same side before switching sides. Perform 10 to 15 reps per side.

Coaching Tips

- As you hinge forward, drive your hips backward; do not allow your back to round out.
- At the bottom of each swing, allow your forearm to touch the inside of your thigh; use your hips to powerfully drive your arm forward off of your thigh to swing the kettlebell back up.
- Once the kettlebell reaches your eye level, pull it back down, keeping a firm grip on the handle.

2. One-Arm Kettlebell Swing Clean

Setup

Stand with your feet slightly wider than shoulder-width apart and hold a kettlebell in one hand.

Action

Slightly bend your knees and hinge at your hips to allow the kettlebell to swing between your legs (see figure a). Quickly reverse this motion by driving your hips forward and your arm upward (see figure b). As the kettlebell moves toward the sky, quickly flip your elbow underneath it and soften your body to accept the kettlebell moving into your body, creating as much of a cushion as you can (see figure c). Perform 10 to 15 reps on each side.

Coaching Tips

- As the kettlebell comes up to your chest, imagine it as an egg that you do not want to break; absorb it as gently as possible by allowing your legs to bend slightly.
- To start the next repetition, push the kettlebell off of your chest and allow it to swing back between your legs.
- Do not allow your lower back to round out at the bottom position.

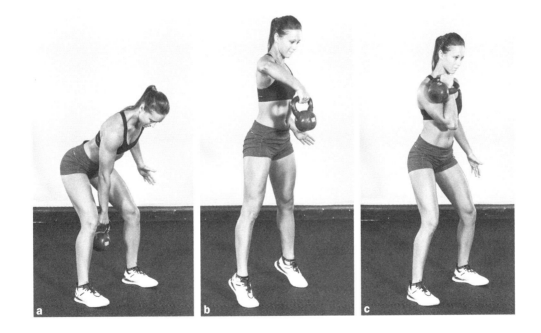

> continued

3. Kettlebell One-Sided Front Squat

Setup

Stand with your feet slightly farther than shoulder-width apart and your toes turned out 10 to 15 degrees. Hold a kettlebell in front of you, resting it on the top of your chest and the outside of your arm with the other arm extended in front of you (see figure *a*). Your hand should be near the center of your chest and your elbow should point down to make a triangle. Stay tall and lift your chest to create a rack for the kettlebell instead of trying to hold it up with only your arm.

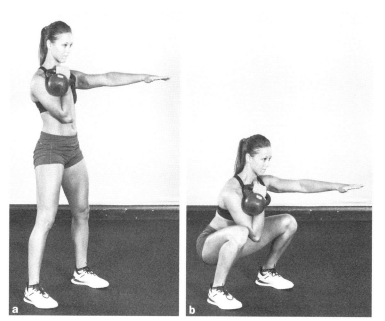

Action

Bend at your knees and hips and lower your body toward the floor; go as low as you can while keeping your other arm extended (see figure *b*). Reverse the motion and return to the standing position to complete a full rep. Perform 10 to 15 reps.

Coaching Tips

- Your heels should not lift off of the ground, and your lower back should not lose its arch as you squat.
- Do not allow your knees to drop in toward the midline of your body; keep your knees in line with your toes on each squat.

4. One-Arm Kettlebell Overhead Push Press

Setup

Stand tall with your feet roughly shoulder-width apart while holding a kettlebell at shoulder level.

Action

Slightly bend your knees (see figure *a*), then quickly reverse the motion, exploding into the kettlebell and driving it overhead with your arm and your legs in a coordinated fashion. Press the kettlebell toward the sky and keep your torso as stable as possible (see figure *b*). Slowly lower the kettlebell back to your shoulder. Perform all repetitions on the same side before switching sides. Perform 6 to 8 reps on each side.

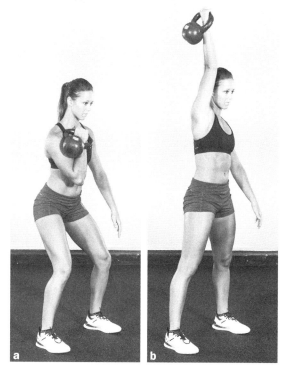

Coaching Tips

- Maintain an upright torso and center your posture by keeping your nose in line with your belly button throughout the exercise.
- At the bottom of each rep, keep your elbow directly underneath the kettlebell.

Bilateral Farmer's-Walk Complex

A farmer's-walk complex consists of a series of dumbbell exercises interspersed between several sets of dumbbell (farmer's) carries. The exercises in this complex are performed back to back (circuit style) without rest until all exercises in a given complex have been completed.

To perform this complex, use a heavier set for the farmer's- portions and a lighter set for the other exercises. The lighter set should be roughly 35 to 40 percent of the weight used for the heavier set. For example, if your heavier set is 80 pounds (about 35 kg) each, then your lighter set should be around 30 pounds (13 kg) each.

To set up for this complex, designate two ends about 20 to 25 yards apart. Place both pairs of dumbbells at one end. If you don't have much free space in your weightroom, just bring the dumbbells into the group fitness room or go outside if the weather is suitable.

1. Farmer's Walk

Setup

Stand next to one end and hold two heavy dumbbells in each hand, with your palms facing your body by your hips (or at your shoulders).

Action

Walk to the other end, then return to your starting point. Keep the dumbbells in position while maintaining a strong upright posture (see figure).

Coaching Tips

- Take normal strides and move as fast as you can without losing control of the weight.
- Maintain a tall, upright posture as you carry the weight.

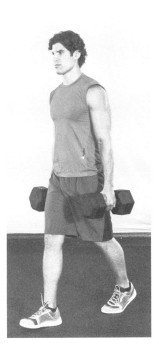

2. Two-Arm Dumbbell Bent-Over Row

Setup

Stand with your feet hip-width apart and hold a dumbbell in each hand. Bend over at your hips, keeping your back straight so that your torso is parallel to the floor. Keep your knees bent 15 to 20 degrees (see figure a).

Action

Row the dumbbells toward you while keeping your arms at a 45-degree angle to your torso (see figure b). Slowly lower the dumbbells back down without allowing them to contact the floor until the set is completed.

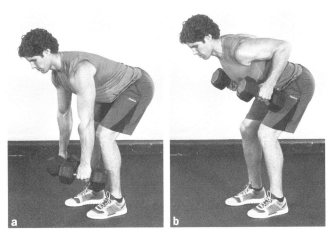

> continued

Coaching Tips

- Do not allow your back to round out at any time.
- Keep your elbows directly above your hands throughout and do not allow your wrists to bend.
- Do not allow the fronts of your shoulders to round forward at the top of each repetition.

3. Farmer's Walk

As described for exercise 1, stand next to one end and hold two heavy dumbbells in each hand with your palms facing your body by your hips (or at your shoulders). Walk to the other end, then return to your starting point. Keep the dumbbells in position while maintaining a strong upright posture.

4. Dumbbell Front-Hold Overhead Press

Setup

Stand tall with your feet shoulder-width apart. Hold a dumbbell in each hand at your shoulders with your elbows directly underneath the handles in front of your torso (see figure *a*).

Action

Press the dumbbells directly overhead until your arms are straight above you, in line with your torso, with the dumbbells parallel to one another at the top (see figure *b*). Slowly reverse the motion, bringing the dumbbells back down to the front of your shoulders.

Coaching Tips

- At the bottom of each repetition, hold the dumbbells parallel with your torso, keeping them directly above your shoulders.
- As you press the dumbbells above you, do not allow your lower back to overextend.

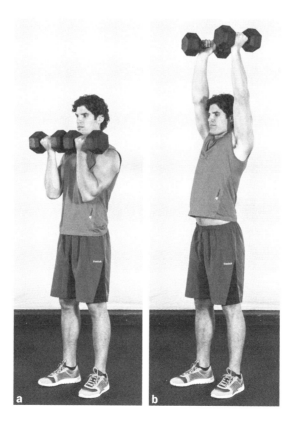

5. Farmer's Walk

As described previously, stand next to one end and hold two heavy dumbbells in each hand with your palms facing your body by your hips (or at your shoulders). Walk to the other end, then return to your starting point. Keep the dumbbells in position while maintaining a strong upright posture.

6. Dumbbell Front Squat

Setup

Stand next to one cone with your feet shoulder-width apart and hold lighter dumbbells in each hand at your shoulders with your elbows directly underneath the handles of the dumbbells (see figure *a*).

Action

Squat as low as you can by bending your knees and sitting your hips back (see figure *b*). Do not allow your heels to rise off of the floor or your lower back to round out. Reverse the motion and return to the tall standing position to complete a rep.

Coaching Tips

- Do not allow your knees to drop in toward the midline of your body; keep your knees tracking in the same direction as your toes.
- The back ends of the dumbbells can rest on the tops of your shoulders on each repetition.

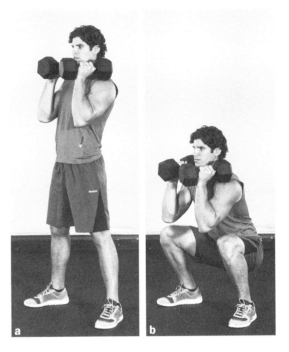

7. Farmer's Walk

As described previously, stand next to one end and hold two heavy dumbbells in each hand with your palms facing your body by your hips (or at your shoulders). Walk to the other end, then return to your starting point. Keep the dumbbells in position while maintaining a strong upright posture.

Unilateral Farmer's-Walk Complex

This complex is performed in the same fashion as the bilateral farmer's walk, except that here you do the entire complex using the same side. In other words, do all of the farmer's walks using your left arm and all of the in-place dumbbell exercises using your left arm. That's half the set. Then switch sides and repeat to complete the set.

To perform this complex, use a heavier dumbbell for the farmer's-walk portions and a lighter dumbbell for the other exercises. The lighter dumbbell should be roughly 35 to 40 percent of the weight used for the heavier dumbbell. For example, if your heavier dumbbell is 80 pounds (about 35 kg), then your lighter dumbbell should be around 30 pounds (13 kg).

To set up for this complex, designate two ends about 20 to 25 yards apart. Place both dumbbells at one end. If you don't have much free space in your weightroom, just bring the dumbbells into the group fitness room or go outside if the weather is suitable.

> continued

1. One-Arm Dumbbell Farmer's Walk

Setup

Stand tall next to one end while holding a heavy dumbbell on the left side of your body, with your palm facing your body by your hip (or at your shoulder).

Action

Walk to the opposite end, then return to your starting point. Keep the dumbbell in position while maintaining a strong upright posture (see figure).

Coaching Tips

- Take normal strides and move as fast as you can without losing control of the weight.
- Maintain a tall, upright posture as you carry the weight.

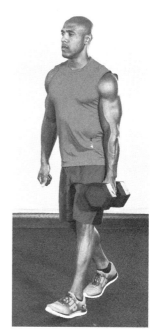

2. One-Arm Freestanding Dumbbell Row

Setup

Assume a split stance with your right leg in front of your left leg and both knees slightly bent. With your left hand, hold the dumbbell in a neutral position so that your palm faces the opposite side of your body; let your other arm hang at your side. Hinge at your hips, keeping your back straight, so that your torso becomes parallel with the floor (see figure *a*).

Action

Perform a row by pulling the dumbbell toward your body, without rotating your shoulders or hips more than a few degrees, while pulling your scapula toward your spine in a controlled manner as your arm moves (see figure *b*). Slowly lower the dumbbell without letting it touch the floor. Perform 6 to 10 reps.

Coaching Tips

- Maintain a stable spinal position, keeping your back straight throughout the exercise.
- Keep your back heel raised off of the ground to ensure that most of your weight is on your front leg.
- Do not allow your rowing-side shoulder to move forward at the end of each rep.

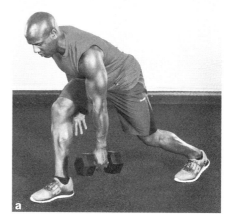

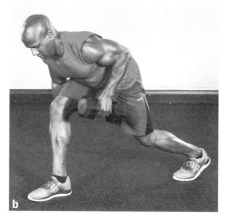

3. One-Arm Dumbbell Farmer's Walk

As described for exercise 1, stand next to one end and hold a heavy dumbbell on the left side of your body, with your palm facing your body by your hip (or at your shoulder). Walk to the other end, then return to your starting point. Keep the dumbbell in position while maintaining a strong upright posture.

4. One-Arm Dumbbell Rotational Push Press

Setup

Stand tall with your feet roughly shoulder-width apart while holding a dumbbell with your left hand in front of your left shoulder.

Action

Slightly bend your knees (see figure *a*), then quickly reverse the motion by pressing the dumbbell straight above your same-side shoulder while rotating to the side opposite the dumbbell (see figure *b*). Perform 4 to 6 reps.

Coaching Tips

- To better allow your hips to rotate in this exercise, raise your same-side heel off of the ground as you turn.
- Begin each repetition with your weight shifted slightly to the leg on the same side as the dumbbell. As you perform each repetition, your weight should shift to the other leg.
- Press the dumbbell and rotate as fast as possible, but lower the dumbbell with deliberate control, which may require you to help with your free hand.

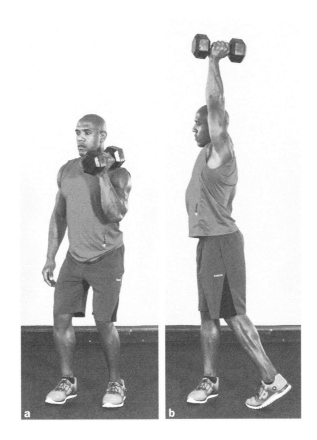

> *continued*

5. One-Arm Farmer's Walk

As described previously, stand next to one end and hold a heavy dumbbell on the left side of your body, with your palm facing your body by your hip (or at your shoulder). Walk to the other end, then return to your starting point. Keep the dumbbell in position while maintaining a strong upright posture.

6. Reverse Lunge With Dumbbell at Shoulder

Setup

Stand tall with your feet about hip-width apart and hold a lighter dumbbell in your left hand at your left shoulder (see figure *a*).

Action

Step backward with your left foot, as you hinge at your hips and lean your torso slightly forward, simultaneously drop your body so that your knee lightly touches the floor (see figure *b*). Reverse the movement by coming out of the lunge and bringing your foot forward so that you are back in the starting position. Perform a series of reverse lunges by stepping back with only this one leg. Perform 6 to 8 reps.

Coaching Tips

- Keep your back straight and your torso centered. Do not lean to one side.
- The back of the dumbbell should rest on top of your shoulder throughout.

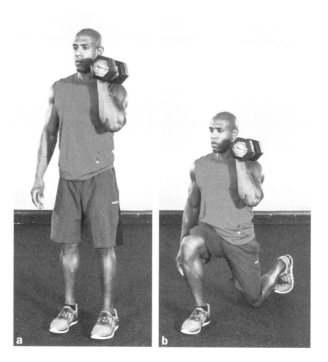

7. One-Arm Farmer's Walk

As described previously, stand next to one end and hold a heavy dumbbell on the left side of your body, with your palm facing your body by your hip (or at your shoulder). Walk to the other end, then return to your starting point. Keep the dumbbell in position while maintaining a strong upright posture.

Plate-Push Complex 1

A plate complex uses a pair of dumbbells approximately 15 to 35 pounds (6 to 15 kg) each depending on your strength level and a 35- to 45-pound (16 to 20 kg) weight plate in a series that alternates dumbbell exercises with weight-plate pushes. These complexes are performed back to back (circuit style) without rest until all exercises in a given complex have been completed. The ideal location for the plate push is a basketball court or turf surface.

To set up for this complex, designate two ends about 20 to 25 yards apart. Place the pair of dumbbells and the weight plate at one end. If you don't have much free space in your weightroom, use a group fitness room or basketball court.

1. Two-Arm Dumbbell Bent-Over Row

Setup

Stand with your feet hip-width apart and hold a dumbbell in each hand. Bend over at your hips, keeping your back straight, so that your torso is parallel to the floor. Keep your knees bent 15 to 20 degrees (see figure *a*).

Action

Row the dumbbells toward you while keeping your arms at roughly a 45-degree angle to your torso (see figure *b*). Slowly lower the dumbbells without allowing them to contact the floor until the set is completed. Perform 10 to 15 reps.

Coaching Tips

- Do not allow your back to round out at any time.
- Keep your elbows directly above your hands throughout and do not allow your wrists to bend.
- Do not allow the fronts of your shoulders to round forward at the top of each repetition.

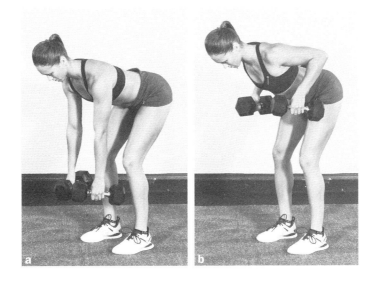

> *continued*

2. Plate Push

Setup

Place a heavy weight plate—try 35 to 45 pounds (about 15 to 20 kg)—on top of a towel so that it glides or on a turf surface. For an additional challenge, you can also place a set of dumbbells (25 to 35 pounds or 11 to 15 kg) inside the weight plate. Get into push-up position with your hands on top of the weight plate.

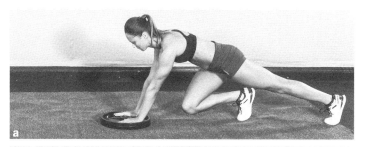

Action

Drive with your legs by bringing your knees up toward your chest in alternating fashion. Push the plate quickly across the floor for 20 to 25 yards up and back for a total of 40 to 50 yards (see figures *a-c*).

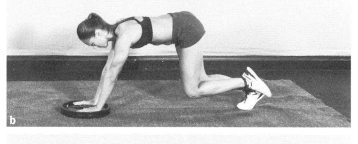

Coaching Tips

- Maximize muscle tension by keeping your elbows straight and your arms at roughly a 45-degree angle above your head.

- Take long strides and keep your hips no higher than your shoulders.

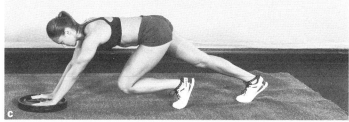

- For an additional challenge, increase the load by placing a pair of heavier dumbbells inside the weight plate.

3. Dumbbell Front-Hold Overhead Press

Setup

Stand tall with your feet shoulder-width apart. Hold a dumbbell in each hand at the same-side shoulder with your elbows directly underneath the handles in front of your torso (see figure *a*).

Action

Press the dumbbells directly overhead until your arms are straight above you, in line with your torso, with the dumbbells parallel to one another at the top (see figure *b*). Slowly reverse the motion by bringing the dumbbells back down to the fronts of your shoulders.

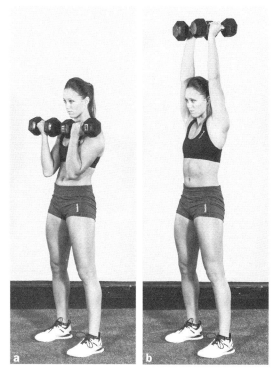

Coaching Tips

- At the bottom of each repetition, hold the dumbbells parallel with your torso, keeping them directly above your shoulders.

- As you press the dumbbells overhead, do not allow your back to overextend.

4. Plate Push

As described in exercise 2, perform a plate push for another 20 to 25 yards down the court or turf surface and back for a total of 40 to 50 yards.

5. One-Leg Dumbbell Romanian Deadlift

Setup

Stand tall and hold a dumbbell in each hand in front of your hips (see figure *a*).

Action

Keeping your back and arms straight, slightly lift the left leg and hinge at your hip. Bend forward toward the floor while extending the left leg back. Keep your weight-bearing knee bent at roughly a 15- to 20-degree angle. As you hinge, allow your non-weight-bearing leg to elevate so that it remains in a straight line with your torso (see figure *b*). Once your torso and non-weight-bearing leg are roughly parallel to the floor, reverse the motion by driving your hips forward to stand tall again, thus completing a full repetition. Alternate legs on each rep. Perform 10 to 14 total reps (5 to 7 per leg).

Coaching Tips

- Do not allow your lower back to round out as you hinge at your hip and lower your torso.
- At the bottom position (when your torso is roughly parallel to the ground), keep your hips and shoulders flat; do not allow them to rotate.
- At the bottom position, the foot of your non-weight-bearing leg should be pointed at the floor.

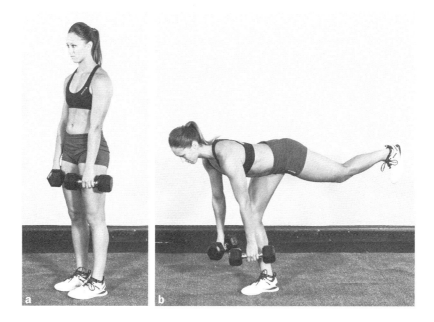

6. Plate Push

As described previously, perform a plate push for another 20 to 25 yards down the court or track surface and back for a total of 40 to 50 yards.

> continued

7. Break-Dancer Push-Up

Setup
Begin in a push-up position with your hands and feet shoulder-width apart (see figure *a*).

Action
Perform a push-up; at the top, rotate your entire body toward your left side, driving your right knee to your left elbow while keeping your left hand in contact with your chin (see figures *b* and *c*). Reverse this motion to perform another push-up and repeat this action on the opposite side, touching your left knee to your right elbow. Perform 5 to 7 reps on each side (10 to 14 total).

Coaching Tips
- Keep your head and hips from sagging toward the floor.
- Rotate your hips and shoulders together at the same rate.

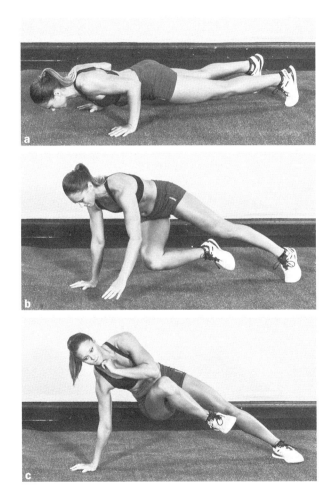

Plate-Push Complex 2

This complex is a variation of plate-push complex 1 and is performed in the same fashion.

1. One-Arm Freestanding Dumbbell Row

Setup

Assume a split stance with your right leg in front of your left leg and both knees slightly bent. With your left hand, hold the dumbbell in a neutral position so that your palm faces the opposite side of your body. Let your other arm hang at your side. Hinge at your hips, keeping your back straight, so that your torso becomes roughly parallel with the floor (see figure *a*).

Action

Perform a row by pulling the dumbbell toward your body, without rotating your shoulders or hips more than a few degrees, while pulling your scapula toward your spine in a controlled manner as your arm moves (see figure *b*). Slowly lower the dumbbell without letting it touch the floor. Complete all reps on one side before switching sides. Perform 8 to 10 reps on each side.

Coaching Tips

- Maintain a stable spinal position, keeping your back straight throughout the exercise.
- Keep your back heel raised off of the ground while performing this exercise to ensure that most of your weight is on your front leg.
- Do not allow your rowing-side shoulder to move forward at the end of each rep.

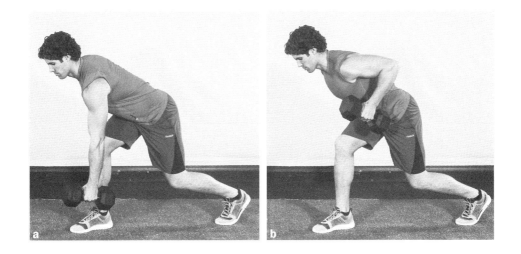

> *continued*

2. Plate Push

Setup

Place a heavy weight plate—try 35 to 45 pounds (about 15 to 20 kg)—on top of a towel so that it glides or on a turf surface. Get into push-up position with your hands on top of the weight plate . For an additional challenge, you can also place a set of dumbbells (25 to 35pounds or 11 to 15 kg) inside the weight plate.

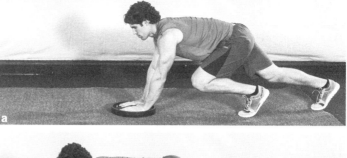

Action

Drive with your legs by bringing your knees up toward your chest in an alternating fashion to push the plate quickly across the floor for 20 to 25 yards up and back for a total of 40 to 50 yards (see figures a-c).

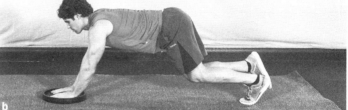

Coaching Tips

- Maximize muscle tension by keeping your elbows straight and your arms at roughly a 45-degree angle above your head.

- Take long strides and keep your hips no higher than your shoulders.

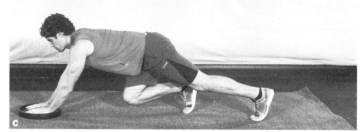

- You can increase the challenge by placing a pair of dumbbells inside the weight plate.

3. One-Arm Dumbbell Rotational Push Press

Setup

Stand tall with your feet roughly shoulder-width apart while holding a dumbbell in front of one shoulder.

Action

Slightly bend your knees (see figure a), then quickly reverse the motion by pressing the dumbbell straight above your same-side shoulder while rotating to the side opposite of the dumbbell (see figure b). Perform all repetitions on the same side before switching sides. Perform 4 to 6 reps per side.

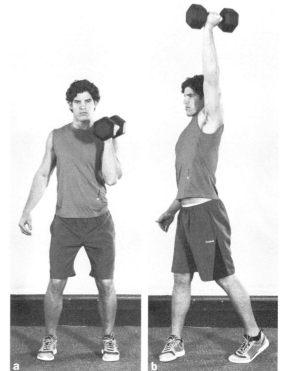

Coaching Tips

- To better allow your hips to rotate in this exercise, raise your same-side heel off of the ground as you turn.

- Begin each repetition with your weight shifted slightly to the leg on the same side as the dumbbell; as you perform each repetition, your weight should shift to the other leg.

- Press the dumbbell and rotate as fast as possible, but lower the dumbbell with deliberate control, which may require you to help with your free hand.

4. Plate Push

As described for exercise 2, perform a plate push for another 20 to 25 yards down the court or turf surface and back for a total of 40 to 50 yards.

5. Dumbbell Anterior Lunge

Setup

Stand tall while holding dumbbells in each hand with your feet hip-width apart (see figure a).

Action

Step forward with one leg, keeping your front knee bent 15 to 20 degrees and your back knee fairly straight. As your front foot hits the ground, lean forward by hinging at your hips and allow your rear heel to come off the ground (see figure b). Your torso should not be lower than parallel to the floor and your back should be straight. Reverse the motion by stepping backward so that your feet are together again and return to an upright position. Then perform the same motion by stepping forward with the other leg. Perform 10 to 14 total reps (5 to 7 reps per side).

Coaching Tips

- Do not let the dumbbells touch the floor at any point during this exercise.
- Do not allow your back to round out at the bottom of each lunge.
- Use good rhythm and timing; perform the step and the hip hinge simultaneously and reverse the motion in the same smooth and coordinated manner.

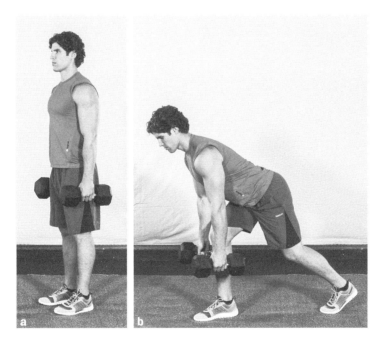

6. Plate Push

As described previously, perform a plate push for another 20 to 25 yards down the court or turf surface and back for a total of 40 to 50 yards.

> continued

7. Dumbbell Plank Row

Setup

Holding a dumbbell in each hand, assume a push-up position with your feet just farther than shoulder-width apart and your wrists directly below your shoulders. (see figure *a*).

Action

While remaining at the top of the push-up position, pick up the dumbbell in your left hand and row it into your body (see figure *b*). Slowly lower it to the floor, then repeat the sequence with your right hand. Continue to alternate hands. Perform 8 to 12 total reps (4 to 6 per side).

Coaching Tips

- Keep your head and hips from sagging toward the floor.
- Do not allow your body to shift from side to side as you perform each row.
- Do not allow your hips to rotate as you perform each row.
- Perform each row in a controlled manner by slowly lowering the dumbbell to the floor on each rep.
- To ensure that the dumbbells do not roll, place your hands directly underneath your shoulders.

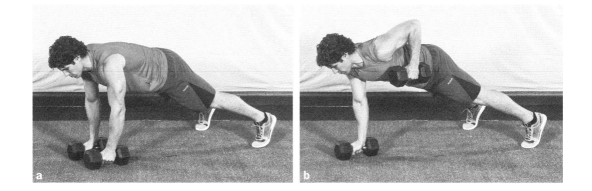

Aside from helping you to be the last person standing when the smoke clears—and providing amazing fitness and physique benefits—the cardio-conditioning methods presented in this chapter test your grit and help you build the fortitude that you need in order to take on any challenge that life throws at you.

4

Upper Body—Pushing

Pushing exercises improve your ability to move something—such as an object or opponent—away from you. Taken as a whole, the exercises presented in this chapter involve pushing horizontally, diagonally, and vertically from a variety of stances and body positions and using both single-arm (unilateral) and double-arm (bilateral) actions.

The Truth About the Bench Press

One of the first pushing exercises that many people, especially guys, think of is the bench press, which has traditionally been considered one of the big lifts. Many guys enjoy benching because it's a great way to get their "man card" from their gym buddies or enjoy a much-needed ego boost every now and then. It's also a must for powerlifters because it accounts for a third of their sport. And if you're training for the American football combine, you'd better be benching to prepare for the much-ballyhooed 225-pound (about 100 kg) rep test.

But what about field, court, and combat athletes—and other athletic-minded individuals—who want to improve their overall performance in a way that transfers outside of the gym? In sport, and in many daily life tasks, we rarely lie back to push on something; instead, when we need to push (or pull), we usually stand. In addition, as established in chapter 1, when you press while standing your movement is limited by the coordination and co-contraction of your shoulders, torso, and hips. In contrast, when you push while lying down, you activate mainly your chest, shoulders, and triceps. Sure, powerlifters use their hips and lower back to aid their bench-press performance, but they're also lying down with their shoulders anchored on the bench, so it's still comparing apples to oranges.

In short, the standing push action is more of a whole-body exercise, whereas the bench press is more of an upper-body exercise. Even so, as established in chapter 2, it's mathematically and physically impossible for anyone to match, or even come close to, his or her bench-press capacity in a push from a standing position. This reality makes it an unnecessary risk to (over) emphasize maximal bench-press efforts for general athletic purposes.

Still, the bench press does have its place in a comprehensive strength-and-conditioning program, but only if it is approached not as some mythic activity but as a general strengthening and size-building exercise. That's why the functional-spectrum training system includes the bench press as a general, compound pressing option—that is, as one option among several compound pushing exercises. And, since a good strength-training program uses both general and specific strength exercises, the general exercises are complemented here by a variety of specific pushing exercises.

Total-Body Power Exercises

These explosive exercises require you to summate force by coordinating all of the muscles in your body, which culminates in an upper-body pushing action. These exercises are classified as specific.

Medicine-Ball Vertical Squat Push Throw

Setup

Stand with your feet roughly shoulder-width apart and hold a medicine ball weighing 3 to 6 kilograms (about 6.5 to 13 lbs.) at your chest with your elbows underneath the ball.

Action

Squat so that your thighs become roughly parallel to the floor while keeping your torso fairly upright (see figure *a*). Explode out of the bottom position by simultaneously extending your arms and legs and launching the ball vertically (see figure *b*).

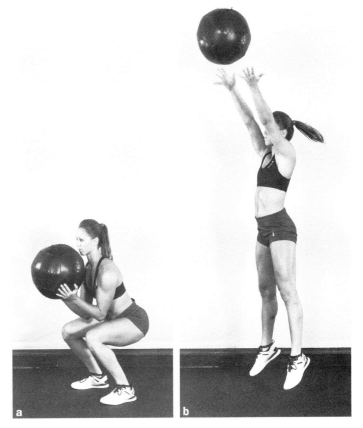

Coaching Tips

- You can use either a rubber (bouncing) medicine ball, a Dynamax-type (minimal-bounce) ball, or a sand-filled (non-bouncing) ball.

- Do not catch the medicine ball in the air; rather, allow it to land after each throw or catch it off the bounce before resetting for the next rep.

- When squatting to prepare for each repetition, do not allow your knees to drop in toward the midline of your body, your heels to lift off of the ground, or your lower back to lose its arch.

- On each throw, explode out of the starting position as fast as you can while throwing the ball as hard as you can.

- At the end of each throw, your feet should leave the ground and your body should be fully extended with your arms overhead.

Medicine-Ball Diagonal Squat Push Throw

Whereas the vertical squat push throw described in the preceding exercise resembles a squat jump, the change in launching angle for this exercise makes it more similar to a broad jump.

Setup

Stand with your feet roughly shoulder-width apart and hold a medicine ball weighing 3 to 6 kilograms (about 6.5 to 13 lbs.) at your chest with your elbows underneath the ball.

Action

Lower your body in a fashion similar to that of a deadlift by shifting your hips backward and bending your knees so that your thighs become roughly parallel to the floor and your torso leans slightly forward (see figure *a*). Explode out of the bottom position by simultaneously extending your arms and legs and launching the ball diagonally as far as you can out in front of you at a 45-degree angle (see figure *b*). As you throw the ball, your forward lean causes you to jump forward, after which you walk to the ball in order to perform the next repetition (unless you're throwing the ball at a tall wall).

Coaching Tips

- On each throw, explode out of the starting position as fast as you can while throwing the ball as hard as you can.
- At the end of each throw, your feet should leave the ground and your body should be fully extended with your arms overhead.

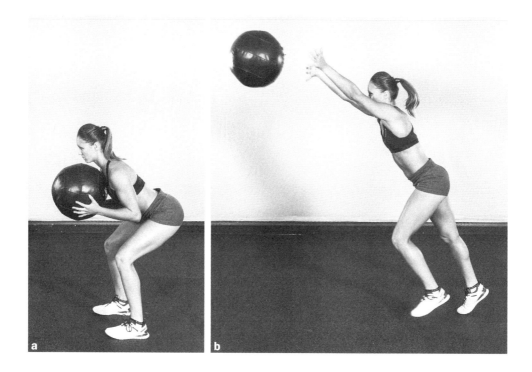

Medicine-Ball Horizontal Punch Throw

Setup

Stand roughly perpendicular to a solid wall with your feet shoulder-width apart and your knees slightly bent. Your front foot—the one closest to the wall—should be at about a 45-degree angle toward the wall, and your back foot should point straight ahead, parallel to the wall. With your torso upright, hold a medicine ball weighing 3 to 6 kilograms (about 6.5 to 13 lbs.) between your hands at chest level with your elbows pointed outward (see figure *a*). Begin each throw with most of your weight shifted away from the wall. Finish each throw with most of your weight on the leg closest to the wall with your rear heel off of the ground.

Action

Explosively rotate your hips and shoulders simultaneously toward the wall while extending your rear arm to throw the ball horizontally as if throwing a punch. Allow your front and back feet to rotate toward the wall as you throw the ball as hard as you can toward the wall (see figure *b*). When the ball bounces back to you, reset your position for the next repetition. Perform all reps on the same side before facing the other direction and performing the exercise on the opposite side.

Coaching Tips

- Keep your rear elbow fairly parallel to the floor before each throw.
- You can use either a rubber (bouncing) medicine ball or a Dynamax-type (minimal-bounce) ball.
- If using a rubber, air-filled ball with a lot of bounce, stand far enough from the wall that you don't feel rushed in catching the ball on the rebound after each throw. Stand far enough away for the ball to bounce at least once before it reaches you.
- If using a Dynamax-type ball, which has limited bounce, you can stand much closer to the wall than if using a rubber medicine ball.
- Stand at a distance from the wall that allows the ball to bounce or roll back to you after each throw without forcing you to feel rushed.

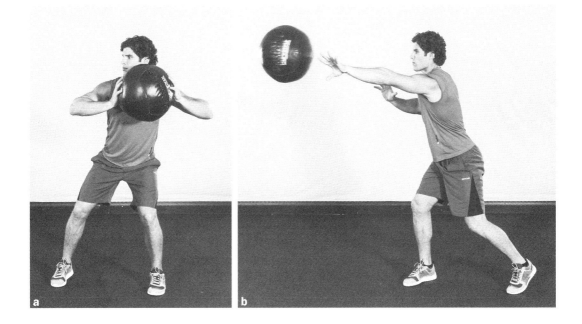

Medicine-Ball Shot-Put Throw

Setup

Stand roughly perpendicular to a solid wall with your feet shoulder-width apart and your knees slightly bent. Your front foot—the one closest to the wall—should be at about a 45-degree angle, and your back foot should point straight ahead. With your torso upright, hold a medicine ball weighing 3 to 6 kilograms (about 6.5 to 13 lbs.) between your hands at chest level with your elbows pointed slightly outward (see figure *a*).

Action

Explosively rotate your hips and shoulders simultaneously toward the wall while extending your legs and your rear arm to throw the ball upward at a 45-degree angle in a shot-put type of action (see figure *b*). On every throw, your feet should leave the ground and the rotation of your body should cause you to land facing the wall. Allow the ball to bounce back to you, then reset your position for the next repetition. Perform all reps on the same side before facing the other direction and performing the exercise on the opposite side.

Coaching Tips

- If using a Dynamax-type medicine ball, which has limited bounce, you can stand much closer to the wall than if using a rubber medicine ball. Stand at a distance from the wall that allows the ball to bounce back to you after each throw without forcing you to feel rushed.
- If using a sand-filled, non-bounce medicine ball, you can throw the ball into open space as far as possible at a 45-degree angle, then walk to where it lands and throw it back to where you started.

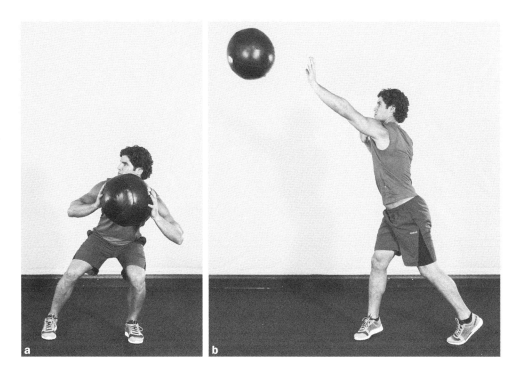

Medicine-Ball Step and Push Throw

Setup

Stand tall with your feet hip-width apart while holding a medicine ball weighing 3 to 6 kilograms (about 6.5 to 13 lbs.) at chest level with your elbows positioned by your sides underneath the ball (see figure a). While holding the ball, your fingers should point toward your target, not up toward the sky.

Action

Lunge forward with your right leg and simultaneously use both hands to explode the ball away from your chest in a pushing action (see figures b and c). Reset and repeat the throwing action while lunging with your left leg. Alternate legs on each rep.

Coaching Tips

- Keep your elbows close to your sides when throwing in order to maximize power and minimize stress in your elbow joints.
- If using a rubber, air-filled ball, which has a lot of bounce, stand at a distance far enough from the wall that you don't feel rushed to catch the ball on the rebound after each throw. Stand far enough away from the wall for the ball to bounce at least once before it reaches you after each throw.
- If using a Dynamax-type medicine ball, which has limited bounce, you can stand much closer to the wall than if using a rubber medicine ball. Stand at a distance from the wall that allows the ball to bounce or roll back to you after each throw without forcing you to feel rushed.

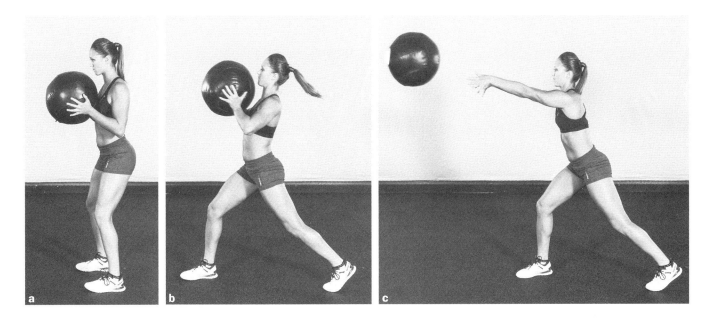

Angled Barbell Press and Catch

Setup

Stand with your feet shoulder-width apart. Place one end of a barbell in a corner or inside a landmine device and hold onto the other end (see figure a).

Action

Explosively press the barbell up and away from you, allowing it to leave your hand by a few inches (see figures b and c), then catch it with your other hand and control it on the way down to your shoulder (see figure d). Explode the barbell up again, throwing it a few inches in front of your hand, then catch it with your other hand and lower it in a controlled motion back to the original side to complete a full repetition.

Coaching Tips

- Each time you catch the barbell, do so as if catching an egg. Use your entire body, simultaneously bending your knees (slightly) and arms to absorb the fall and keep the egg from breaking.
- It's ok to allow your torso to rotate a bit each time you catch and throw the barbell.

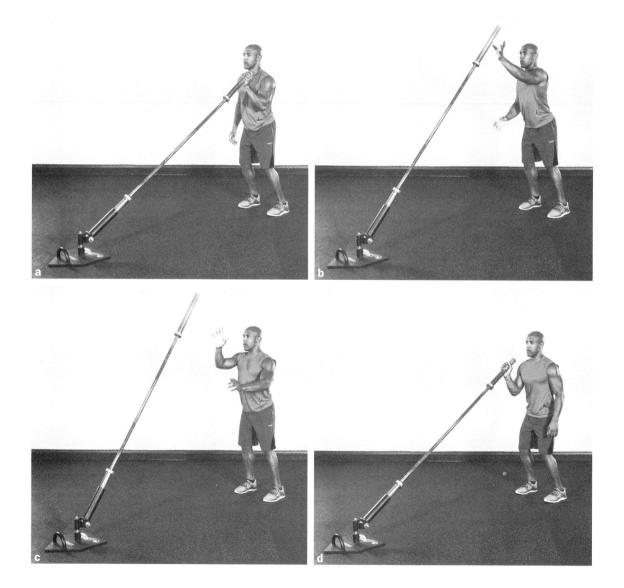

Barbell Overhead Push Press

Setup

Stand with your feet shoulder-width apart and hold the barbell at the top of your chest with your hands just outside shoulder-width apart.

Action

Slightly bend your knees (see figure *a*), then quickly reverse the motion, exploding into the bar and driving it overhead with your arms and legs in a coordinated fashion (see figure *b*). Once the bar is completely overhead, slowly reverse your motions to complete a full repetition.

Coaching Tips

- Keep your wrists straight; do not allow them to bend backward at any time.
- Do not allow your lower back to overextend as you press the barbell overhead.

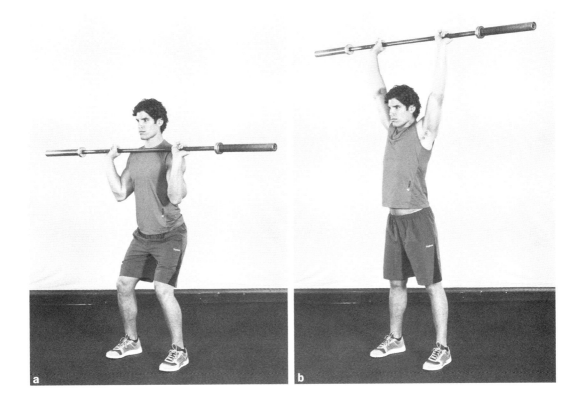

Cross-Body Exercises

These exercises train the X-factor relationships, which coordinate the leg and hip on one side of the body with the torso and upper body on the other side. They also emphasize the upper-body pushing musculature, which consists primarily of the chest, shoulders, and triceps.

One-Arm Dumbbell Rotational Push Press

Setup

Stand tall with your feet roughly shoulder-width apart while holding a dumbbell in front of one shoulder.

Action

Slightly bend your knees (see figure a), then quickly reverse the motion and press the dumbbell straight above your same-side shoulder while rotating to the side opposite of the dumbbell (see figure b). Perform all repetitions on the same side before switching sides.

Coaching Tips

- To better allow your hips to rotate, raise your same-side heel off of the ground as you turn.
- Begin each repetition with your weight shifted slightly to the leg on the same side as the dumbbell. As you perform each repetition, your weight should shift to the other leg.
- Press the dumbbell and rotate as fast as possible, but lower the dumbbell with deliberate control, which may require you to help with your free hand.
- You can also perform this exercise without the torso rotation.

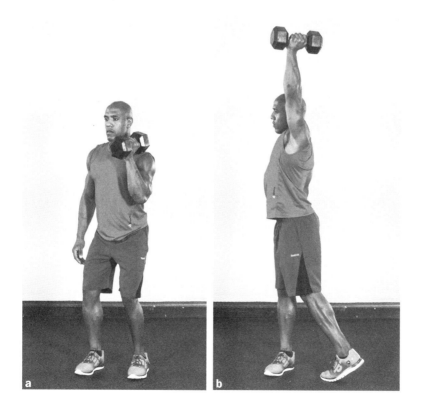

Dumbbell Rotational Shoulder Press

Setup

Stand tall with your feet roughly shoulder-width apart while holding a dumbbell in front of each shoulder (see figure a).

Action

Press one dumbbell into the air as you rotate to the opposite side (see figure b). Reverse the motion and press the other dumbbell while rotating to the other side.

Coaching Tips

- To better allow your hips to rotate, raise your heel off of the ground as you turn.
- Press the dumbbell directly over your same-side shoulder.
- Lower the dumbbell in a smooth, controlled manner as you bring your torso back to facing straight ahead before you begin turning to the opposite side to perform the rep with the other arm.

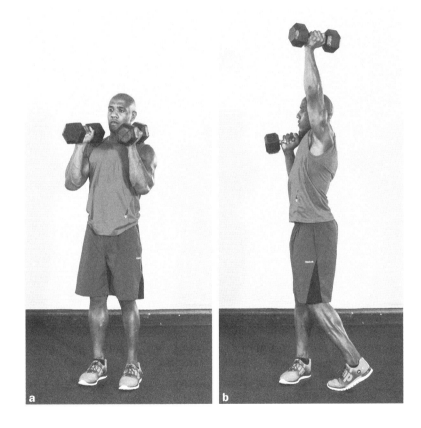

Angled Barbell Press

Setup

Stand with one leg in front of the other, splitting your stance. Place one end of a barbell in a corner or inside a landmine device and hold onto the other end of the barbell (see figure a). If the barbell is in your right hand, your right leg is your back leg.

Action

Press the barbell up and away from you while keeping your torso upright and stable (see figure b). Slowly reverse the motion and lower the barbell back in front of your shoulder.

Coaching Tips

- Do not press the barbell toward the midline of your body; keep it in line with your same-side shoulder as you press it up and out.

- At the bottom of each repetition, your forearm should form a 90-degree angle with the barbell.

- Do not allow your wrist to bend backward at any time; keep your wrist straight throughout this exercise.

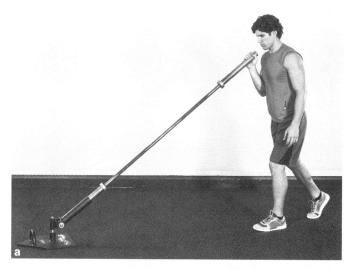

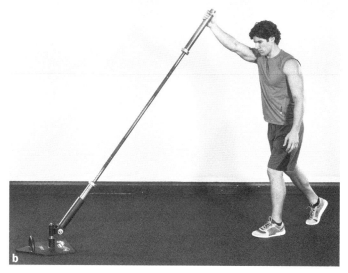

Angled Barbell Rotational Push Press

Setup

Place one end of a barbell in a corner or inside a landmine device and hold onto the other end of the barbell. Holding the bar at your chest, stand roughly parallel to the barbell with your feet shoulder-width apart and your knees bent (see figure *a*).

Action

Rotate your body (hips and torso) toward the barbell's anchor point as you extend your legs and push the barbell away from you by extending your arm straight (see figure *b*). Slowly reverse the motion to lower the barbell to your chest as you allow your knees to bend, thus completing a full rep.

Coaching Tips

- Begin each repetition with your weight shifted slightly to your rear leg—the one on the same side as the hand underneath the barbell. As you perform each repetition, your weight should shift to the front leg, and you should finish each rep with your rear heel off of the ground and rotated toward the barbell.

- At the bottom of each repetition, keep the barbell close to your body, with your elbow directly underneath your wrist.

- It's okay to use your free hand to help lower the barbell and to help keep it in place at the beginning of each repetition.

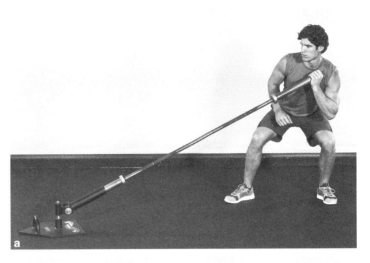

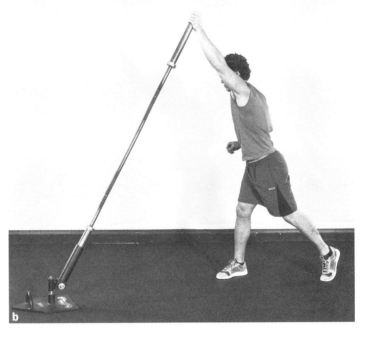

One-Arm Cable Press

Setup

Stand facing away from an adjustable cable column while holding a handle at roughly shoulder height. With the cable handle in your left hand, split your stance with your left leg behind your right leg.

Action

Press the cable straight out in front of you (see figure a). Slowly reverse the motion and bring the handle back in to your body as you bring your left arm back toward you in a row-like motion while extending the opposite arm and without allowing your shoulders or hips to rotate more than a few degrees (see figure b).

Coaching Tips

- Keep your rear foot straight and your back heel off of the ground throughout this exercise.
- Lean your torso slightly forward to allow you to move heavier loads.
- Keep your elbow at roughly a 45-degree angle from your body at the beginning of each repetition.
- To prevent the cable attachment from digging into your arm, you can use an extender strap (which can be purchased at a store that sells rock-climbing gear) between the handle and the cable attachment.

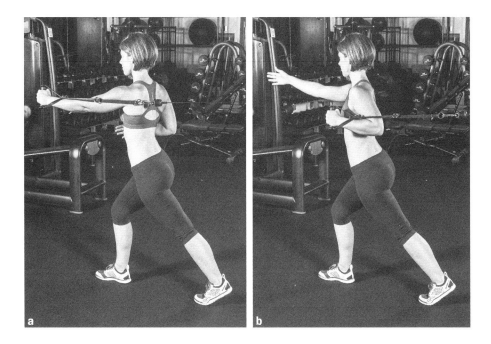

One-Arm Push-Up

Setup

Assume a one-arm plank position with your feet spread several inches wider than your shoulders (see figure *a*). Your weight-bearing arm should be positioned so that your wrist is directly under the same-side shoulder. Your non-weight-bearing arm should be on the opposite hip or behind your back.

Action

Drop into a one-arm push-up, allowing your torso to rotate a few degrees away from your weight-bearing arm while keeping your elbow on the working side tight to your body (see figure *b*). Drive into the floor and push your body back to the top of the push-up to complete a full rep. Perform all repetitions on one side before switching to the other arm.

Coaching Tips

- Turn your weight-bearing hand out slightly so that your fingers point at roughly a 45-degree angle away from your body.
- Do not allow your lower back to sag toward the floor at any time.

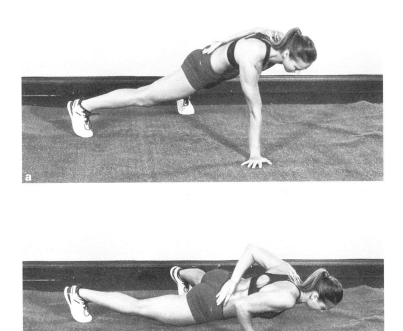

Push-Up Lock-Off

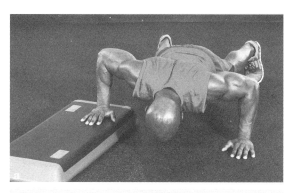

Setup
Begin in a push-up position with your feet shoulder-width apart, one hand on top of a medicine ball or platform, and your other hand on the floor.

Action
Perform a push-up with one hand on top of the platform or medicine ball (see figure a). At the top of the push-up, lock off by fully straightening the elbow of the arm resting on the platform or ball. Place the other arm at your chest (see figure b). Perform half of the repetitions with your right arm elevated and the other half with your left arm elevated.

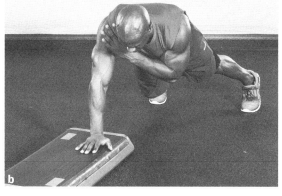

Coaching Tips
- Do not allow your shoulders or hips to rotate at any time; keep your torso parallel to the ground throughout.
- Pause for one or two seconds at the top of each repetition, then slowly lower yourself.

Box Crossover Push-Up

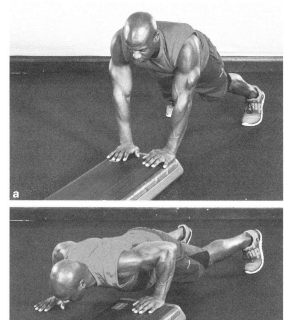

Setup
Begin in a push-up position with both hands on top of a medicine ball or platform and your feet just outside shoulder-width apart (see figure a).

Action
Step one hand off of the box or ball to the floor while performing a push-up (see figure b). As you come out of the push-up, bring your hand back to the platform or ball. Repeat the same action to the other side.

Coaching Tips
- Do not allow your head or hips to sag toward the floor at any time.
- Do not move your feet.

Compound Exercises

These pushing exercises integrate efforts by the chest, shoulder, and triceps muscles to perform the movement.

Barbell Bench Press

Setup

Lie on a weight bench with your feet flat on the floor, pressing them firmly into the ground to keep you stable. Hold an Olympic-type barbell using a grip that places your hands outside your shoulders (see figure *a*).

Action

Slowly lower the bar toward your chest until your elbows reach just below your torso. Keep your elbows at roughly a 45-degree angle relative to your torso (see figure *b*). Press the bar up to the sky above your chest.

Coaching Tips

- Do not allow your wrists to bend backward at any time.
- Keep your elbows directly under your wrists throughout.

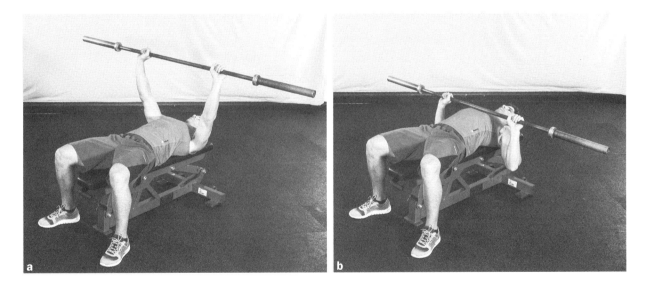

Incline Barbell Bench Press

Setup

Lie on a weight bench angled at about 45 degrees with your feet flat on the floor, pressing them firmly into the ground to keep you stable. Hold an Olympic-type barbell using a grip that places your hands outside your shoulders (see figure *a*).

Action

Slowly lower the bar toward your chest until your elbows reach just below your torso; keep your elbows at roughly a 45-degree angle relative to your torso (see figure *b*). Press the bar up to the sky above your chest.

Coaching Tips

- Do not allow your wrists to bend backward at any time.
- Keep your elbows directly under your wrists throughout.

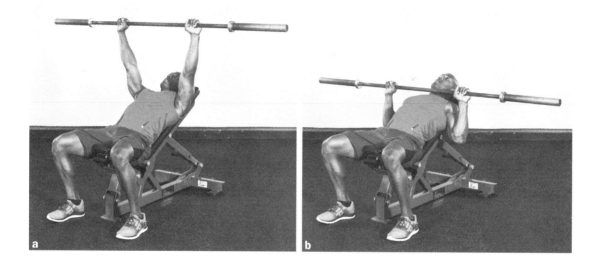

Dumbbell Bench Press

Setup

Lie on a weight bench with your feet flat on the floor, pressing them firmly into the ground to keep you stable. Hold a dumbbell in each hand above your shoulders with your arms straight (see figure *a*).

Action

Slowly lower the dumbbells outside your body until your elbows go just below your torso (see figure *b*). Press the dumbbells back up toward the sky above your shoulders.

Coaching Tips

- You can also perform the dumbbell bench press in an alternate-arm style by pressing one arm while the other arm remains straight.
- When performing the alternate-arm version, do not begin lowering one arm until the opposite arm (which just performed the press) is fully straight.

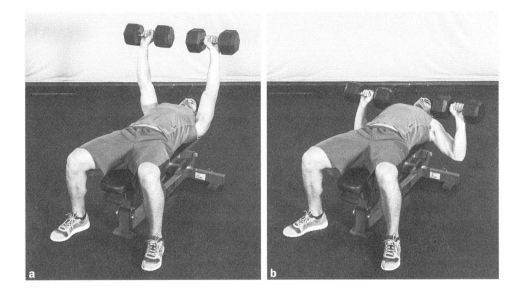

Incline Dumbbell Bench Press

Setup

Lie on a weight bench angled at about 45 degrees with your feet flat on the floor, pressing them firmly into the ground to keep you stable. Hold a pair of dumbbells above your head outside your shoulders (see figure a).

Action

Slowly lower the dumbbells outside your body until your elbows reach just below your torso (see figure b). Reverse the motion and press the dumbbells back up.

Coaching Tips

- You can also perform the incline dumbbell bench press in an alternate-arm style by pressing one arm while the other arm remains straight.
- When performing the alternate-arm version, do not begin lowering one arm until the opposite arm (which just performed the press) is fully straight.

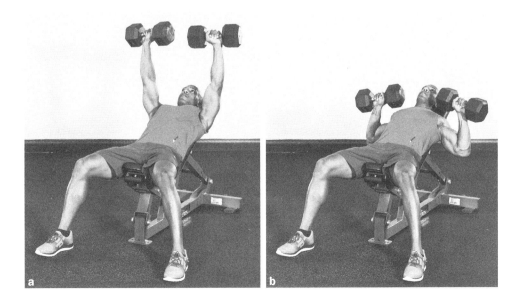

Dumbbell Overhead Press

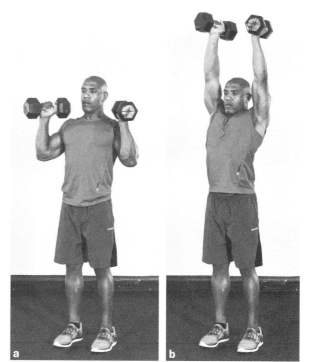

Setup

Stand tall with your feet hip-width apart. Hold a dumbbell in each hand just above the shoulder with your elbows at roughly a 45-degree angle to your torso (see figure a).

Action

Press the dumbbells directly overhead until your arms are almost straight (see figure b). Slowly reverse the motion, bringing the dumbbells back down to the starting position outside your shoulders.

Coaching Tips

- At the bottom of each repetition, your elbows should be directly underneath the dumbbells; your forearms should remain perpendicular to the floor.
- Do not allow your wrists to bend backward at any time.

Dumbbell Front-Hold Overhead Press

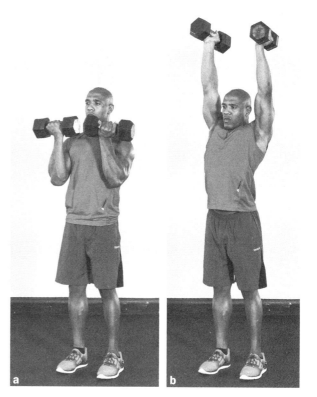

Setup

Stand tall with your feet shoulder-width apart. Hold a dumbbell in each hand at shoulder height with your elbows directly underneath and in front of your torso (see figure a).

Action

Press the dumbbells directly overhead until just before your arms are straight above you, in line with your torso and with the dumbbells parallel to one another at the top (see figure b). Slowly reverse the motion, bringing the dumbbells back down to the fronts of your shoulders.

Coaching Tips

- At the bottom of each repetition, hold the dumbbells parallel to your torso.
- Do not allow your lower back to overextend as you press the weight overhead.

Kettlebell Shoulder-to-Shoulder Overhead Press

Setup

Stand tall with your feet parallel to one another and a little farther than shoulder-width apart. Hold onto the round part of a kettlebell with both hands and with your thumbs inside the handle above one shoulder (see figure *a*).

Action

Press the kettlebell overhead so that when your arms reach full extension, the kettlebell is directly in line with the center of your body (see figure *b*). Slowly reverse the motion and lower the kettlebell to your opposite shoulder (see figure *c*). Press it up again so that it ends up in the middle of your body, then lower it back to the other shoulder.

Coaching Tips

- Do not allow your shoulders or hips to rotate.
- Do not allow your torso to side-bend; maintain your upright torso position throughout.

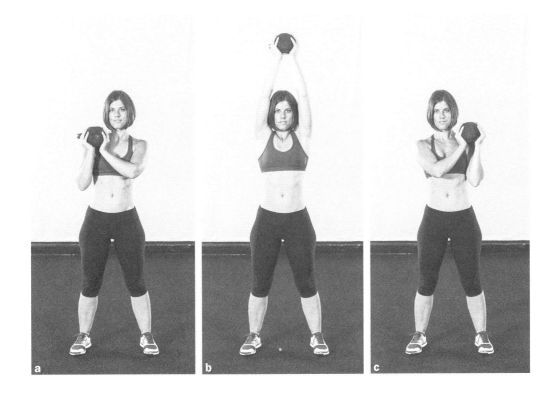

Kettlebell Bottom's-Up Overhead Press

Setup
Stand tall with your feet roughly hip-width apart while holding a kettlebell upside-down in front of your shoulder (see figure *a*).

Action
Press the kettlebell toward the sky while keeping it balanced; stop just before your elbow is fully straightened (see figure *b*). Slowly reverse the motion, bringing the kettlebell back to the starting position in front of your shoulder. Repeat all reps on one side before switching to the other side.

Coaching Tips
- Do not allow the kettlebell to flip to the side of your pressing arm. If it does flip, reset it back to the correct position and restart the repetition.
- Keep your elbow directly underneath the kettlebell throughout.

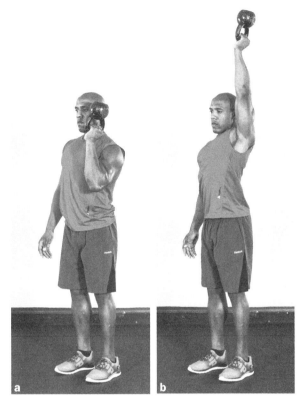

Push-Up

Setup
Place your hands on the floor just farther than shoulder-width apart with your elbows straight (see figure *a*). Turn your hands outward so that your fingers point at roughly 45 degrees.

Action
Perform a push-up by lowering your body to the floor while keeping your elbows directly above your wrists (see figure *b*). Once your elbows reach an angle just below 90 degrees, reverse the motion by pushing your body up so that your elbows are straight again.

Coaching Tips
- At the top of each push-up, do not finish with your shoulder blades pinched together; instead, protract (push apart) your shoulder blades while keeping your body in a straight line.
- At the bottom of each push-up, position your arms at a 45-degree angle to your torso.

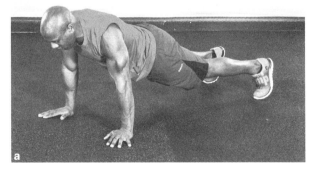

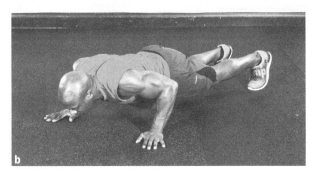

Superband Push-Up

Setup

Place a superband around your upper back and place your fingers (but not your thumbs; see inset) inside the bands from the bottom up. Position your hands on the floor shoulder-width apart with your elbows straight (see figure a). Turn your hands outward so that your fingers point at roughly 45 degrees.

Action

Perform a push-up by lowering your body to the floor while keeping your elbows directly above your wrists (see figure b). Once your elbows reach an angle just below 90 degrees, reverse the motion by pushing your body up so that your elbows are straight again.

Coaching Tips

- At the top of each push-up, do not finish with your shoulder blades pinched together; instead, protract (push apart) your shoulder blades while keeping your body in a straight line.
- At the bottom of each push-up, position your arms at a 45-degree angle to your torso.

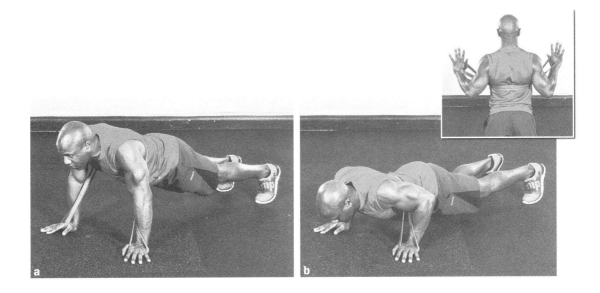

Feet-Elevated Push-Up

Setup

Begin in a push-up position with your hands shoulder-width apart on the floor and your feet elevated on top of a weight bench or chair (see figure a).

Action

Perform a push-up by lowering your chest toward the floor until your elbows reach an angle just below 90 degrees (see figure b). Then press yourself away from the floor until your elbows are straight.

Coaching Tips

- Keep your body in a straight line, from your head to your hips to your ankles; do not allow your head or hips to sag toward the floor.
- Position your arms and hands in the same manner described for the basic push-up.

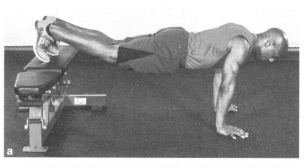

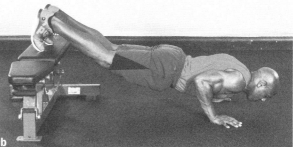

Clap Push-Up

Although this exercise involves an explosive action, it does not require force summation from the entire body. For this reason, it is categorized as a compound exercise rather than a total-body explosive exercise.

Setup

Place your hands shoulder-width apart on the floor with your elbows straight (see figure a). Turn your hands outward so that your fingers point at roughly 45 degrees.

Action

Lower yourself to the floor while keeping your elbows directly above your wrists and at a 45-degree angle to your torso (see figure b). Once your elbows reach an angle just below 90 degrees, quickly reverse the motion by explosively pushing your body up so that your hands leave the floor (see figure c). Quickly clap your hands once, then return them back to the floor and land as gently as possible as you lower to begin the next repetition.

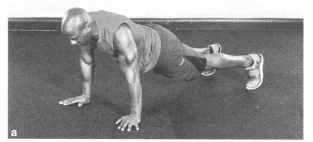

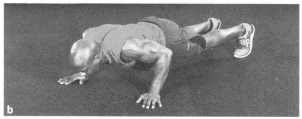

Coaching Tips

- Do not allow your hips to elevate before the rest of your body; keep your body in a straight line throughout.
- At the bottom of each push-up, position your arms at a 45-degree angle to your torso.

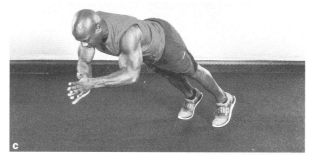

Close-Grip Push-Up

Setup

Begin in a push-up position with both hands on top of a medicine ball or platform and your feet shoulder-width apart (see figure a).

Action

Perform a push-up by lowering your chest toward the medicine ball or platform until your elbows reach an angle just below 90 degrees (see figure b). Then press yourself away from the floor until your elbows are straight.

Coaching Tips

- Turn your hands outward so that your fingers point down toward the floor.
- At the bottom of each push-up, your elbows should be against your sides.

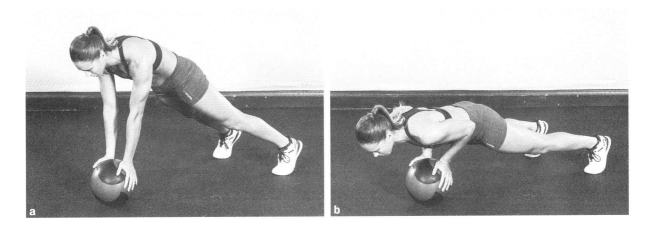

Standing Cable Chest Press

Setup

Stand tall in a split stance, just in-front of the middle of a cable cross-over machine. Hold the handles in each hand at your shoulder level with arms out to your sides and your elbows bent to 90-degrees (see figure a).

Action

Press into the handles by extending your arms and bringing them together towards the midline of your body (see figure b). Slowly reverse the motion until your arms are back out to yours sides and your elbows are bent.

> continued

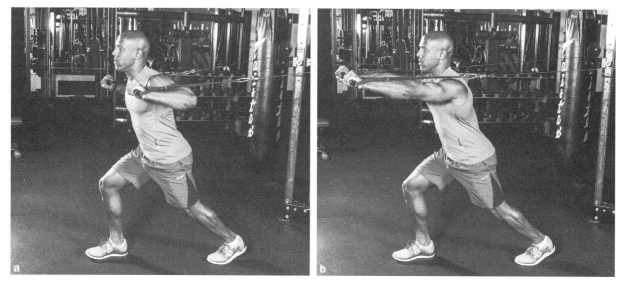

Coaching Tips

- The wider the cables are apart, the farther in-front of the apparatus you'll need to stand to properly perform this exercise.
- Keep your rear heel elevated off of the floor throughout.
- A slight forward torso lean is okay to use if needed to perform this exercise.

Heavy-Band Step and Press

Setup

Face away from a heavy-duty resistance band attached at roughly shoulder height to a stable structure or inside a doorjamb (many resistance bands come with a doorjamb attachment). With your knees slightly bent and your feet roughly hip-width apart, hold a handle in each hand with your arms at a 45-degree angle to your sides and your forearms parallel to the floor. The band should create enough tension that it forces you to lean your torso slightly forward (see figure *a*).

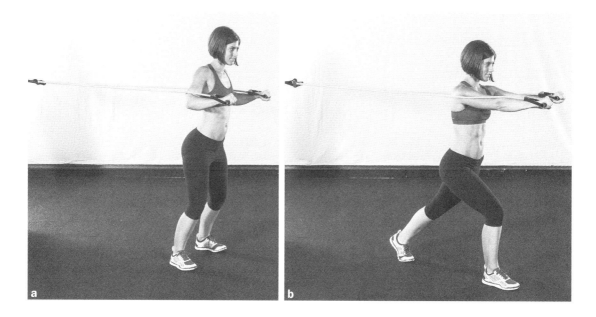

Action

Step forward with one leg while performing a chest press with both arms; maintain your slight forward torso lean with your rear heel off of the ground (see figure b). Step your lead leg back to the starting position while allowing your arms to come back as well. Alternate legs on each repetition.

Coaching Tips

- Explode into each repetition as if you were shoving someone.
- Use a resistance band that creates enough tension to make you work to hold your position *from the start* of each repetition—not just at the end, when your arms are extended.

Isolation Exercises

These are single-joint movements that focus on individual muscle groups. These exercise applications consist primarily of classic bodybuilding exercises that target the chest, shoulders, and triceps musculature.

Cable Pec Fly

Setup

Stand tall, in either a split stance or a parallel stance, just in front of the middle of a cable crossover machine. In each hand, hold handles attached at shoulder level. Your arms extend out to your sides with a slight bend in the elbows (see figure a).

Action

Bring your arms together in front of you while keeping a soft bend in your elbows, as if you were hugging a tree, until your palms touch in the center (see figure b). Slowly reverse the motion until your arms are back out to your sides and your elbows are just behind your shoulders.

Coaching Tips

- When setting up to perform this exercise, stand just in front of the cables.
- If necessary, a slight forward torso lean is acceptable.

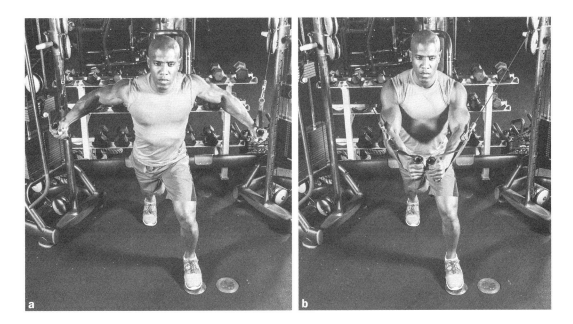

Dumbbell Pec Fly

Setup

Lie on a weight bench with your feet flat on the floor, pressing them firmly into the ground to keep you stable. Hold a dumbbell in each hand above your shoulders with your arms straight and your palms facing each other (see figure *a*).

Action

Keeping your elbows slightly bent, slowly open your arms out to your sides until your elbows go just below your torso (see figure *b*). Reverse the motion by driving the dumbbells back up in a motion similar to that of hugging a tree.

Coaching Tips

- For additional isometric work, you can squeeze the dumbbells together for one or two seconds at the top of each rep.
- Lower the dumbbells in a controlled fashion on each rep.

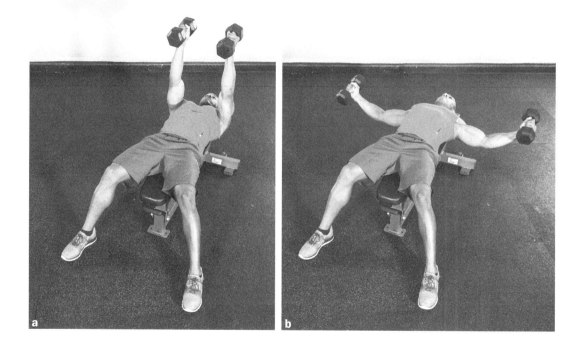

Dumbbell Side Shoulder Raise

Setup

Stand tall with your feet hip-width apart while holding a pair of dumbbells at your sides (see figure a).

Action

With your elbows slightly bent, raise your arms out to the sides at roughly a 30-degree angle until the dumbbells reach just above your shoulders (see figure b). Slowly lower the dumbbells back to your sides.

Coaching Tips

- At the bottom position, do not allow the dumbbells to rest against your hips; keep your hands just outside your hips to maintain some tension in your shoulders throughout.
- Keep the dumbbells parallel to the floor, which, combined with the arm angle of the raises, makes the exercise safer for the shoulder joint.

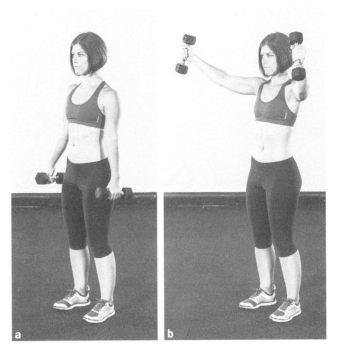

Dumbbell Front Shoulder Raise

Setup

Stand tall with your feet hip-width apart while holding a pair of dumbbells at your sides (see figure a).

Action

With your elbows slightly bent, raise your arms out in front of your body until the dumbbells reach just above your shoulders (see figure b). Slowly lower the dumbbells back to your sides.

Coaching Tips

- Do not swing the weight up. Use deliberate control on the lifting and lowering portion of each rep.
- Keep the dumbbells parallel to one another throughout.

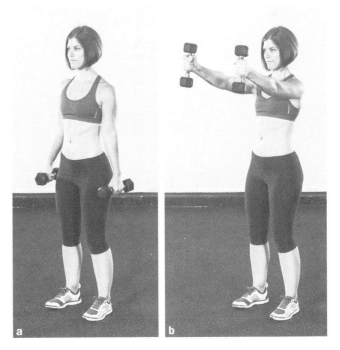

Dumbbell Wide-Arm Upright Row

Setup

Stand tall with your feet hip-width apart while holding a pair of dumbbells resting on your thighs (see figure a).

Action

Pull the dumbbells toward the sky, outside of your torso, until your elbows reach shoulder height (see figure b). Then lower the dumbbells back to your thighs in a controlled fashion to reset and begin your next repetition.

Coaching Tips

- To make the exercise safer for the shoulder joints, keep the dumbbells wider than in the traditional manner (in which the hands are close together).
- Keep your wrists fairly straight throughout.

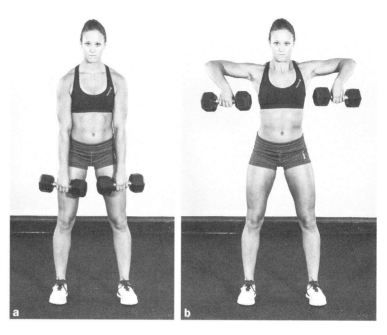

Dumbbell Triceps Skull Crusher

Setup

Lie supine on a weight bench while holding a dumbbell in each hand with your arms outstretched above your shoulders toward the sky (see figure a).

Action

Bend your elbows, lowering the dumbbells toward your forehead while keeping your palms facing one another (see figure b). Once your elbows reach just below a 90-degree angle, reverse the motion and extend your elbows until they're almost straight again to complete the rep.

Coaching Tips

- To avoid getting hit in the head by the dumbbells, lower them slowly with deliberate control.
- You can also perform this exercise with an EZ bar.

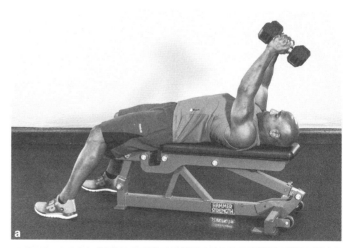

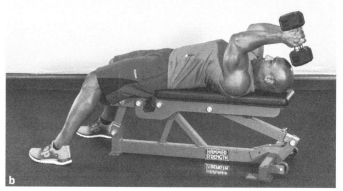

Cable Triceps Rope Extension

Setup

Stand in front of an adjustable cable column with a rope attached above your eye level. Hold one side of the rope in each hand with your arms by your sides and your elbows bent above 90 degrees (see figure a).

Action

With your knees slightly bent, straighten your elbows toward the sides of your body until your arms are straight (see figure b).

Coaching Tips

- Do not allow your shoulders to round forward as you press the rope downward on each repetition.
- Keep your elbows by your sides throughout.

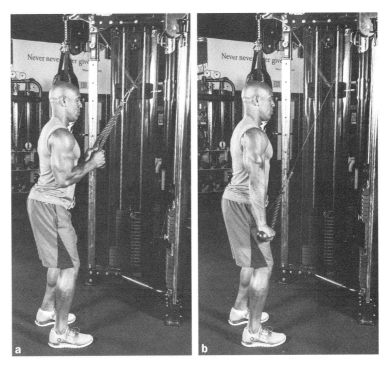

Suspension Triceps Skull Crusher

Setup

Using a suspension trainer, face away from the anchor point, grab the handles, and lean your weight forward with your arms extended at roughly a 45-degree angle above your head (see figure a).

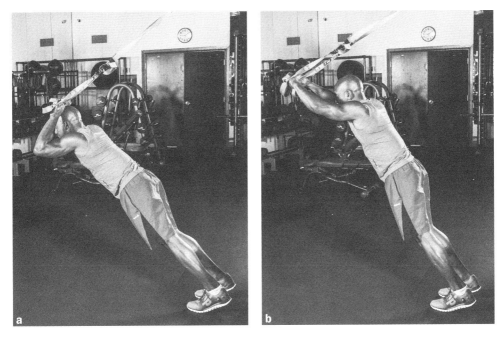

> continued

Action

Bend at your elbows and lower your forehead to your wrists (see figure *b*). Reverse direction and extend your elbows, as in a triceps extension, to complete the rep.

Coaching Tips

- Keep your entire body straight throughout the action.
- To increase the difficulty, lower your body closer to the floor; the closer your shoulders come to being under the anchor point, the tougher the exercise is.
- To decrease the difficulty, use a higher body angle.

Overhead Cable Triceps Rope Extension

Setup

You'll need an adjustable cable column to perform this exercise. Stand in front of the cable column with a rope attached above your head. Facing away from where the rope is attached, in a split stance with a slight forward lean of your torso, hold each side of the rope in each hand with your arms by your ears and your elbows bent beyond 90 degrees (see figure *a*).

Action

Keeping your body in the starting position, extend your elbows until your arms are straight (see figure *b*). Slowly reverse the motion and repeat.

Coaching Tips

- Do not drive your shoulders downward as you extend your arms on each rep.
- Keep your rear heel off of the ground throughout.

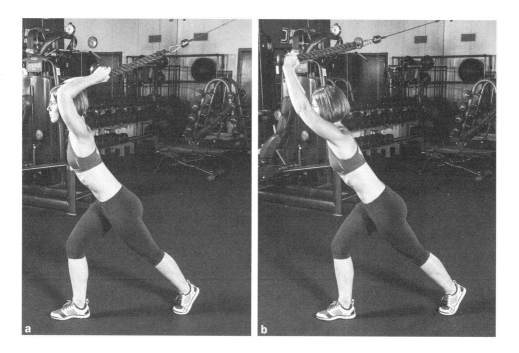

If every action has a reaction, then pushing work requires a corresponding amount of pulling—particularly for desk jockeys. That's what the next chapter is all about!

5

Upper Body—Pulling

Pulling exercises improve your ability to move something—such as an object or opponent—closer to you in order to better control it or hold it. Although the upper-body pulling motion is the opposite of pushing, these two movements are often used together—for example, in actions such as sawing and punching (e.g., a one–two combination in which a left jab is followed immediately by a right cross). As with the pushing exercises presented in chapter 4, the exercises provided here involve pulling horizontally, diagonally, and vertically from a variety of stances and body positions and using both single-arm (unilateral) and double-arm (bilateral) actions.

Total-Body Power Exercises

These explosive exercises require you to summate force by coordinating all of the muscles in your body, which culminates in an upper-body pulling action. These exercises are classified as specific.

Medicine-Ball Step and Overhead Throw

Setup

Standing with your feet roughly hip-width apart, hold the medicine ball weighing 2 to 5 kilograms (about 4.5 to 11 lbs.) over your head (see figure *a*) and lean backward slightly to stretch your abdominal region (see figure *b*).

Action

Step forward with one foot as you explosively throw the ball at the wall in the manner of a soccer throw (see figure *c*). Aim for a target on the wall that's roughly at your torso height. Stand far enough from the wall to allow the ball to bounce at least once before you catch it and reset for the next rep. Alternate the leg that you step with on each rep.

Coaching Tips

- In starting each rep, do not lean back so far as to overextend your lower back; lean back just enough to initiate a stretch in the front of your torso.
- If using a Dynamax-type medicine ball, which has limited bounce, you can stand much closer to the wall than if using a rubber medicine ball. Stand at a distance from the wall that allows the ball to bounce or roll back to you after each throw without forcing you to feel rushed.

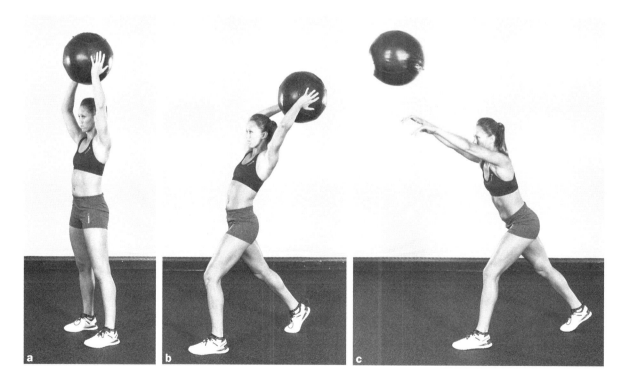

Medicine-Ball Rainbow Slam

Setup

Stand with your feet shoulder-width apart while holding a medicine ball weighing 3 to 6 kilograms (about 6.5 to 13 lbs.) above your head with your elbows slightly bent (see figure a). Shift your weight slightly to the side on which you're holding the ball.

Action

Slam the ball to the ground at roughly a 45-degree angle, just outside your opposite foot, while shifting your weight to the same side (see figure b). Allow the ball to take a very small bounce, catch it, and reverse the motion to perform the next repetition on the other side by moving your arms around your head in a rainbow-like arc. Perform all reps on the same side before switching sides.

Coaching Tips

- As you slam the ball, allow your shoulders and hips to rotate slightly.
- To avoid getting hit in the face when the ball bounces, do *not* keep your face directly above where the ball is being slammed.
- At the top of the range of motion, when your arms are overhead, reach as high as possible to create a stretch in your torso musculature.

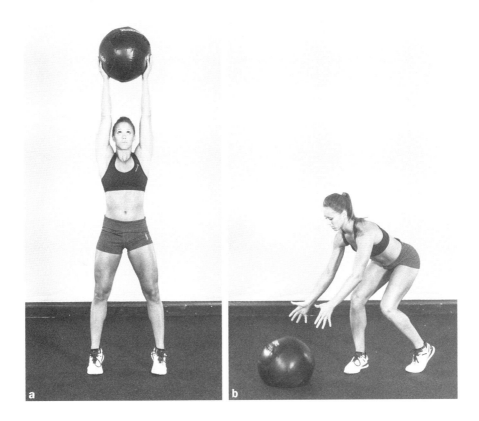

Barbell Hang Clean

Setup

Stand with your feet shoulder-width apart and hold a barbell with your hands just outside shoulder-width apart. Hinge slightly at your hips, keeping the bar against your thighs (see figure a).

Action

Explode your hips into the bar as you pull it upward (see figure b). Once the bar reaches shoulder level, quickly flip your elbows underneath the bar to catch it at the top of your chest (see figure c).

Coaching Tips

- Your heels will leave the ground as you drive the bar upward, but do not allow your entire foot to leave the ground (doing so reduces your potential for power production).
- To initiate the movement, use your lower body, not your arms.

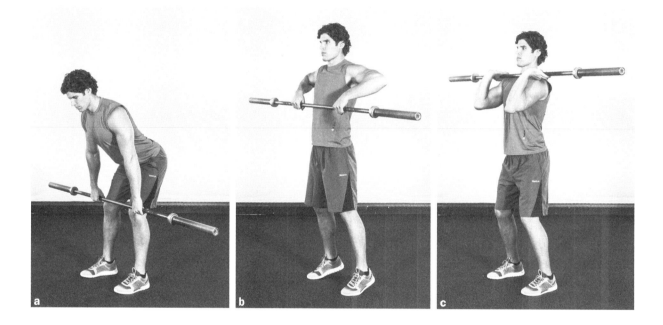

Barbell High Pull

Setup

Stand with your feet shoulder-width apart and hold a barbell with your hands a few inches outside shoulder-width apart. Slightly bend your knees and hinge forward at your hips with the barbell resting on your thighs (see figure a).

Action

Explode your body upward, using your arms and legs to pull the bar toward the sky until your elbows reach shoulder height (see figure b). Then lower the bar back to your thighs in a controlled fashion to reset and begin your next repetition.

Coaching Tips

- When you lift the bar, do not allow your lower back to over extend.
- To initiate the movement, use your lower body, not your arms.

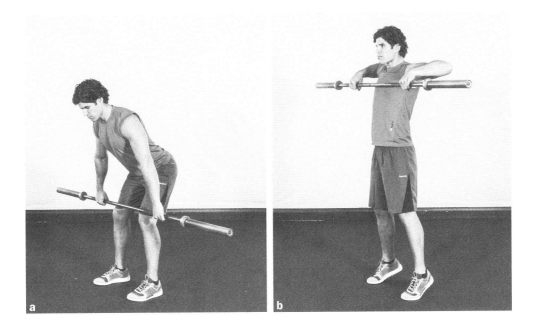

Dumbbell High Pull

Setup

This exercise is performed in the same way as the barbell high pull except that the dumbbells allow your arms to begin closer and then move apart at the top of each rep. Stand with your feet shoulder-width apart and hold a dumbbell in each hand just in front of your thighs. Slightly bend your knees and hinge forward at your hips with the dumbbell handles resting on your thighs (see figure *a*).

Action

Explode your body upward, using your arms and legs to pull the dumbbells slightly outward and toward the sky until your elbows reach shoulder height (see figure *b*). Then lower the dumbbells back to your thighs in a controlled fashion to reset and begin your next repetition.

Coaching Tips

- When you lift the dumbbells, do not allow your lower back to overextend.
- To initiate the movement, use your lower body, not your arms.

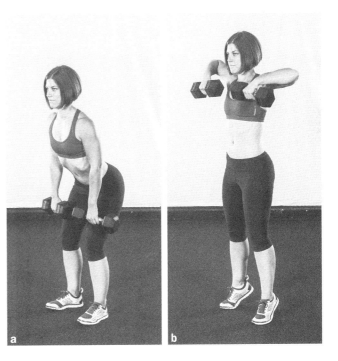

Kettlebell Swing

Setup

Stand with your feet roughly hip-width apart and hold a kettlebell with both hands.

Action

Keeping your back and arms straight, drive the kettlebells between your legs as if hiking a football and hinge forward at your hips. Keep your knees bent at roughly a 15- to 20-degree angle (see figure *a*). Once your forearms come into contact with your thighs, explosively reverse the motion by simultaneously driving your hips forward and swinging the kettlebell up to eye level (see figure *b*).

Coaching Tips

- As you hinge forward, drive your hips backward; do not allow your back to round out.

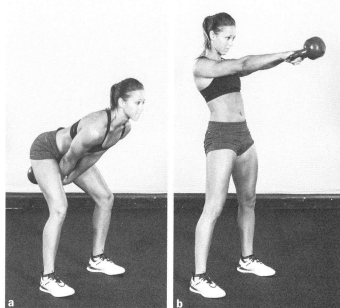

- At the bottom of each swing, allow your arms to touch the insides of your thighs.
- On each rep, use your hips to powerfully drive your arms forward off of your thighs to swing the kettlebells back up.
- Once the kettlebells reach your eye level, pull them back down, keeping a firm grip on the handles.

One-Arm Kettlebell Swing

Setup

Stand with your feet roughly hip-width apart, hold a kettlebell in one hand with your arm straight.

Action

Keeping your back and arm straight, drive the kettlebell between your legs as if hiking a football and hinge forward at your hips. Keep your knees bent at roughly a 15- to 20-degree angle (see figure *a*). Once your forearm comes into contact with your thigh, explosively reverse the motion by simultaneously driving your hips forward and swinging the kettlebell up to roughly eye level (see figure *b*). Perform all reps on the same side before switching sides.

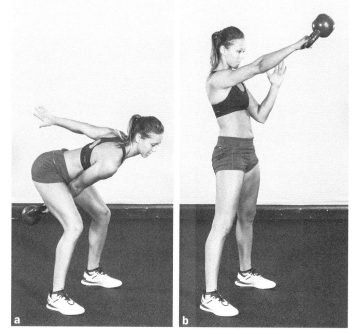

Coaching Tips

- As you hinge forward, drive your hips backward; do not allow your back to round out.
- On each rep, use your hips to powerfully drive your arm forward off of your thigh to swing the kettlebell back up.

Double Kettlebell Swing Clean

Setup

Stand with your feet farther than shoulder-width apart and hold a kettlebell in each hand.

Action

Slightly bend your knees and hinge at your hips to allow the kettlebells to swing between your legs (see figure a). Quickly reverse this motion by driving your hips forward and moving your arms upward (see figure b). As the kettlebells move toward the sky, quickly flip your elbows underneath them and soften your body to accept the motion of the kettlebells into your body, creating as much cushion as you can (see figure c).

Coaching Tips

- As the kettlebells come up to your chest, imagine them as eggs that you do not want to break; absorb them as gently as possible by allowing your legs to bend slightly.
- To start the next repetition, push the kettlebells off of your chest and allow them to swing back between your legs.
- At the bottom position, do not allow your lower back to round out.

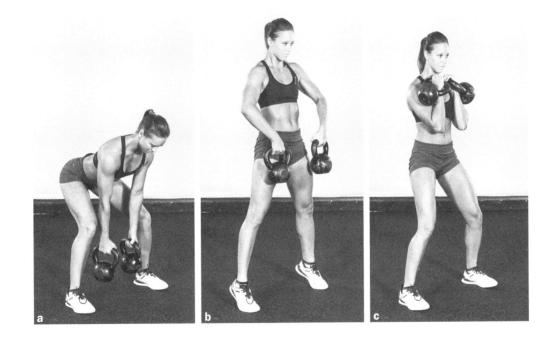

One-Arm Kettlebell Swing Clean

Setup

Stand with your feet farther than shoulder-width apart and hold a kettlebell in one hand.

Action

Slightly bend your knees and hinge at your hips to allow the kettlebell to swing between your legs (see figure *a*). Quickly reverse this motion by driving your hips forward and your arm upward (see figure *b*). As the kettlebell moves toward the sky, quickly flip your elbow underneath it and soften your body to accept the motion of the kettlebell into your body, creating as much cushion as you can (see figure *c*).

Coaching Tips

- As the kettlebell comes up to your chest, imagine it as an egg that you do not want to break; absorb it as gently as possible by allowing your legs to bend slightly.
- To start the next repetition, push the kettlebell off of your chest and allow it to swing back between your legs.
- At the bottom position, do not allow your lower back to round out.

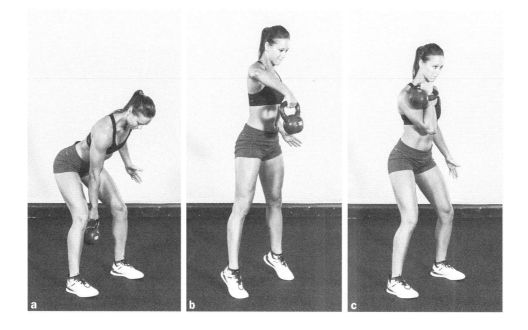

Rope Slam

Setup

Stand tall with your feet hip-width apart while holding one end of a rope in each hand. Keeping your elbows slightly bent, raise your arms in front of you until they're above your head (see figure a).

Action

Slam the rope to the floor by explosively driving both arms down while slightly bending your knees and hips (see figure b) and then back up (see figure c).

Coaching Tips

- On each repetition, focus only on producing maximal force dedicated to the downward slam.
- This exercise does not involve exerting yourself each time you elevate the rope to start the next repetition; therefore, lift the rope in a normal fashion and allow yourself to set up correctly in order to execute each slam as forcefully as possible.

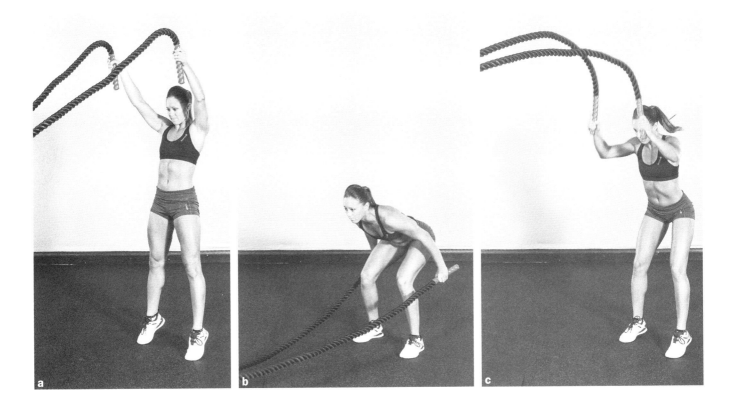

Cross-Body Exercises

These exercises train the X-factor relationships, which coordinate the leg and hip on one side of the body with the torso and upper body on the other side. They also emphasize the upper-body pulling musculature, which consists primarily of the lats, midback, posterior shoulders, and biceps.

One-Arm Freestanding Dumbbell Row

Setup

Assume a split stance with your right leg in front of your left leg and both knees slightly bent. With your left hand, hold the dumbbell in a neutral position so that your palm faces the opposite side of your body; your right hand hangs near the front (right) knee. Hinge at your hips, keeping your back straight so that your torso becomes roughly parallel with the floor (see figure a).

Action

Perform a row by pulling the dumbbell toward your body, without rotating your shoulders or hips more than a few degrees, while pulling your scapula toward your spine in a controlled manner as your arm moves (see figure b). Slowly lower the dumbbell without letting it touch the floor. Complete all reps on one side before switching sides.

Coaching Tips

- Maintain a stable spinal position, keeping your back straight throughout the exercise.
- Keep your back heel raised off of the ground to ensure that most of your weight is on your front leg.
- Do not allow your rowing-side shoulder to move forward at the end of each rep.

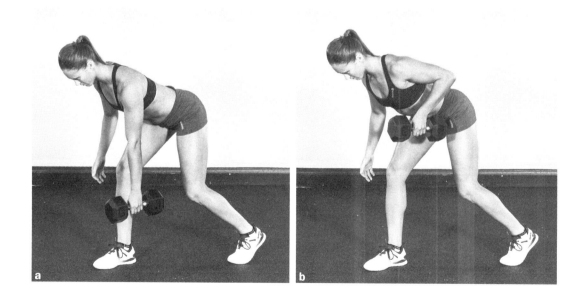

One-Arm One-Leg Dumbbell Bench Row

Setup

Stand facing a traditional weight bench with your feet hip-width apart, your knees slightly bent, your right hand on top of the bench, and a dumbbell in your left hand. Keeping both of your knees slightly bent, lift your right leg until it's roughly in line with your torso, which is roughly parallel to the floor (see figure a).

Action

Perform the row by pulling the dumbbell toward your body so that your left elbow ends up at roughly a 90-degree angle while you drive your left shoulder blade toward your spine (see figure b). Slowly lower the dumbbell toward the floor until your arm straightens without allowing the dumbbell to touch the floor.

Coaching Tips

- Keep your hips level with the floor throughout.
- Do not straighten your down leg at any time; keep the knee of your base leg bent about 20 degrees.
- Do not allow your rowing-side shoulder to move forward at the end of each rep.

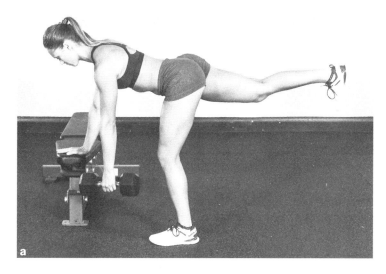

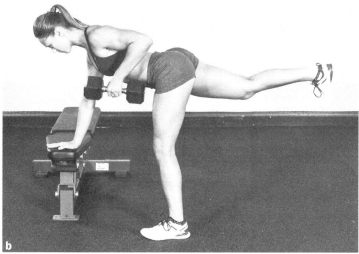

One-Arm Dumbbell Bench Row

Setup

Stand facing a traditional weight bench with your right hand on top of the bench and a dumbbell in your left hand. Keep a straight back that is roughly parallel to the floor (see figure a). Stand in a slightly staggered stance, with your left leg behind your right leg, or in a parallel stance (shown) with your feet hip-width apart, and your knees slightly bent.

Action

Perform the row by pulling the dumbbell toward your body so that your left elbow ends up at roughly a 90-degree angle while you drive your left shoulder blade toward your spine (see figure b). Slowly lower the dumbbell toward the floor until your arm straightens without allowing the dumbbell to touch the floor.

Coaching Tips

- Keep your hips level with the floor throughout.
- Do not allow your rowing-side shoulder to move forward at the end of each rep.

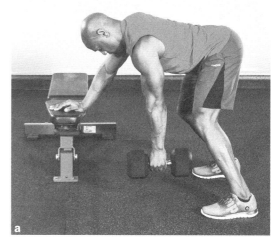

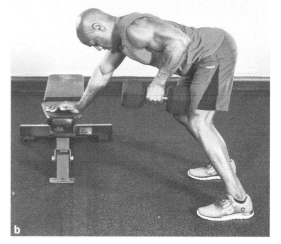

One-Arm Cable Row

Setup

Stand tall with your spine straight and your knees slightly bent while facing an adjustable cable column adjusted to roughly shoulder height. With your right hand, grab the handle in a neutral grip (i.e., with your palm facing the opposite side of your body) and split your stance so that your right leg is behind your left leg (see figure a).

Action

Perform a row by pulling the cable toward your body, driving your shoulder blade back so that it's retracted at the end of the row (see figure b). Maintain a stable spine without allowing your shoulders and hips to rotate more than a few degrees. Slowly reverse the motion by allowing your scapula to protract while your arm straightens. Perform all reps on one side before doing the other side.

Coaching Tips

- Keep your rear heel off of the ground to ensure that most of your weight remains on your front leg.
- Do not allow your rowing-side shoulder to move forward at the end of each rep.

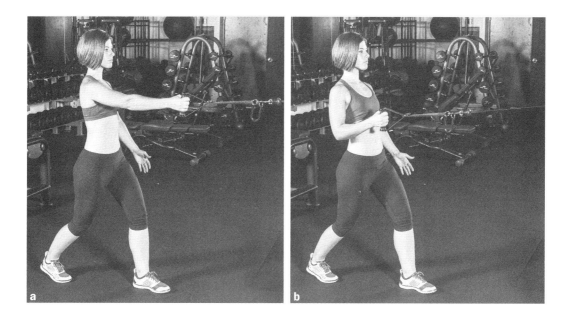

One-Arm Cable Row With Hip Rotation

Setup

Stand facing an adjustable column that's set at your mid torso level with you back straight, your feet roughly shoulder-width apart, and your knees slightly bent. Hold the handle in your right hand with your arm extended out in front of your shoulder (see figure a).

Action

Perform a row by pulling the cable toward your body, driving your shoulder blade back so that it's retracted at the end of the row. As you reach the end of the row, rotate your hips toward the rowing side (in this case, your right

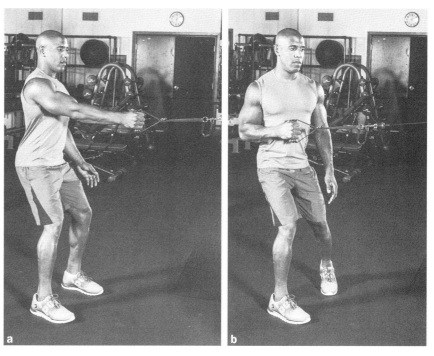

side) by allowing your left heel to elevate and pivoting on the ball of your left foot (see figure b). Slowly reverse the motion as you extend your arm, maintaining control, while straightening your feet back to face the cable. Perform all reps on one side before switching to the other side.

Coaching Tips

- At the end of each row, rotate your hips and torso no more than 45 degrees from the cable or band.
- As you pull the cable or band, shift your weight to the rowing side; as your arms extend back out, shift your weight back to being centered.

One-Arm Compound Cable Row

Setup

Stand facing an adjustable cable column that's set at your mid torso level with your feet roughly shoulder-width apart in a split stance with your left leg in front and your knees slightly bent. Hold the handle in your right hand using a neutral grip (i.e., with your palm facing the opposite side of your body).

Action

Hinge at your hips, reaching your right arm in front of you toward the origin of the cable (see figure a). Reverse this motion while performing a row. Finish the row at the same time that you return to the upright standing position (see figure b). Slowly reverse the motion, hinging at your hips and reaching out; use good rhythm and timing. Perform all reps on one side before switching to the other side.

Coaching Tips

- Keep your rear heel off of the ground to ensure that most of your weight remains on your front leg.
- Do not allow your rowing-side shoulder to move forward at the end of each rep.

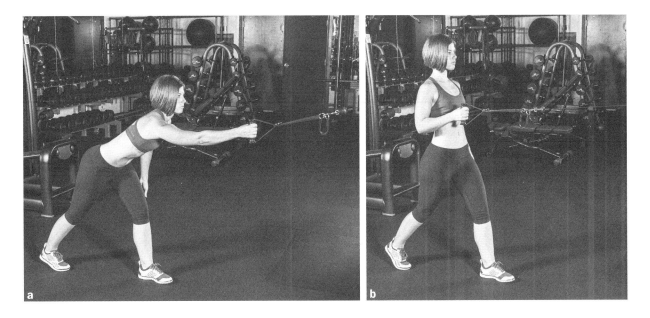

Bent-Over One-Arm Cable Row

Setup

Stand facing an adjustable cable column with your feet roughly hip-width apart. Take a big step backward with your right leg and hinge forward at your hips so that your torso is at roughly a 45-degree angle to the floor. Your left knee should be bent slightly and your right (back) leg straight with the heel off of the ground. With your right hand, hold the cable handle, which is attached low, in a neutral grip (i.e., with your palm facing the opposite side of your body) (see figure a).

Action

Perform a row by pulling the cable toward your body, driving your shoulder blade back so that it's retracted at the end of the row (see figure b). Maintain a stable spine without allowing your shoulders and hips to rotate more than a few degrees. Slowly reverse the motion by allowing your scapula to protract while your arm straightens. Perform all reps on one side before switching to the other side.

Coaching Tips

- Your torso and back leg should form a straight line, which should remain constant throughout the exercise.
- Most of your weight should be on your front leg.
- You can position your free hand either on your same-side hip or on top of your front leg.

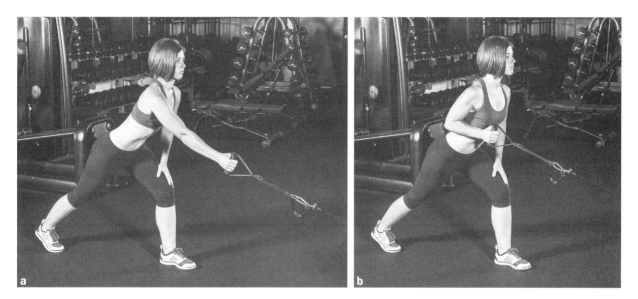

One-Arm Anti-Rotation Suspension Row

Setup

Face the anchor point of a suspension trainer and hold a handle in your right hand. Lean backward, away from the anchor point, with your body forming a straight line and extend your left arm by your side (see figure *a*).

Action

Without allowing your body to rotate at any point, perform rows by pulling your body toward the handle (see figure *b*) and going back down. Each time that you pull yourself toward the handle, keep your elbow (on the rowing side) tight to your body.

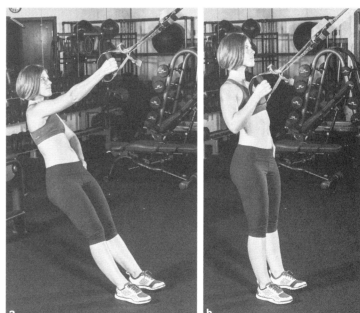

Coaching Tips

- Keep your body in a straight line throughout; keep your shoulders and hips parallel to the floor and do not allow your hips to sag toward the floor.
- To increase the difficulty, walk your feet farther out to increase your body angle and bring you lower.
- To decrease the difficulty, decrease your body angle by walking your feet in so that they're more underneath you.

Cable-Rope Tug-of-War Row

Setup

Attach a triceps rope to an adjustable cable column at your midtorso level. Stand at a 45-degree angle to the cable with your feet slightly farther than shoulder-width apart and your right leg back. Grab the rope with a baseball-bat type of grip, keeping your right hand behind your left. With your knees bent to roughly 15 to 20 degrees, hinge at your hips leaning your torso forward so that it's parallel to the floor and your arms are outstretched above you toward the origin of the cable (see figure a).

Action

Slowly reverse this motion by bringing your torso upright while leaning backward slightly with your upper body. Plant your feet on the ground and pull the rope into your body until your right wrist contacts your ribs on your right side (see figure b). Perform half of the repetitions with the same leg forward, then switch your stance and grip and perform the other half.

Coaching Tips

- Each time you perform the row, use your legs as anchors to drive your torso backward slightly.
- At the beginning of each repetition, allow your arms and upper back to stretch forward without rounding your lower back.
- As you perform the exercise, your weight should shift from front to back.

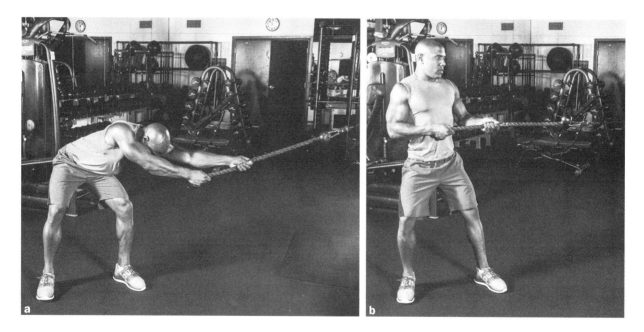

Compound Exercises

These pulling exercises integrate efforts by the lats, midback, posterior shoulders, and biceps muscles.

Chin-Up

Setup
Hang from a pull-up bar using an underhand grip (see figure *a*).

Action
Bring yourself up so that your chin goes above the bar without swinging your body (see figure *b*). Slowly lower yourself with control.

Coaching Tips
- Grip the bar at a width that feels comfortable for you.
- Pause for one second at the top of each rep before lowering yourself.

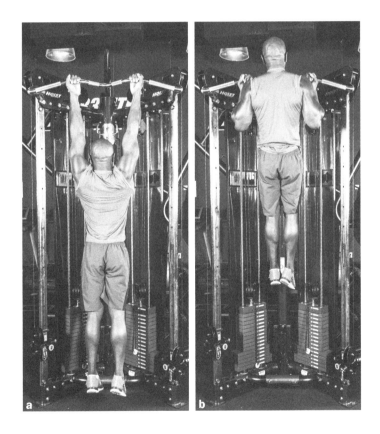

Compound Chin-Up

Setup
Hang from a pull-up bar using an under-hand grip (see figure a).

Action
Bring your chest up to the bar while simultaneously leaning your torso backward slightly so it forms roughly a 45-degree angle with the ground (see figure b). Slowly reverse the motion, lowering yourself and allowing your torso to return to a position perpendicular to the floor once your arms are fully straight.

Coaching Tips

- As you pull yourself up, do not allow your lower back to overextend.
- You can keep your knees slightly bent throughout this exercise.

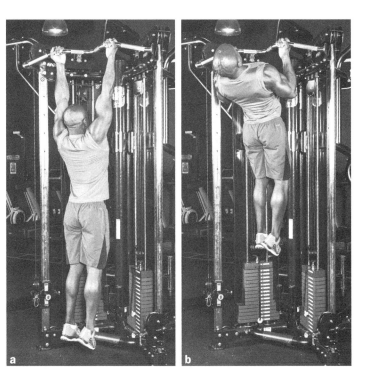

Pull-Up

Setup
Hang from a pull-up bar using an overhand grip (see figure a).

Action
Bring yourself up so that your chin goes above the bar without swinging your body (see figure b). Slowly lower yourself with control.

Coaching Tips

- Of the two grips, the underhand (chin-up) grip is the strongest for most people.
- Another great option is the neutral grip, in which your palms face one another (thus you need a bar that allows for this positioning). Some people who experience shoulder discomfort when performing pull-ups find a neutral grip to be more comfortable. And regardless of shoulder issues, many people simply find the neutral grip to be a stronger option.

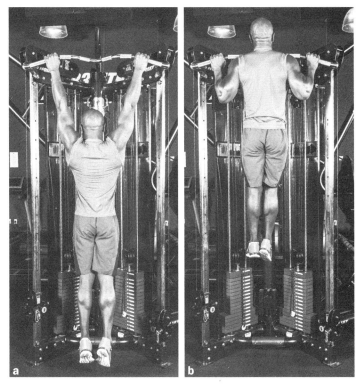

Lateral Pull-Up

Setup

Hang from a pull-up bar with an overhand grip and your hands farther than shoulder-width apart (see figure *a*).

Action

As you pull yourself up, move your body toward one hand so that your shoulder moves in front of the same-side hand (see figure *b*). Reverse the motion by moving back to the center as you allow your arms to straighten. Repeat by pulling yourself up to the other side.

Coaching Tips

- The overall motion of the exercise resembles an inverted triangle.
- Do not allow your shoulders to roll forward at the top of each repetition; keep your chest elevated at the top.

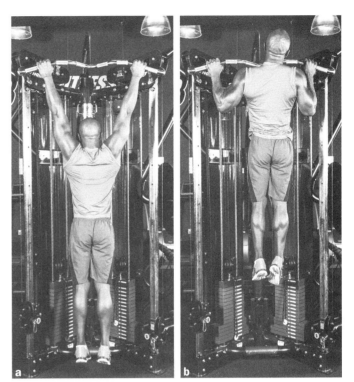

Lat Pull-Down

Setup

Position yourself just behind a traditional lat pull-down bar and hold it with an overhand grip over your head (see figure *a*).

Action

Pull the bar down to the top of your chest while keeping your back straight and your elbows following a straight line (see figure *b*). Slowly reverse the motion under control.

Coaching Tips

- Find a grip width somewhere outside of shoulder width that feels most comfortable to you.
- For variety, you can use an underhand grip.

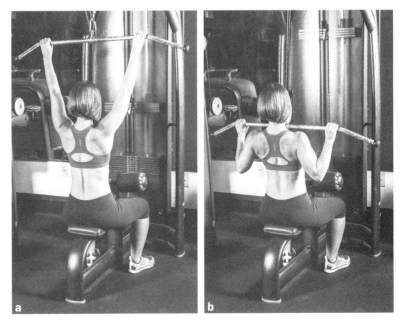

- You can also use a neutral grip by exchanging the straight bar for a handle that allows your palms to face one another spaced roughly shoulder-width apart. Many people who have minor shoulder issues find the neutral grip to be more comfortable.
- You can also add variety to this exercise by varying your torso position; a subtle backward lean can be mixed in with a fairly vertical torso.

Leaning Lat Pull-Down

Setup

This exercise is performed in the same manner as the lat pull-down except that you lean your torso backward slightly instead of remaining upright. Position yourself just behind a traditional lat pull-down bar and hold it with an overhand grip over your head (see figure a).

Action

While leaning your torso backward at roughly 25 degrees from upright, pull the bar down to the top of your chest while keeping your elbows pointed in the same direction as your line of pull (see figure b). Slowly reverse the motion with control.

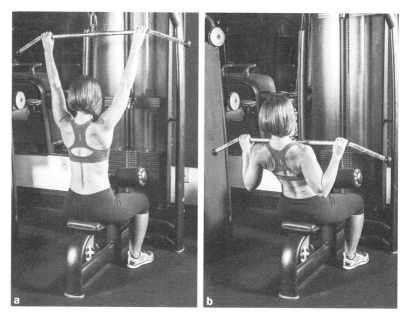

Coaching Tips

- Find a grip width somewhere outside of shoulder width that feels most comfortable to you.
- For variety, you can use an underhand grip.
- You can also use a neutral grip by exchanging the straight bar for a handle that allows your palms to face one another spaced roughly shoulder-width apart. Many people who have minor shoulder issues find the neutral grip to be more comfortable.

Fighter's Cable Lat Pull-Down

Setup

You'll need a dual adjustable cable machine for this exercise. Assume a half-kneeling position directly between a set of cables above you. Hold a handle in each hand with your arms straight at roughly a 45-degree angle to your torso (see figure a).

Action

Pull one arm toward your body, bringing your elbow all the way down to your hip bone, and combining the pull-down motion with a small side crunch in a motion (similar to that of a fighter blocking a body strike) (see figure b). Reverse the motion in a controlled fashion. Once your arm becomes straight, repeat the action with the other arm.

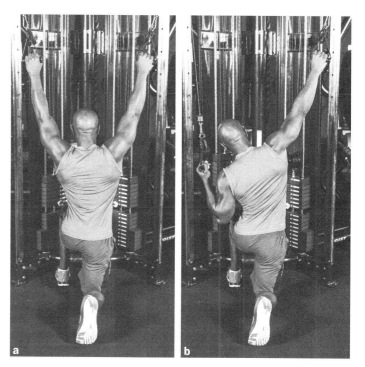

Coaching Tips

- Do not twist your torso.
- Keep your forearms perpendicular to the floor throughout.

Barbell Bent-Over Row

Setup

Stand with your feet roughly hip-width apart. Hold the barbell with an underhand grip and your hands just outside shoulder-width apart. Bend over at your hips, keeping your back straight so that your torso is roughly parallel to the floor and keeping your knees bent 15 to 20 degrees (see figure a).

Action

Row the bar into your body just above your belly button, pinching your shoulder blades together at the top (see figure b). Slowly lower the bar to complete the rep.

Coaching Tips

- You can also perform bent-over rows with an overhand grip, which many people find to be a less-strong gripping option.
- At the top of each repetition, pause for one second, keeping the barbell against your midtorso.
- Do not allow your back to round out at any time.
- Do not allow the fronts of your shoulders to round forward at the top of each repetition.

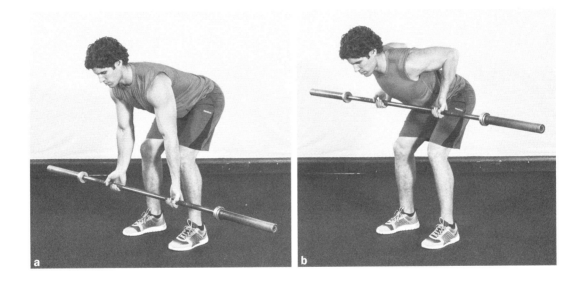

Wide-Grip Barbell Bent-Over Row

Setup

Stand with your feet shoulder-width apart and hold a barbell with your hands roughly one foot (0.3 m) outside your hips. Bend over at your hips, keeping your back straight so that your torso is roughly parallel to the floor and keeping your knees bent 15 to 20 degrees (see figure a).

Action

Row the bar into the middle of your torso just below your chest, pinching your shoulder blades together at the top (see figure b). Slowly lower the bar without allowing it to contact the floor until the set is completed.

> continued

Coaching Tips

- At the top of each repetition, pause for one second, keeping the barbell as close to the lower part of your chest as possible.
- Do not allow your back to round out at any time.
- Keep your elbows directly above your hands and do not allow your wrists to bend.
- Do not allow the fronts of your shoulders to round forward at the top of each repetition.

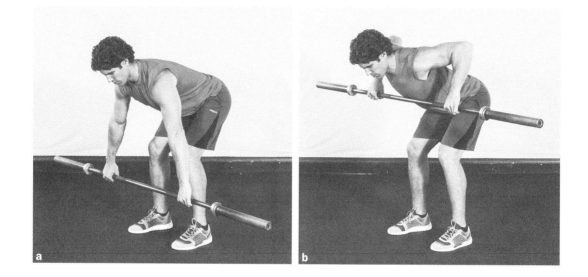

Two-Arm Dumbbell Bent-Over Row

Setup

Stand with your feet hip-width apart and hold a dumbbell in each hand. Bend over at your hips, keeping your back straight so that your torso is roughly parallel to the floor and keeping your knees bent 15 to 20 degrees (see figure *a*).

Action

Row the dumbbells toward you while keeping your arms at a 45-degree angle to your torso; at the top, pinch your shoulder blades together (see figure *b*). Slowly lower the dumbbells without allowing them to contact the floor until the set is completed.

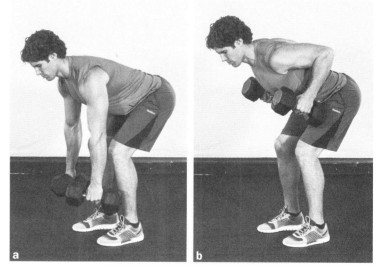

Coaching Tips

- Pause for one second at the top of each repetition.
- Do not allow your back to round out at any time.
- Do not allow your wrists to bend.
- Do not allow the fronts of your shoulders to round forward at the top of each repetition.

Seated Row

Setup

This exercise usually requires a specially designed seated-row apparatus that is available in most gyms. It can also be done by sitting on the floor in front of a low cable with your feet braced against two dumbbells (pictured). Sit with your feet hip-width apart against the platform or dumbbells, your knees slightly bent, and your back straight. Hold the handles with a neutral grip and your hands about shoulder-width apart (see figure a).

Action

Pull the handles into your body at midtorso level, pinching your shoulder blades together at the end (see figure b). Slowly reverse the movement.

Coaching Tips

- Pause for one second at the top of each repetition, keeping the handles as close to your torso as possible.
- Do not overarch your lower back as you row.
- Do not allow the fronts of your shoulders to round forward at the end of each repetition.

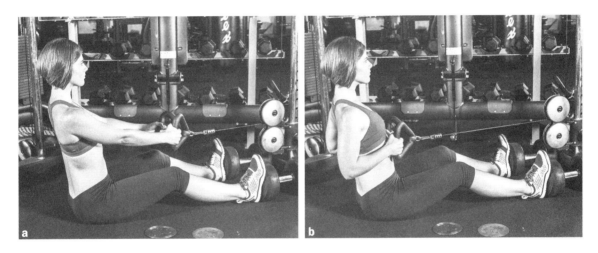

Wide-Grip Seated Row

Setup

This exercise usually requires a specially designed seated-row apparatus that is available in most gyms. It can also be done by sitting on the floor in front of a low cable with your feet braced against two dumbbells (pictured). Sit with your feet hip-width apart against the platform or dumbbells, your knees slightly bent, and your back straight. Hold a lat bar in an overhand grip with your hands roughly 10 inches (25 cm) outside your chest (see figure *a*).

Action

Pull the bar into your body at chest level, pinching your shoulder blades together at the end (see figure *b*). Slowly reverse the movement.

Coaching Tips

- Pause for one second at the top of each repetition, keeping the bar as close to your chest as possible.
- Do not allow your wrists to bend as you pull the bar; keep your elbows directly behind your hands throughout.
- Do not allow the fronts of your shoulders to round forward at the end of each repetition.

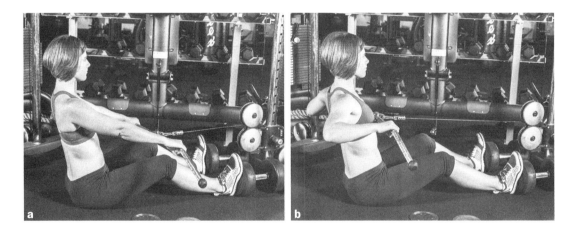

Suspension Row

Setup

Using a suspension trainer, face the anchor point and hold onto the handles with your palms either facing each other or facing the sky and with your arms extended straight in front of your shoulders (see figure a for an example with the palms facing each other). Lean back with your body in a straight line from head to toe.

Action

Pull yourself up toward your hands by bending at your elbows. Keep your elbows tight to your sides and perform a rowing motion until the insides of your wrists are close to your bottom ribs, thus ensuring a full range of motion (see figure b). Pause at the top for one second, then slowly lower yourself until your elbows are straight.

Coaching Tips

- Keep your body in a straight line and do not lead with your hips when pulling yourself up.
- Do not allow your wrists to bend as you pull yourself up; keep your elbows directly behind your hands throughout.
- Do not allow the fronts of your shoulders to round forward at the end of each repetition.
- To increase the difficulty, start the exercise from a more severe backward lean, bringing your body closer to the floor.

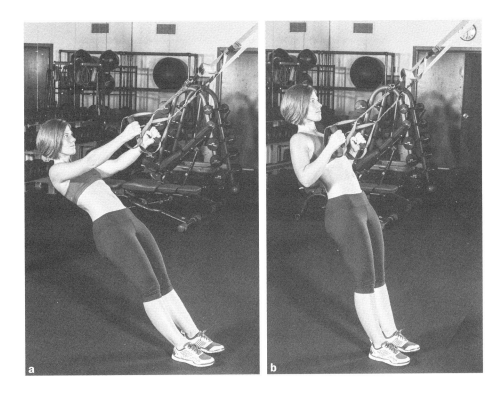

Smith-Bar Underhand-Grip Row

Setup

This exercise is an alternative version of the suspension row. Using a Smith machine, face a barbell positioned at belly-button height. Hold onto the bar using an underhand grip with your arms extended straight in front of your shoulders (see figure *a*). Lean back with your body in a straight line from head to toe.

Action

Pull yourself up toward the bar by bending at your elbows, keeping your elbows tight to your sides, and performing a rowing motion until your midtorso contacts the bar (see figure *b*). Pause at the top for one second, then slowly lower yourself until your elbows are straight.

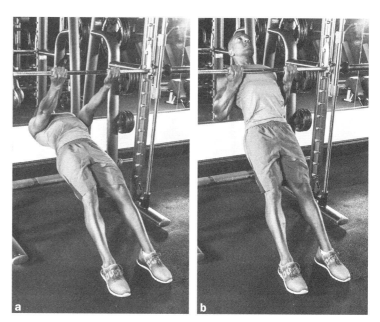

Coaching Tips

- Keep your body in a straight line; do not lead with your hips when pulling yourself up.
- Do not allow the fronts of your shoulders to round forward at the end of each repetition.
- To increase the difficulty, start the exercise from a more severe backward lean by lowering the bar, thus bringing your body closer to the floor.

Wide-Elbow Suspension Row

Setup

Using a suspension trainer, face the anchor point and hold onto the handles with your thumbs facing each other and your arms extended straight in front of your shoulders (see figure *a*). Lean back with your body in a straight line from head to toe.

Action

Pull yourself up toward your hands by bending at your elbows and performing a rowing motion while flaring out your elbows (see figure *b*). Pause at the top for one second, then slowly lower yourself until your elbows are straight.

Coaching Tips

- Keep your body in a straight line; do not lead with your hips when pulling yourself up.
- Do not allow your wrists to bend as you pull yourself up; keep your elbows directly behind your hands throughout.
- Your elbows should be at a 90-degree angle to your torso at the top of each repetition.
- Do not allow the fronts of your shoulders to round forward at the end of each repetition.
- To increase the difficulty, start the exercise from a more severe backward lean, thus bringing your body closer to the floor.

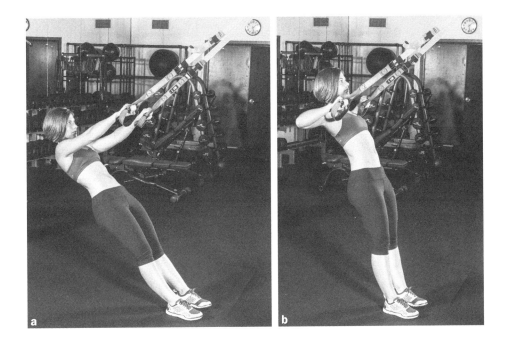

Wide-Elbow Smith-Bar Row

Setup

This exercise is an alternative version of the wide-elbow suspension row. Using a Smith machine, face a barbell positioned at belly-button height and hold onto the bar using an overhand grip with your hands placed about 5 inches (13 cm) outside of your shoulders. Keeping your arms straight and extended in front of your shoulders, lean back with your body in a straight line from head to toe (see figure a).

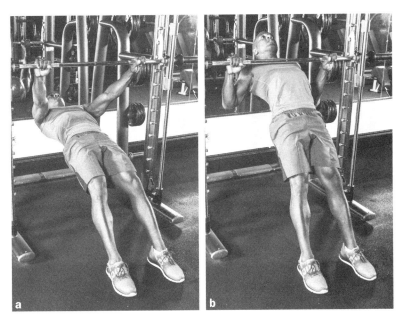

Action

Pull yourself up toward the bar by bending at your elbows and performing a rowing motion while flaring out your elbows (see figure b). Pause at the top for one second, then slowly lower yourself until your elbows are straight.

Coaching Tips

- Keep your body in a straight line; do not lead with your hips when pulling yourself up.
- Do not allow your wrists to bend as you pull yourself up; keep your elbows directly behind your hands throughout.
- Your elbows should be at a 90-degree angle to your torso at the top of each repetition.
- To increase the difficulty, start the exercise from a more severe backward lean by lowering the bar, thus bringing your body closer to the floor.

Isolation Exercises

These are single-joint movements that focus on individual muscle groups. These exercise applications consist primarily of classic bodybuilding exercises that target the lats, midback, posterior shoulders, and biceps.

Bent-Over Dumbbell Shoulder Fly

Setup

Stand with your feet hip-width apart and hold a dumbbell in each hand. Bend over at your hips, keeping your back straight so that your torso is at roughly a 45-degree angle to the floor and keeping your knees bent 15 to 20 degrees (see figure a).

Action

Keeping a small bend in your elbows, raise your arms out to your sides until they become parallel with the floor; pinch your shoulder blades together at the top. Your arms should be at a 90-degree angle relative to your torso at the top of each repetition (see figure b). Slowly lower the dumbbells in front of your torso.

Coaching Tips

- Pause for one second at the top of each repetition.
- Do not allow your back to round out at any time.
- Do not swing the dumbbells up.

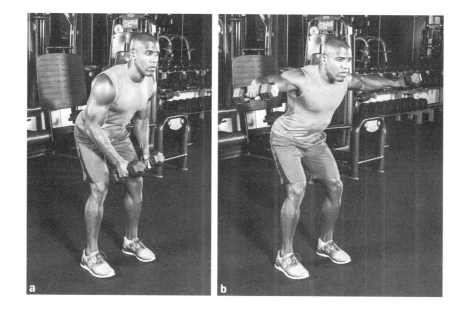

Dumbbell Shoulder Y

Setup

Stand with your feet hip-width apart and hold a dumbbell in each hand. Bend over at your hips, keeping your back straight so that your torso is parallel to the floor and keeping your knees bent 15 to 20 degrees (see figure a).

Action

Keeping a small bend in your elbows, raise your arms out to shoulder height, pointing your thumbs toward the sky. Your arms should be at a 45-degree angle relative to your torso at the

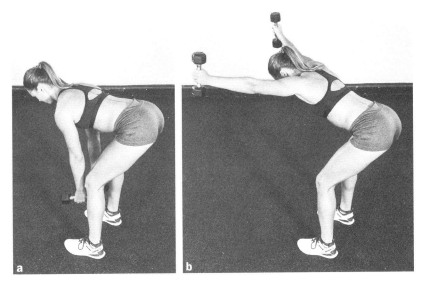

top of each repetition, thus forming a Y shape with your torso (see figure b). Pause for one second at the top of each repetition, then slowly lower the dumbbells in front of your torso.

Coaching Tips

- Do not allow your back to round out at any time.
- Do not swing the dumbbells up.

Dumbbell Shoulder A

Setup

Stand with your feet hip-width apart and hold a dumbbell in each hand. Bend over at your hips, keeping your back straight so that your torso is parallel to the floor and keeping your knees bent 15 to 20 degrees (see figure a).

Action

Keeping a small bend in your elbows, raise your arms out to your sides, just outside your hips, pointing your thumbs toward the floor. Your arms should be at a 15-degree angle relative to your

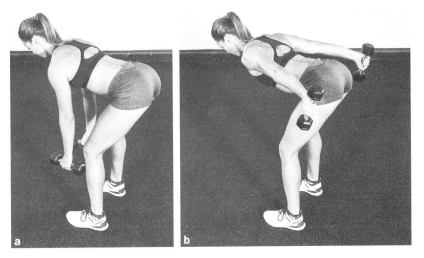

torso at the top of each repetition, thus forming an A shape with your torso (see figure b). Pause for one second at the top of each repetition, then slowly lower the dumbbells in front of your torso.

Coaching Tips

- Do not allow your back to round out at any time.
- Do not swing the dumbbells up.
- Pinch your shoulder blades together at the top of each rep.

Dumbbell Shoulder T

Setup

Stand with your feet hip-width apart and hold a dumbbell in each hand. Bend over at your hips, keeping your back straight so that your torso is parallel to the floor and keeping your knees bent 15 to 20 degrees (see figure *a*).

Action

Keeping a small bend in your elbows, raise your arms out to your sides, pointing your thumbs toward the sky. Your arms should be at a 90-degree angle relative to your torso at the top of each repetition, thus forming a T shape with your torso (see figure *b*).

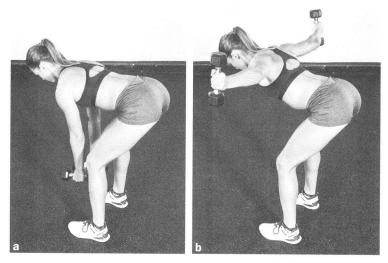

Pause for one second at the top of each repetition, then slowly lower the dumbbells in front of your torso.

Coaching Tips

- Do not allow your back to round out at any time.
- Pinch your shoulder blades together at the top of each rep.
- Do not swing the dumbbells up.

Shoulder W

Setup

Stand with your feet hip-width apart. Bend over at your hips, keeping your back straight so that your torso is parallel to the floor and your knees bent 90 degrees. Your arms are bent against your torso with the top of your hands at roughly shoulder-height (see figure *a*).

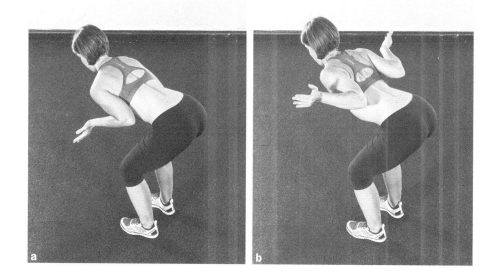

Action

Raise your arms out to your sides just outside your torso, pointing your thumbs toward the sky. At the top of each repetition, your arms should form a W-shape (see figure b). Pause for one second at the top of each repetition and then slowly lower your arms back down in front of your torso.

Coaching Tips

- Do not allow your back to round out at any time.
- Hold dumbbells to add load and increase the difficulty of this exercise.
- Pinch your shoulder-blades together at the top of each rep.

Suspension Y-Pull

Setup

Using a suspension trainer, face the anchor point and hold onto the handles with your palms facing the floor and your arms extended straight out in front of your shoulders (see figure a). Lean back with your body in a straight line from head to toe.

Action

Without bending your elbows, open your arms out diagonally to form a Y (see figure b). At the top of each rep, your body should end up being even with your arms. Pause at the top for one second before reversing the motion and slowly lowering yourself to the starting position to complete the rep.

Coaching Tips

- Keep your body in a straight line; do not lead with your hips when pulling yourself up.
- Do not allow your wrists to bend as you pull yourself up.
- Maintain tension against the handles throughout, especially at the top of each rep.
- To increase the difficulty, start the exercise from a more severe backward lean, thus bringing your body closer to the floor.

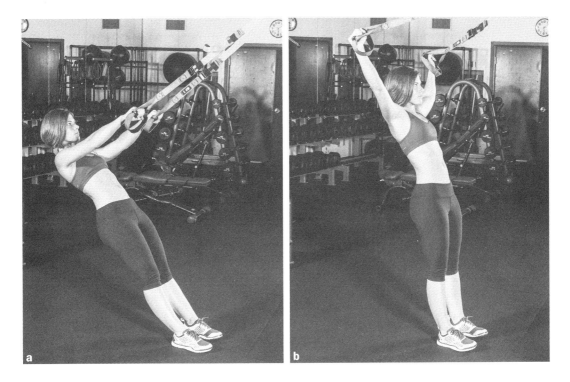

Rope Face Pull

Setup

Stand in front of an adjustable cable column with a rope attached at or above your eye level. Hold one end of the rope in each hand with your palms facing one another and your elbows pointed out to the sides (see figure a).

Action

Pull the rope toward your face as you drive your arms apart so that your hands end up just outside your ears (see figure b). Slowly reverse the movement back to the starting position.

Coaching Tips

- Do not overarch your lower back.
- Your elbows should be slightly higher than your shoulders at the end of each repetition.
- The middle of the rope should end up just in front of your forehead at the end of each repetition.

Cable Reverse Shoulder Fly

Setup

Stand tall with your spine straight, your feet hip-width apart, and your knees slightly bent while facing an adjustable cable column at roughly shoulder height. With your right hand, grab the handle on the left and with your left hand grab the handle on your right. Your arms will be crossed in front of your body with your palms facing down to the floor (see figure a).

Action

Keeping your elbows slightly bent, pull the handles horizontally by opening your arms out to the sides of your body. Pinch your shoulder blades together at the end (see figure b). Slowly reverse the movement back to the starting position.

Coaching Tips

- Keep a stable spine and minimize any overarching in your lower back.
- Your arms should be at a 90-degree angle to your torso throughout the exercise.

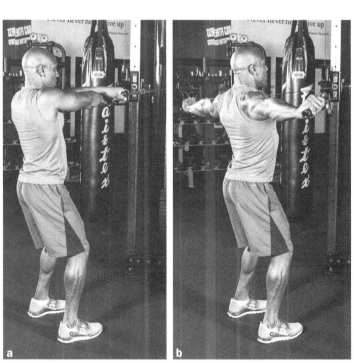

Cable Compound Straight-Arm Pull-Down

Setup

Stand facing an adjustable cable column with your feet roughly hip-width apart and a rope attached to a cable column above your eye level. Hold one end of the rope in each hand with your palms facing one another. Hinge at your hips with a slight bend at your knees and your arms extended above your head (see figure a).

Action

At the same time you raise your torso to an upright position, pull the rope down, keeping a small bend in your elbows, until the handles touch just outside of your hips (see figure b). Slowly reverse the motion, hinging at your hips and reaching your arms back above your head; use good rhythm and timing.

Coaching Tips

- Do not round your shoulders forward at the top of each repetition.
- Perform the exercise smoothly with your arms going down as your torso goes up and vice versa.

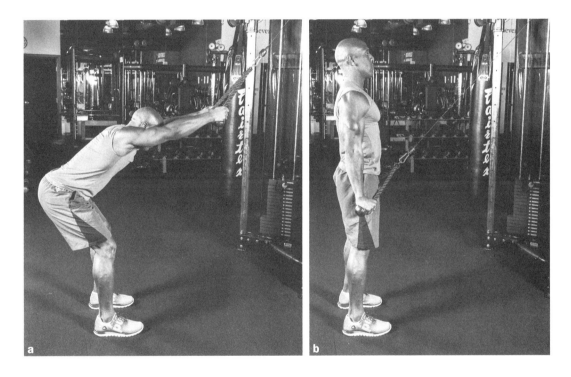

Cable Rotational Straight-Arm Pull-Down

Setup

You'll need an adjustable cable column to perform this exercise. Stand facing the cable column with your feet roughly hip-width apart with a rope attached above eye-level, your arms around shoulder-level, and your elbows slightly bent (see figure a).

Action

Pull the rope downward and slightly to the right while lifting your left heel and rotating your left foot so the torso rotates to the right (see figure b). Slowly reverse the motion returning to the middle position, and repeat this same action by pulling the rope to down to your left side while pivoting on your right foot and rotating your torso to the left.

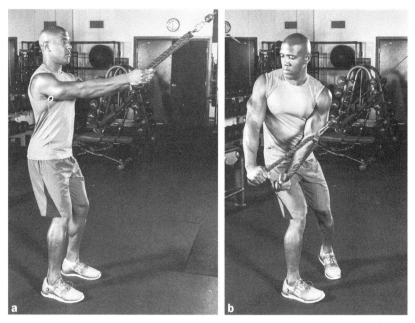

Coaching Tips

- Do not round your shoulders forward at the top of each repetition.
- This exercise should be done in a smooth manner using good rhythm and timing between the arm pull and the torso rotation.

Dumbbell Biceps Curl

Setup

Stand tall with your feet hip-width apart and hold a dumbbell in each hand by your hips (see figure a).

Action

Curl one dumbbell up toward your shoulders by bending at your elbow without allowing your elbow to move forward (see figure b). Once your hand is up in front of your shoulder, reverse the motion by slowly lowering the dumbbell to your side. Repeat the same action with the other arm and continue alternating arms.

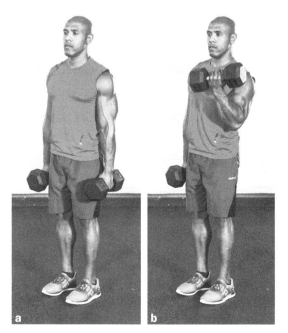

Coaching Tips

- Do not swing the weight up by overextending at your lower back.
- This exercise can also be done by curling both arms simultaneously.
- You can also perform dumbbell hammer curls by keeping the handles of the dumbbells vertical.

EZ-Bar Biceps Curl

Setup

Stand tall with your feet hip-width apart, holding an EZ-Bar with both hands by your hips with an underhand grip (see figure a).

Action

Curl the bar up toward your shoulders by bending at your elbows without allowing your elbows to move forward (see figure b). Once your hands are up in front of your shoulders, reverse the motion by slowly lowering the bar back down.

Coaching Tips

- Do not swing the weight up by over-extending at your lower back.
- You can also perform this exercise with an overhand grip.

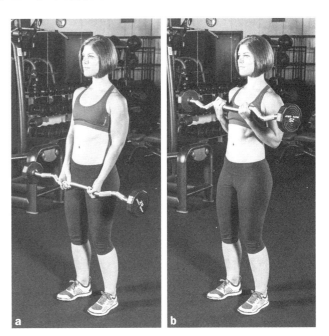

Cable Biceps Curl

Setup

Stand tall in front of an adjustable cable column with a rope handle attached to a cable column below your knees. Hold each side of the handle using a neutral grip with your palms facing each other, your arms by your sides, and your elbows slightly bent (see figure a).

Action

Curl the rope up toward your shoulders by bending at your elbows without allowing your elbows to move forward (see figure b). Once your hands are up in front of your shoulders, reverse the motion by slowly lowering the rope until your arms are almost straight.

Coaching Tips

- For additional training variety, you can use an EZ-Bar handle attachment.
- You can also perform reverse cable curls with an EZ-Bar by grabbing the handle with your palms facing down.

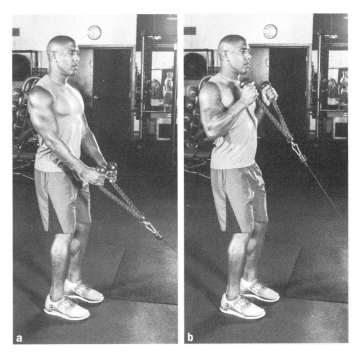

Suspension Biceps Curl

Setup

Using a suspension trainer, face the anchor point and hold onto the handles with your palms facing the ceiling. Lean back with your body in a straight line from head to toe, your elbows straight, and your arms extended out in front of your shoulders (see figure a).

Action

Bending only at your elbows, perform a biceps curl and pull yourself up so that your knuckles touch your forehead (see figure b). Reverse the action to complete the rep.

Coaching Tips

- Keep your body straight throughout the exercise.
- To increase the difficulty, start the exercise from a more severe backward lean, thus bringing your body closer to the floor.

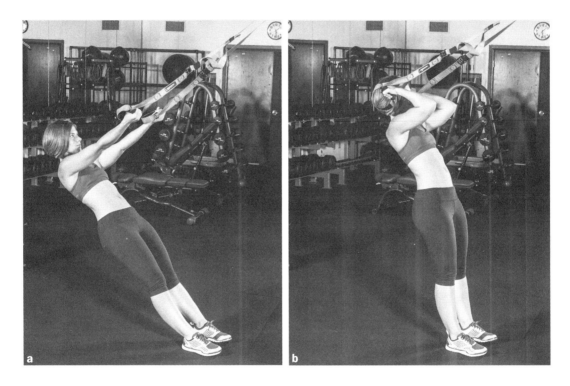

Now that we've covered a variety of pushing and pulling movements focused on the upper body, the next chapter provides you with a variety of exercises for building a stronger, better-looking, and high-performance lower body.

6

Lower Body

Field, court, and combat sports—as well as everyday activities—rely on specific movements for performance. When it comes to the lower body, all of these movements involve some type or combination of squat, hip hinge, lunge, step, run, or jump. The lower-body exercises featured in this chapter help you improve your ability to perform these fundamental human actions.

The exercises presented here challenge your lower body in a three-dimensional manner from either a parallel stance, a split stance, or a single-leg stance to ensure that you're strong in all positions and capable of moving in any direction. That's what increasing your functional capacity is all about; it's not just about upping your conventional deadlift numbers and thinking that takes care of everything. Remember, as my friend and iron-game legend Richard Sorin says, "athletes (and athletic-minded individuals) are *not* in the gym to become weightlifters; they're there to be athletes made stronger in the weightroom."

These groups—field, court, and combat athletes, as well as athletic-minded folks who also have bodybuilding-related goals—are the ones for whom this book is written. For these people, the conventional barbell deadlift, squat, and bench press aren't simply exercises; they're tools in a box that also contains many other tools to help them achieve their goals. To powerlifters (i.e., weightlifters), however, the conventional deadlift, squat, and bench press are not tools; they are events—ends in themselves. It's disappointing that this difference goes unacknowledged by so many coaches, trainers, and gym goers. As a result, they fail to apply the principle of specificity: Different training goals require different training approaches.

So, let's talk about lower-body training as it relates to those of you who *aren't* in the gym to be competitive powerlifters. If you're not trying not be a powerlifter, then there is no single exercise that you must do; when it comes to performing exercises like conventional barbell deadlifts, you need only use them in a way that's safe and helps you improve your overall strength and muscle. You do need to possess basic competence in the lifts you're performing; however, you do not need to learn or practice the powerlifting-specific skills required to be a master deadlifter.

Nor does it matter what you can lift, because nonweightlifters don't chase certain lifting numbers—they chase *progress*. Doing that doesn't mean lifting a specific amount of weight that would impress the powerlifting community; it simply means getting stronger than you were without sacrificing your overall health or physical capacity to participate in the other physical activities and sports you enjoy. Similarly, when it comes to building muscle size (i.e., hypertrophy), progress is judged not by lifting an impressive amount of weight in the gym but by the quality of the *way* in which you perform the lift and by the resulting changes in your physique—the effects that show outside of the gym.

Single-Leg Versus Double-Leg Training

Elsewhere in this book, I said that pitting free weights against machines is like pitting fruits against vegetables. Similarly, debate about single-leg versus double-leg exercise is like arguing about whether one should eat only carrots or only broccoli. In reality, each vegetable offers a unique flavor and provides a certain set of nutrients, so just include them both in your diet to make it more tasty and nutritious!

As for single-leg and double-leg exercises, the double-leg exercises (e.g., squats, deadlifts) place you in a wider base of support and force you to use both your legs and your hips, together, to coordinate many muscles in order to move big loads, which is very metabolically taxing. In contrast, unilateral leg-training exercises force you into a *narrow* base of support, which works your legs and hips in a slightly different manner; a manner that's often closer to how your legs work during sports since many athletic actions (i.e., running and cutting) are single-leg dominant. Of course, they also force you to focus on controlling and using one side at a time, which is great for strengthening your weaker, less coordinated side.

Therefore, using both types gives you a wider range of benefits; in addition, having both types to choose from provides a much larger pool of exercise options for adding variety to your lower-body workouts. In summary, since both unilateral and bilateral leg training help you improve muscle and strength—and since both offer unique, complementary benefits—it makes sense to incorporate both into your lower-body workouts in order to make them more well-rounded and effective.

Total-Body Power Exercises

These explosive exercises require you to summate force by coordinating all of the muscles in your body with emphasis on the lower body.

25-Yard Dash

Setup
Place two cones roughly 25 yards apart.

Action
Jog up to the first cone, then sprint as fast as you can to the other cone. Once you pass the second cone, jog several steps before you stop. Walk back to the start cone and repeat.

Coaching Tips
- While sprinting, keep your elbows bent at roughly a 90-degree angle and drive with your arms.
- The jog-up start is recommended (rather than a quick-start from a still position) as a way to maximize the safety of the exercise.
- Do not take short, choppy steps; allow your legs to take powerful strides without overstriding (striding beyond your ability).

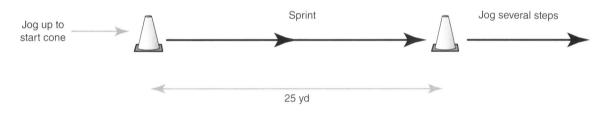

30-Yard Shuttle

This exercise includes changes of direction, thus posing a greater agility challenge than does the 25-yard dash.

Setup
Place three cones five yards apart in a straight line.

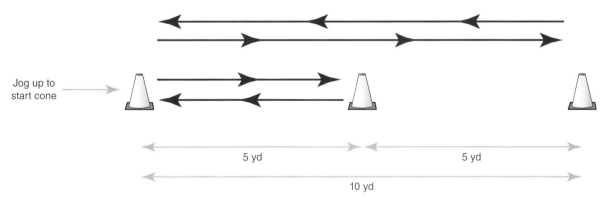

> continued

Action

Jog up to the first cone, then sprint as fast as you can to the middle cone. Sprint back to the first cone, then sprint to the far cone. Turn around again and sprint back to the starting cone. Along the way, touch each cone every time you get to one. This drill requires that you cut (change direction) four times, and you end up sprinting for a total of 30 yards: 5 yards up, 5 yards back, 10 yards up, and 10 yards back.

Use a work-to-rest ratio of 1:3 or 1:4 between rounds, depending on your fitness level. For example, using a 1:3 ratio, if it takes you 15 seconds to complete a 30-yard shuttle, then rest for 45 seconds before starting the next round.

Coaching Tips

- You can also perform this drill in reverse order: 10 yards up and back, then 5 yards up and back.
- Drive with your arms while running.
- When changing direction at each cone, be aware of your lower-body alignment and control.

Power Skip

Setup

Designate two ends about 30 to 40 yards apart.

Action

Jog up to the first end, then perform the power skip. To do so, keep your torso upright while bending your right knee to raise your leg until your thigh is horizontal to the ground; simultaneously, extend your left leg and drive it hard into the ground to explode your body as far forward as possible (see figure). Land lightly, then quickly perform the same action on the opposite side. Once you pass the second end, stop and walk back to the start end, then repeat. Try to cover as much ground as possible, getting to the second end in as few strides as you can.

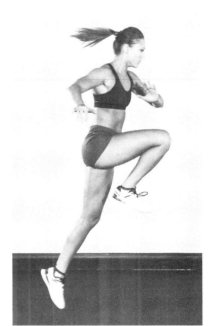

Coaching Tips

- Similar to the action of rope jumping, the stride used in this exercise requires a double-foot strike pattern each time you contact the ground.
- Coordinate the pumping of your arms with the double-foot strikes.
- If you're working in a small space, designate two ends about 15 to 20 yards apart and perform a full lap between them to cover a total of 30 to 40 yards.

Lateral Power Shuffle

Setup

Designate two ends about 20 to 30 yards apart. Assume an athletic stance with your feet shoulder-width apart and your knees and hips slightly bent (see figure *a*).

Action

Shift your weight toward your right, picking up your left foot and explosively pushing your right foot into the ground to start moving to your left (see figures *b-d*). Continue to move to your left in this manner: picking up your left foot and placing it to the left while pushing your right foot into the ground to generate force and momentum for the sideways movement. Your feet should remain fairly parallel with one another, and your toes should face forward. Once you reach the other end, reverse direction by shifting your weight off of your *right* leg, then push off with your *left* foot and begin shuffling back to the starting point. Try to cover as much ground as possible, getting to the second point in as few strides as you can.

Coaching Tips

- Do not allow your feet to touch one another; keep a few inches between your feet.
- Land as softly as possible on each stride, allowing your legs to bend slightly on each landing.

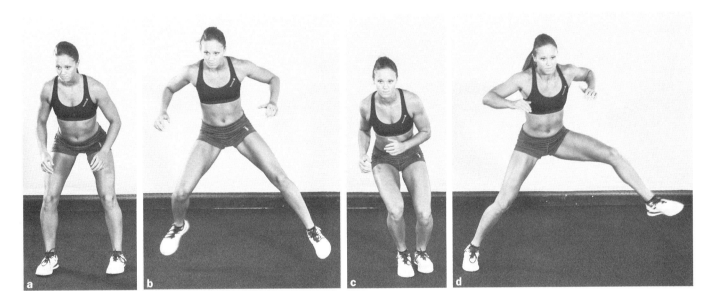

Squat Jump With Arm Drive

Setup
Stand with your feet roughly shoulder-width apart.

Action
Squat by bending at your knees and hips so that your thighs are just above parallel to the ground. Reach your arms slightly behind your hips, keeping your elbows slightly bent (see figure a). Jump straight up by simultaneously extending your legs and swinging your arms above you (see figure b). Land as lightly and quietly as possible, thus returning to the starting position.

Coaching Tips
- Jump as high as you can on each repetition.
- Each time you squat, keep your knees in the same line as your toes; your knees should not come toward one another at any time.
- Do not allow your back to round out at the bottom of each repetition.
- To add load to the exercise, wear a weight vest.

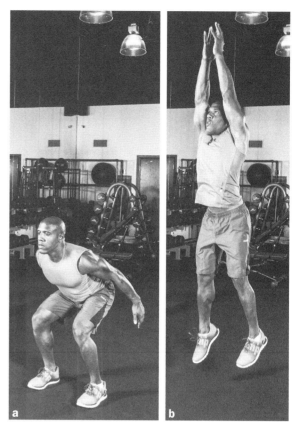

180-Degree Squat Jump With Cross-Arm Drive

Setup
Stand with your feet roughly shoulder-width apart.

Action
Squat by bending at your knees and hips so that your thighs are just above parallel to the ground. Reach both of your arms across your body to just outside your right knee (see figure a). Jump up and turn your body in the air 180 degrees to the left by simultaneously extending your legs and swinging your arms above you (see figure b). Land as lightly and quietly as possible, facing the other direction, while lowering your body into a squat and lowering your arms down across your body to just outside your left knee (see figure c). Repeat the action by jumping up and turning 180 degrees to your right.

Coaching Tips
- Jump as high as you can on each repetition.
- Each time you squat, keep your knees in the same line as your toes; your knees should not come toward one another at any time.
- Do not allow your back to round out at the bottom of each repetition.

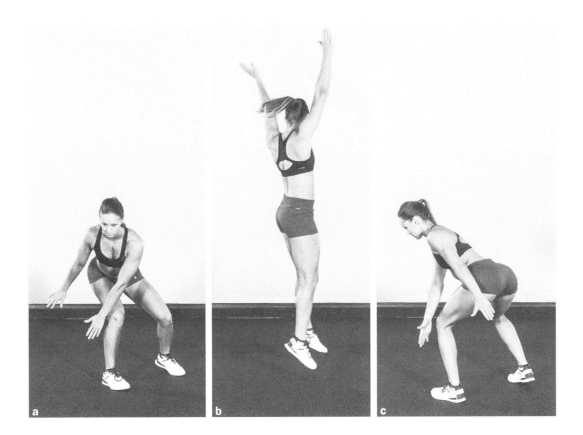

Deadlift Jump With Arm Drive

Setup

With your feet roughly shoulder-width apart, hinge at your hips and bend forward toward the floor. Keep your back straight and your knees bent at a 15- to 20-degree angle. Let your arms hang in front of your body by your knees, keeping your elbows slightly bent (see figure *a*).

Action

Jump straight up by simultaneously extending your hips and knees and swinging your arms above you (see figure *b*). Land as lightly and quietly as possible, thus returning to the starting position.

Coaching Tips

- Jump as high as you can on each repetition.
- Do not allow your back to round out at the bottom of each repetition.
- Each time you set up for the next jump, keep your knees in the same line as your toes; your knees should not come toward one another at any time.
- To add load to the exercise, wear a weight vest.

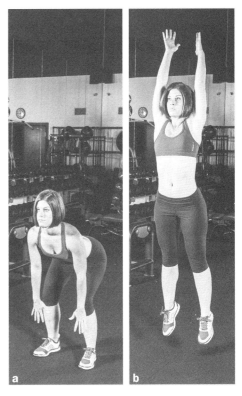

Broad Jump

Setup

With your feet roughly shoulder-width apart, hinge at your hips and bend forward toward the floor. Keep your back straight and your knees bent at a 15- to 20-degree angle. Reach your arms slightly behind your hips, keeping your elbows slightly bent (see figure a).

Action

Allow your weight to shift forward. Just before you feel as though you're going to fall, jump forward as far as possible by simultaneously extending your hips and knees and swinging your arms above you (see figures b and c). Land as lightly as possible (see figure d). Reset your position to perform the next repetition.

Coaching Tips

- Do not allow your back to round out at the bottom of each repetition.
- Each time you drop down to perform the next jump, keep your knees in the same line as your toes; your knees should not come toward one another at any time.
- If you're working in a small space, turn around after each repetition and jump back to where you were instead of continuing to jump in the same direction.

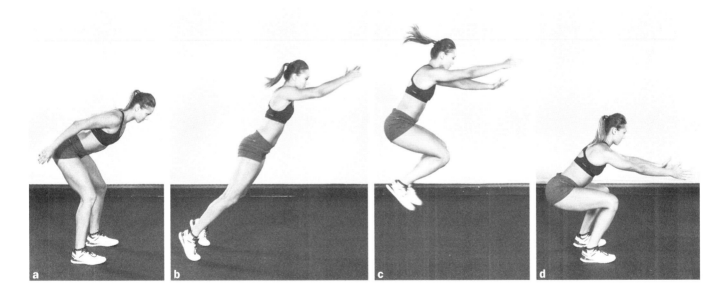

Anterior-Leaning Lunge Scissor Jump

Setup

Assume a split stance with your legs hip-width apart and your rear heel off of the ground, thus putting most of your weight on your front leg.

Action

Lean your torso forward by hinging at your hips and reach your arms down, keeping them just behind your toes (see figure a). Jump as high as possible while scissoring your legs (see figure b) so that you land in the same position but with the opposite leg forward (see figure c). Jump again, repeating the action.

Coaching Tips

- Land as quietly and lightly as possible, using each landing to load the next jump.
- Each time you land, keep your knees in the same line as your toes; your knees should not come toward your body's midline at any time.
- Each time you land, hinge forward at your hips, keeping your spine straight.
- Each time you explode back up, raise your torso.

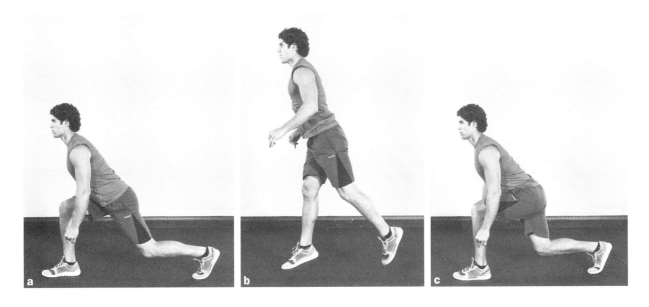

Lateral Bound

Setup

Balance on your right leg with your left leg held off of the ground by bending your knee and lifting your heel behind you (see figure *a*). Squat and reach across your body with your left arm.

Action

Explode toward your left side, jumping as far you can at a 45-degree angle (see figure *b*). Land softly on your left leg in a single-leg squat position, reaching across your body with your right arm (see figure *c*). Repeat by jumping back to the right side.

Coaching Tips

- Land with a soft knee into a squat position to ensure maximal force absorption and maximal power production on the next jump.
- Each time you land, keep your knees in the same line as your toes; your knees should not come toward your body's midline at any time.
- Jump at a 45-degree angle and make an all-out effort on each repetition.

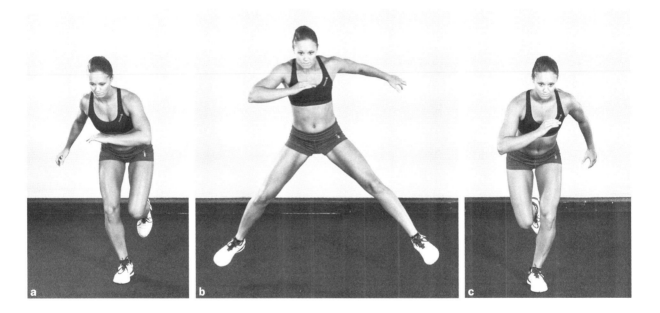

Cross-Body Exercises

The cross-body exercises presented here emphasize the lower-body musculature—which consists primarily of the glutes, hamstrings, quadriceps, and calves—while integrating the torso and upper body on the side opposite that of the working leg.

One-Leg One-Arm Dumbbell Romanian Deadlift

Setup
Stand on one leg and hold a dumbbell in the opposite hand at your hip (see figure a).

Action
Keeping your back and arm straight, hinge at your hip and bend forward toward the floor; keep your weight-bearing knee bent at roughly a 15- to 20-degree angle. As you hinge, allow your non-weight-bearing leg to elevate so that it remains in a straight line with your torso (see figure b). Once your torso and non-weight-bearing leg are roughly parallel to the floor, reverse the motion by driving your hips forward to stand tall again, thus completing the rep. Perform all repetitions on one side before switching sides.

Coaching Tips
- Do not allow your lower back to round out as you hinge your hips and lower your torso.
- At the bottom position (when your torso is roughly parallel to the ground), keep your hips and shoulders flat and do not allow them to rotate.
- At the bottom position, the foot of your non-weight-bearing leg should point at the floor.

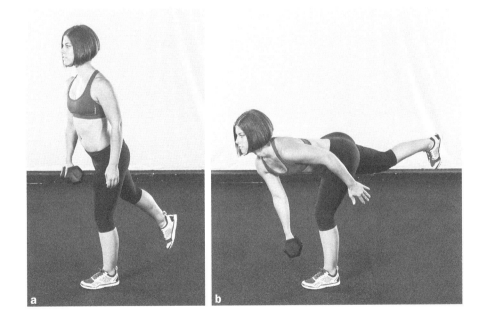

One-Leg 45-Degree Cable Romanian Deadlift

Setup

This exercise is performed exactly like the one-leg one-arm Romanian deadlift with a dumbbell, except that it uses a cable column on the low setting to change the vector of resistance to a 45-degree angle. Stand tall on one leg, holding the cable handle in your opposite hand (see figure a).

Action

Keeping your back and arm straight, hinge at your hip and bend forward toward the floor; keep your weight-bearing knee bent at a 15- to 20-degree angle. As you hinge forward, allow your non-weight-bearing leg to elevate so that it remains in a straight line with your torso (see figure b). Once your torso and non-weight-bearing leg are at about a 45-degree angle to the floor, reverse the motion by driving your hips forward toward the cable to stand tall again, thus completing the rep. Perform all repetitions on one side before switching sides.

Coaching Tips

- Do not allow your lower back to round out as you hinge your hips and lower your torso.
- At the bottom position (when your torso is roughly at a 45-degree angle to the ground), keep your hips and shoulders flat and do not allow them to rotate.
- At the bottom position, the foot of your non-weight bearing leg should point at the floor.
- The range of motion is shorter when using the cable than when using the dumbbell because the force you're working against is at a higher point. Whereas the dumbbell pulls you toward the floor, the cable pulls you toward its anchor point at a 45-degree angle.

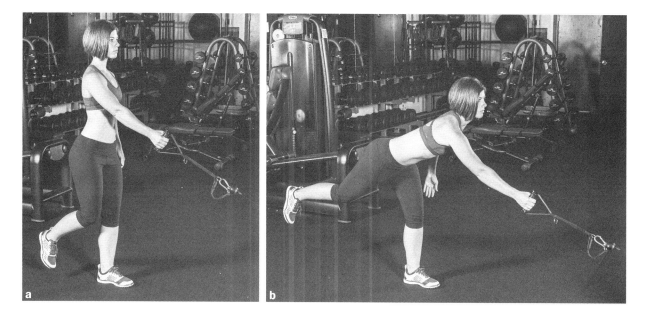

One-Leg One-Arm Angled Barbell Romanian Deadlift

Setup

Place one end of a barbell in a corner or inside a landmine device. Stand at the non-corner end of the barbell with the corner or landmine device to your right side. Hold onto the top of the weighted end of the barbell (above where the weight plates are loaded) with your right hand in front of your right thigh while standing on your left leg (see figure a).

Action

Keeping your back and arm straight, hinge at your left hip and bend forward toward the floor, keeping your left knee bent at roughly a 15- to 20-degree angle. As you hinge, allow your non- weight-bearing leg to elevate so that it remains in a fairly straight line with your torso (see figure b). Once your torso becomes roughly parallel with the ground, reverse the motion by driving your hips forward and lifting the barbell off of the ground. Perform all repetitions on one side before standing on the other side of the barbell to switch legs.

Coaching Tips

- At the bottom position (when your torso is roughly parallel to the ground), keep your hips and shoulders flat and do not allow them to rotate.
- Unlike when using the dumbbell or the cable, in this exercise you can lean slightly into the barbell by pushing into it as you elevate it, thus adding a small hip abduction element to the exercise.

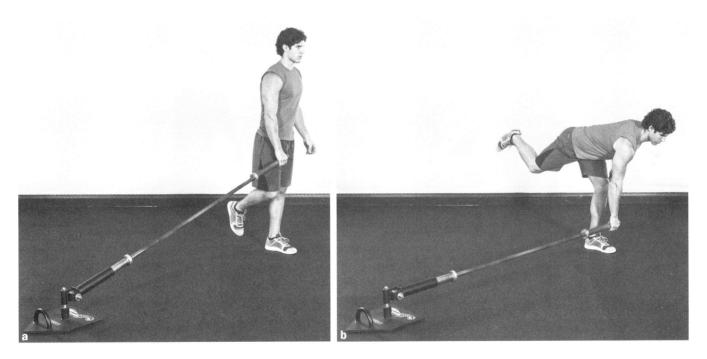

Lateral Lunge With Cross-Body Reach

Setup

Stand tall with your feet hip-width apart while holding a dumbbell in your left hand by your side (see figure *a*).

Action

Step out laterally with your right leg, allowing your right knee to bend 20 degrees. Simultaneously shift your weight to your right leg as you reach your left arm in front of your right shin or ankle, hinging at your hip joint without rounding your back as you lean forward and reach across your body (see figure *b*). Once your torso is roughly parallel to the ground, explode out of this position and return to the starting position. Perform all reps on one side before switching hands with the dumbbell and stepping with the other leg.

Coaching Tips

- Your trailing leg should be straight each time you step laterally and drop into the lunge.
- Keep both feet pointed straight ahead on each rep.
- Do not over-rotate your shoulders to perform the cross-reach. Your shoulders should rotate just enough to bring the dumbbell in front of your shin or ankle on the side to which you stepped.

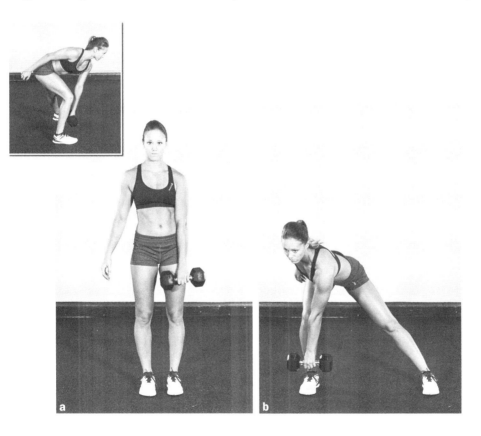

One-Leg Elevated Offset Reverse Lunge

Setup

Stand on the flat side of an Olympic-style weight plate or on an aerobic step platform with your feet hip-width apart. Hold a dumbbell in your right hand at your shoulder (see figure a).

Action

Step your right leg backward and place the ball of that foot on the floor while bending both knees and lowering your body into a lunge (see figure b). Once your back knee lightly touches the floor, reverse the motion by stepping back onto the platform. Perform all reps on the same leg before switching sides with the dumbbell and stepping back with your left leg.

Coaching Tips

- Do not allow your shoulders to rotate or tilt toward the heavier side; keep your shoulders even throughout.
- Use a platform low enough that you can touch your back knee to the floor on each repetition.
- If your lower-body strength demands you use a weight-load that's greater than what you're able to hold with one hand, this exercise can also be done holding two unevenly loaded dumbbells at your hips, with the heaviest of the two dumbbells held on the opposite side of the working leg. So, if you're stepping back with your right leg, you would hold the heavier dumbbell on your right side.
- If you're using two unevenly loaded dumbbells, there should be approximately a 35 to 65 light dumbbell to heavy dumbbell loading distribution. So, the heavier of the two dumbbells makes up roughly 65 percent of the total weight you're holding.

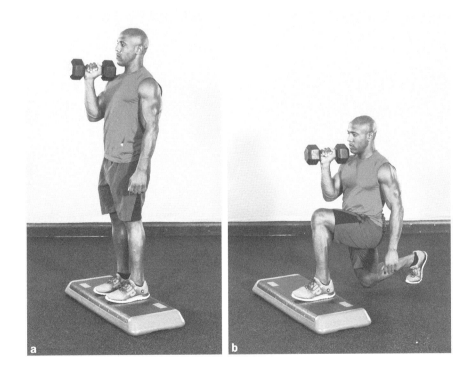

One-Leg Offset Traveling Lunge

Setup

Stand tall with your feet hip-width apart while holding a dumbbell in in your right hand at your shoulder (see figure *a*).

Action

Lunge forward with your left leg, simultaneously bending your knees (see figure *b*). Once your back knee lightly touches the floor, stand back up tall while bringing your rear leg forward to meet your front leg and repeat this action by lunging forward again with your left leg (see figures *c* and *d*). Perform all reps on the same leg while traveling down the room before switching sides.

Coaching Tips

- Do not allow your shoulders to rotate or tilt toward the heavier side; keep your shoulders even throughout.
- Do not step so far out on each lunge that you're unable to perform the exercise in a smooth, controlled fashion.
- If your lower-body strength demands you use a weight-load that's greater than what you're able to hold with one hand, this exercise can also be done holding two unevenly loaded dumbbells at your hips, with the heaviest of the two dumbbells held on the opposite side of the working leg. So, if you're stepping back with your right leg, you'd hold the heavier dumbbell on your left side.
- If you're using two unevenly loaded dumbbells, there should be approximately a 35 to 65 light dumbbell to heavy dumbbell loading distribution. So, the heavier of the two dumbbells makes up roughly 65 percent of the total weight you're holding.

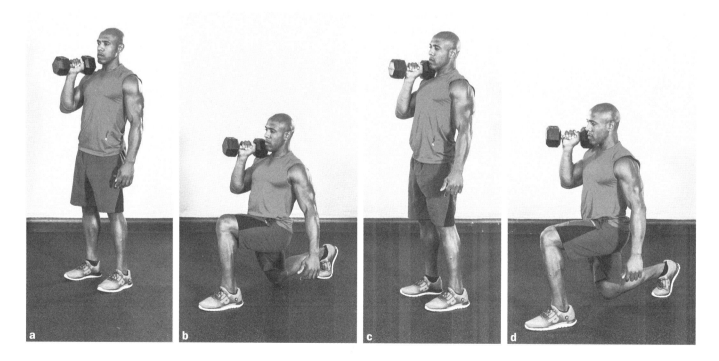

Angled Barbell Cross-Shoulder Reverse Lunge

Setup

Place one end of a barbell in a corner or inside a landmine device. With the barbell in front of you, stand tall with your feet hip-width apart. Hold onto the end of the barbell with both hands, stacked one over the other, and with the bar against the front of your right shoulder (see figure a).

Action

Step backward with your right foot and drop your body into a reverse lunge so that your back knee lightly touches the floor (see figure b). Reverse the movement by coming out of the lunge and bringing your right foot forward so that you are back in the starting position. Perform all reps on the same side before switching sides and placing the barbell in front of your other shoulder.

Coaching Tips

- Keep your hands against your chest while holding the end of the barbell throughout.
- You can also perform this exercise in an alternating fashion by shifting the barbell over to the same side of the leg you're stepping back with on each rep.

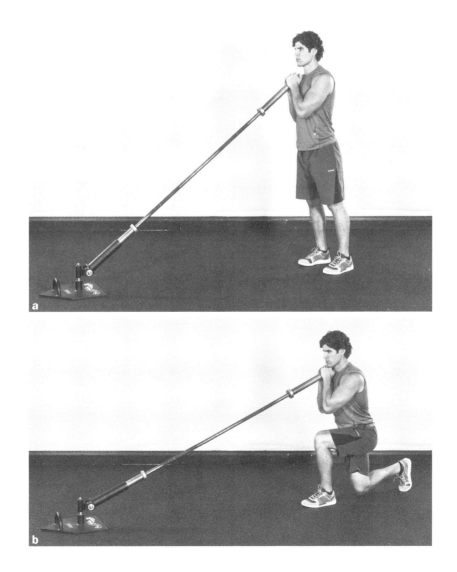

Compound Exercises

These lower-body exercises integrate efforts by the glutes, hamstrings, quadriceps, calves, and lower-back musculature to perform the movement.

Barbell Romanian Deadlift

Setup

Standing tall with your feet hip-width apart, hold a barbell in front of your thighs with your arms straight; grip the bar just outside your hips (see figure a).

Action

Keeping your back straight, hinge at your hips and bend forward toward the floor; keep your knees bent at a 15- to 20-degree angle (see figure b). Once your torso is roughly parallel to the floor, drive your hips forward toward the barbell, reversing the previous motion to stand tall again and thus complete the rep.

Coaching Tips

- As you hinge forward, drive your hips backward and do not allow your back to round out.
- Lift the bar by extending your hips, not by overextending at your lower back.
- Keep the barbell close to you throughout; it should touch your shins at the bottom and track against the fronts of your legs as you perform each repetition.

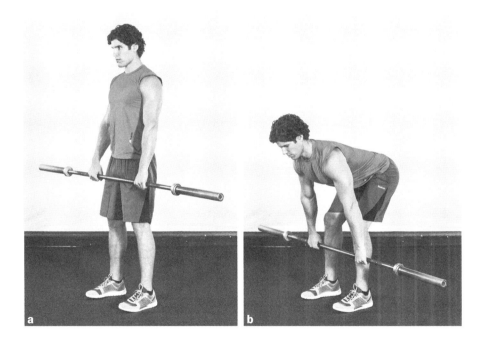

Barbell Sumo Deadlift

Setup

Stand in front of a barbell with your feet about 1 foot (0.3 m) farther than shoulder-width and turned out roughly 45 degrees. Keeping your back straight and maintaining an arch in your lower back, hinge at your hips and bend your knees. Lower your torso to about a 45-degree angle and grab the bar with your hands at shoulder width (see figure a).

Action

Keeping your back straight, drive your hips forward toward the barbell and lift it off of the ground until your legs straighten (see figure b). Reverse the motion and slowly lower the barbell back to the floor to complete the rep.

Coaching Tips

- As you hinge your torso forward and bend your knees, drive your hips backward and do not allow your back to round out.
- Lift the bar by extending your hips, not by overextending at your lower back.
- Keep the barbell close to you throughout; it should touch your shins at the bottom.
- You can also use a mixed grip, with one hand in an overhand position and the other in an underhand position, which is especially helpful when lifting heavier loads.

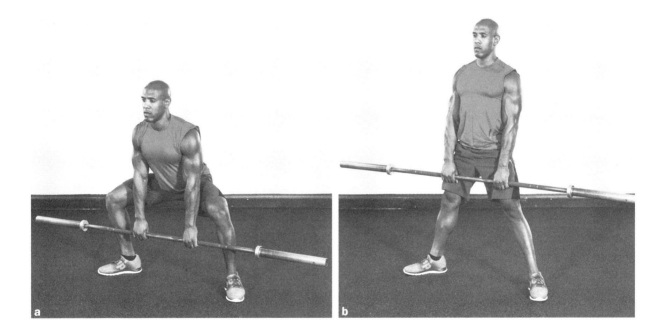

Barbell Hybrid Deadlift

Setup

This exercise combines the Romanian and sumo deadlifts. Stand in front of a barbell with your feet slightly farther than shoulder-width apart and turned out 15 degrees. Keeping your back straight and maintaining an arch in your lower back, hinge at your hips and bend your knees. Lower your torso to about a 45-degree angle and grab the bar with your hands at shoulder width (see figure a).

Action

Keeping your back straight, drive your hips forward toward the barbell and lift it off of the ground while straightening your legs (see figure b). Reverse the motion and slowly lower the barbell back to the floor to complete the rep.

Coaching Tips

- As you hinge forward, drive your hips backward and do not allow your back to round out.
- Lift the bar by extending your hips, not by overextending at your lower back.
- Keep the barbell close to you throughout; it should touch your shins and track against the fronts of your legs as you perform each repetition.
- Your arms should be close to touching the insides of your legs at the bottom of each lift.

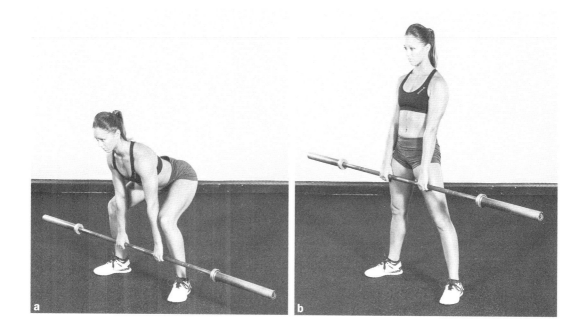

Barbell Back Squat

Setup

Place a barbell across your shoulders (not on your neck) and stand with your feet just farther than shoulder-width apart and your toes turned out 10 to 15 degrees (see figure *a*).

Action

Bend at your knees and hips and lower your body toward the floor; go as low as you can without losing the arch in your lower back (see figure *b*). Once you've gone as deep as you can, reverse the motion and stand up.

Coaching Tips

- Your heels should not lift off of the ground, and your lower back should not lose its arch.
- Do not allow your knees to drop in toward the midline of your body; keep your knees tracking in the same direction as your toes.
- You may have to adjust your stance a bit to find the position that best suits you.

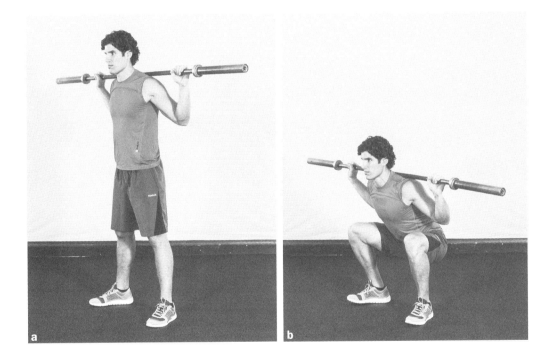

Barbell Squat and Calf Raise

Setup

This exercise is performed using the same mechanics as the barbell back squat; it differs only in how you finish at the top of each rep. Place a barbell across your shoulders (not on your neck) and stand with your feet just farther than shoulder-width apart and your toes turned out 10 to 15 degrees (see figure a).

Action

Bend at your knees and hips and lower your body toward the floor; go as low as you can without losing the arch in your lower back (see figure b). Once you've gone as deep as you can, quickly reverse the motion and stand up. At the top of reach rep, perform a calf raise by pushing your toes into the ground and lifting your heels as high as you can, thus ending up on the balls of your feet (see figure c). Slowly lower yourself by first allowing your heels to touch the floor and then returning to the squat position to complete the rep.

Coaching Tips

- Your heels should not lift off of the ground when you drop into the squat position; lift them only at the top of each rep when you're standing tall.
- Perform the exercise in one smooth action, up and down.
- Do not allow your knees to drop in toward the midline of your body; keep your knees tracking in the same direction as your toes.
- You may have to adjust your stance a bit to find the position that best suits you.

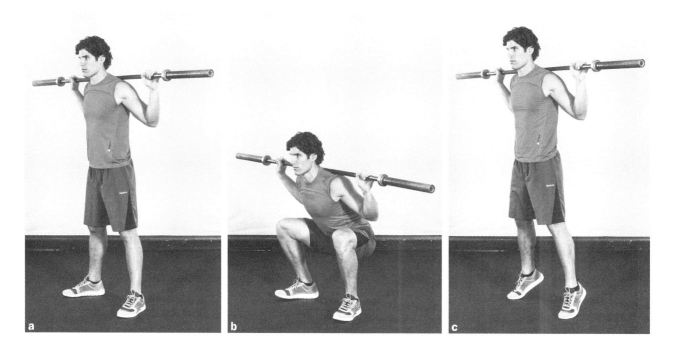

Barbell Front Squat

Setup

The front squat is performed using the same mechanics as the back squat; the only difference involves the bar placement. Rest an Olympic-type barbell on the top of your chest and stand with your feet just farther than shoulder-width apart and your toes turned out 10 to 15 degrees (see figure a). Stay tall and lift your chest to create a rack for the bar instead of trying to hold it up with only your arms.

Action

Bend at your knees and hips and lower your body toward the floor as far as you can go without losing the arch in your lower back (see figure b). Once you've gone as deep as you can control, reverse the motion by extending your legs and returning to the standing position to complete the rep.

Coaching Tips

- As you drop into the squat, keep your elbows lifted high toward the sky.
- Your heels should not lift off of the ground, and your lower back should not lose its arch.
- Keep your knees wide and tracking in the same direction as your toes; do not allow your knees to drop in toward the midline of your body.

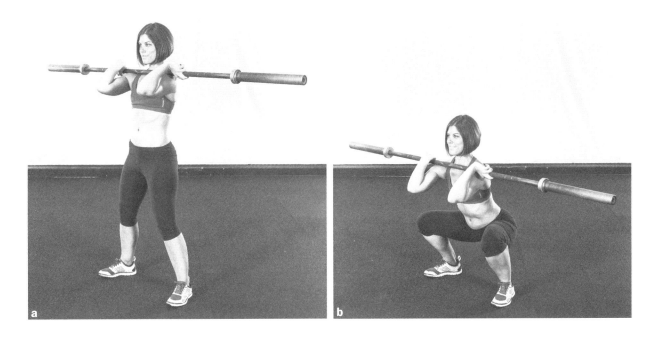

Barbell Good Morning

Setup

Stand tall with your feet hip-width apart and place a barbell across your shoulders behind your head, grabbing the barbell outside your shoulders (see figure a).

Action

Keeping your back straight, hinge at your hips and bend forward toward the floor; keep your knees bent at roughly a 15- to 20-degree angle (see figure b). As you hinge forward, drive your hips backward. Once your torso is roughly parallel to the floor, drive your hips forward toward the barbell, reversing the previous motion to stand tall again and complete the rep.

Coaching Tips

- Do not allow your back to round out.
- Lift the bar by extending your hips, not by overextending at your lower back.
- Except for holding the barbell in a different position, this exercise uses essentially the same motion as the Romanian deadlift. Therefore, it's contradictory to categorize it as an isolation exercise while categorizing the Romanian deadlift as a compound exercise.

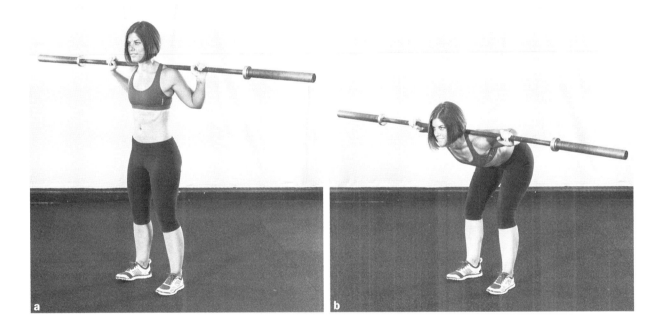

Elevated Barbell Reverse Lunge

Setup

Stand on the flat side of an Olympic-type weight plate or on an aerobic step platform (shown here) with your feet hip-width apart. Hold a barbell across your shoulders behind your head, grabbing the barbell outside your shoulders (see figure *a*).

Action

Step your right leg backward, placing the ball of your foot on the floor while bending both knees and lowering your body into a lunge (see figure *b*). Once your back knee lightly touches the floor, reverse the motion by stepping back up to the platform. Perform the same action with the other leg.

Coaching Tips

- When performing this exercise, as your knees bend, you can hinge at your hips and lean your torso forward while keeping your back straight to better recruit your glute musculature and make the exercise more knee friendly.

- Use a platform low enough that you can touch your back knee to the floor on each repetition.

- If a reduction in range is needed, you can perform this exercise without standing on top of a platform.

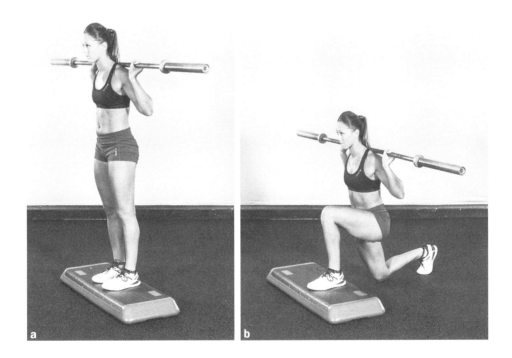

Trap-Bar Squat

Setup

To perform this exercise, you need a specially designed bar commonly known as a trap bar. Stand inside the bar with your hands holding onto the handles and your feet roughly shoulder-width apart (see figure a).

Action

Keep your feet flat and your knees in line with your toes and maintain a strong inward arch in your lower back while lowering into a squatting position (see figure b). Stand up tall so that your hands end up directly outside of your hips. Slowly lower back into the squat until the weight plates you have loaded on the bar touch the floor.

Coaching Tips

- At the bottom position, your heels should not lift off of the ground and your lower back should not lose its arch.
- Do not allow your knees to drop in toward the midline of your body; keep your knees tracking in the same direction as your toes.
- Although some people refer to this exercise as a deadlift rather than a squat, the torso and hip position more closely resemble those of a barbell squat than of a barbell deadlift. Having said that, the exercise can also be performed with slightly less knee bend and a more forward torso position, thus resembling the deadlift; that version is what I refer to as a trap-bar deadlift.

Goblet Squat

Setup

The goblet squat is performed using the same mechanics as the back squat; the only difference is that in this case you hold a dumbbell with both hands in front of your chest. With both hands on one end of a dumbbell, place the dumbbell against the top of your chest with your elbows clamped down on the bottom end of the dumbbell. Stand with your feet just farther than shoulder-width apart and your toes turned out 10 to 15 degrees (see figure a).

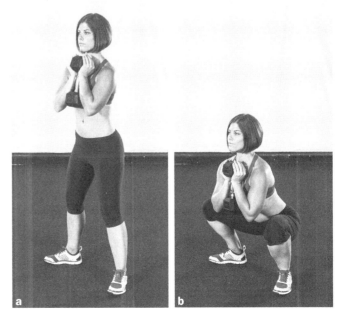

Action

Bend at your knees and hips and lower your body toward the floor as low as you can without losing the arch in your lower back (see figure b). Once you've gone as deep as you can control in the squat, reverse the motion by extending your legs and returning to the standing position to complete the rep.

Coaching Tips

- Your heels should not lift off of the ground, and your lower back should not lose its arch.
- Keep your knees wide and tracking in the same direction as your toes; do not allow your knees to drop in toward the midline of your body.
- You can also perform a body-weight squat by interlacing your fingers behind your head.

Machine Leg Press

Setup

To perform this exercise, you'll need to use the machine that's commonly known as the leg press machine. Sit upright and place your feet flat around the middle of the platform at roughly shoulders width apart (see figure a).

Action

Bend at your knees and hips as far as you can while keeping your feet flat on the platform and maintaining your starting alignment (see figure b). Once you've gone as deep as you can control, reverse the motion by extending your legs and finishing each rep without locking out your knees.

Coaching Tips

- Keep your knees wide and tracking in the same direction as your toes. Do not allow your knees to drop in toward the midline of your body.
- Adjust the foot width to best fit your body.
- You can change the muscular focus of this exercise by adjusting your foot placement on the platform.
- A higher foot placement stresses the glutes and hamstrings more, whereas a lower foot placement tends to place more stress on the quadriceps.

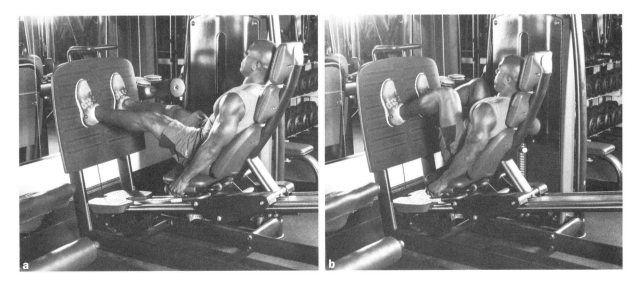

One-Leg Knee-Tap Squat

Setup

Stand in front of a pad that is 2 to 3 inches (about 8 to 13 cm) thick, a small stack of weight plates with a mat on top, or a workout step. Stand on your left leg and lift the right foot off the floor with the knee bent and slightly behind your left leg. Your hands are outstretched in front of you to serve as a counterbalance (see figure a).

Action

Slowly lower yourself toward the floor by bending your weight-bearing knee and sitting back at your hips until you lightly tap your back knee on the object (see figure b). Reverse the motion and stand up again. Perform all reps on the same side before switching sides.

Coaching Tips

- Do not allow your back (non-weight-bearing) foot to touch the floor.
- You can also perform the exercise while holding a dumbbell at each shoulder.

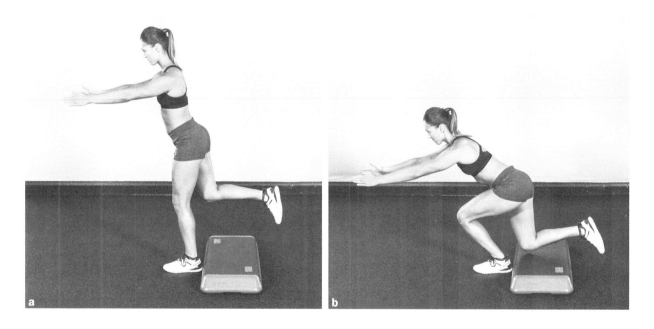

Bulgarian Split Squat

Setup

Stand tall while holding a dumbbell in each hand by your sides. Assume a split-squat stance by placing your left foot on top of a bench or chair behind you (see figure a).

Action

Lower your body toward the floor without allowing your back knee to rest on the floor (see figure b). As you lower your body, keep your back straight and lean your torso forward at about a 45-degree angle. Drive your heel into the ground to raise your body to the starting position, thus completing the rep. Perform all reps on one side before switching to the other leg.

Coaching Tips

- At the bottom of each rep, the dumbbells should be on each side of your front foot.
- Keep your weight on your front foot throughout the exercise.
- Your front leg should be far enough in front of the bench that your shin can stay fairly vertical as you drop into each rep.
- You can also perform this exercise using only body weight by placing your hands on your hips.

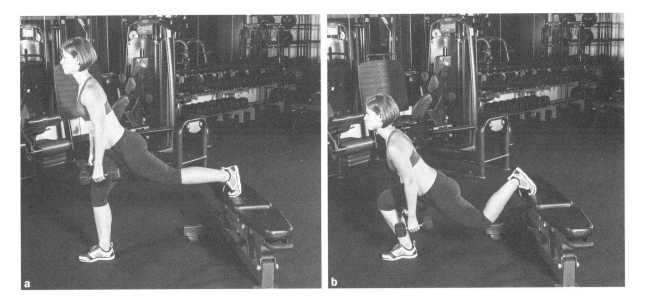

Bulgarian Split Squat and Romanian Deadlift Combination

Setup

Stand tall while holding a dumbbell in each hand by your sides. Assume a split-squat stance by placing your left foot on top of a bench or chair behind you (see figure a).

Action

Lower your body toward the floor without allowing your back knee to rest on the floor. As you lower your body, keep your back straight and lean your torso forward at about a 45-degree angle (see figure b). Drive your heel into the ground to raise your body to the starting position (see figure c) Then, keeping your back straight, hinge at your hips and bend forward toward the floor; keep your front knee bent at roughly a 15- to 20-degree angle. Once your torso is roughly parallel to the floor (see figure d), reverse the previous motion to stand tall again and complete the rep. Perform all repetitions on the same side before switching sides.

Coaching Tips

- Keep your weight on your front foot throughout the exercise.
- Do not allow your back to round out at any point.

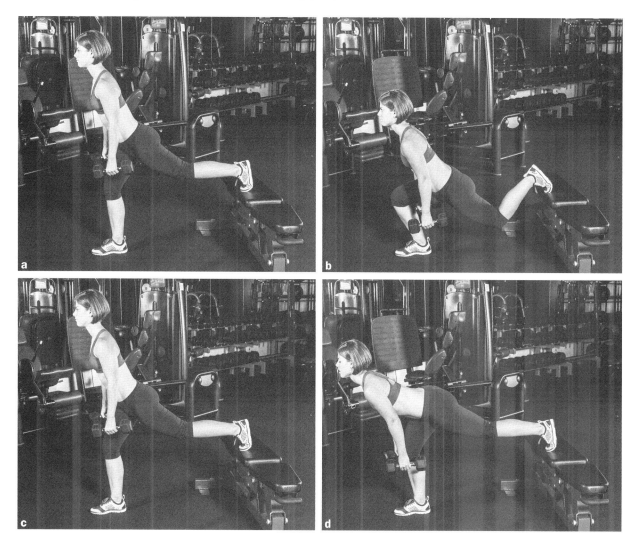

Dumbbell Reverse Lunge

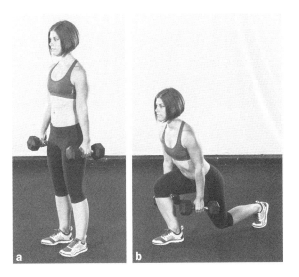

Setup

Stand with your feet hip-width apart while holding a dumbbell in each hand at your sides (see figure *a*).

Action

Step your left leg backward, placing the ball of your foot on the floor while bending both your knees and lowering your body into a lunge. As your knees bend, hinge forward at your hips, allowing the bottom of your ribs to touch the top of your front thigh (see figure *b*). Once your back knee lightly touches the floor, reverse the motion by stepping back up and returning to the starting position. Perform the same motion by stepping back with your other leg.

Coaching Tips

- Keep your back straight as you hinge at your hips and lean your torso forward to better recruit the glute musculature and make the exercise more knee friendly.
- At the bottom of each lunge, the dumbbells should end up at each side of your front foot due to the forward torso lean.
- You can also perform this exercise using only body weight by placing your hands on your hips.

Elevated Dumbbell Reverse Lunge

Setup

Stand on the flat side of an Olympic-type weight plate or on a workout step with your feet hip-width apart while holding a dumbbell in each hand at your sides (see figure *a*).

Action

Step your right leg backward, placing the ball of your foot on the floor while bending both your knees and lowering your body into a lunge (see figure *b*). As your knees bend, hinge forward at your hips, allowing your ribs to touch the top of your front thigh. Once your back knee lightly touches the floor, reverse the motion by stepping back up to the platform. Perform the same action with your other leg.

Coaching Tips

- When performing this exercise, as your knees bend, you can also hinge at your hips and lean your torso slightly forward while keeping your back straight to better recruit the glute musculature and make the exercise more knee friendly.
- Use a platform low enough that you can touch your back knee to the floor on each repetition.
- If a reduction in range is needed, you can perform this exercise with standing on top of a platform.
- At the bottom of each lunge, the dumbbells end up at each side of your front foot due to the forward torso lean.
- You can also perform this exercise using only body weight by placing your hands on your hips.

Dumbbell Fighter's Lunge

Setup

This exercise got its name because it resembles the motion of a fighter throwing a knee strike. Stand tall with your feet hip-width apart while holding a dumbbell in each hand. The dumbbell in your left hand should be outside of your left hip, and the dumbbell in your right hand should be in front of your right thigh (see figure *a*).

Action

Perform a reverse lunge by stepping backward with your right leg, allowing your right knee to gently touch the ground and your torso to lean slightly forward (see figure *b*). As you return to the standing position, allow your right thigh to meet the center handle of the dumbbell. With the dumbbell against the middle of your right thigh, flex your hip and raise your knee just above a 90-degree angle with the floor, as if throwing a knee strike (see figure *c*). Step backward again with your right leg and repeat. Perform all reps on one side before switching to the other side.

Coaching Tips

- As your rear leg comes forward to meet the dumbbell, the dumbbell should be at about midthigh level as you flex your hip.
- As you flex your hip, lift your knee just above your hip joint before returning your leg back for the next rep.
- Lift the dumbbell with your hip—not your arm.
- Your thigh should meet the dumbbell gently rather than smashing into it and making the exercise uncomfortable to perform.

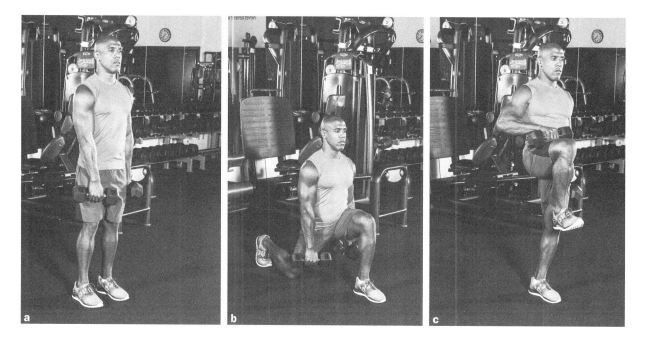

Traveling Lunge

Setup

Stand tall with your feet hip-width apart while holding a dumbbell in each hand at your sides (see figure *a*).

Action

Take a large step forward and drop your body so that your back knee lightly touches the floor while allowing your torso to lean slightly forward (see figure *b*). Stand back up tall while bringing your rear leg forward to meet your front leg (see figure *c*) and step forward with the opposite leg—the one that was behind you on the last rep (see figure *d*). Repeat as you travel down the room.

Coaching Tips

- Keep your back straight as you hinge at your hips and lean your torso forward to better recruit the glute musculature and make the exercise more knee friendly.
- At the bottom of each lunge, the dumbbells end up at each side of your front foot due to the forward torso lean.
- Do not step so far out on each lunge that you're unable to perform this exercise in a smooth, controlled fashion.
- You can also perform this exercise using only body weight by placing your hands on your hips.

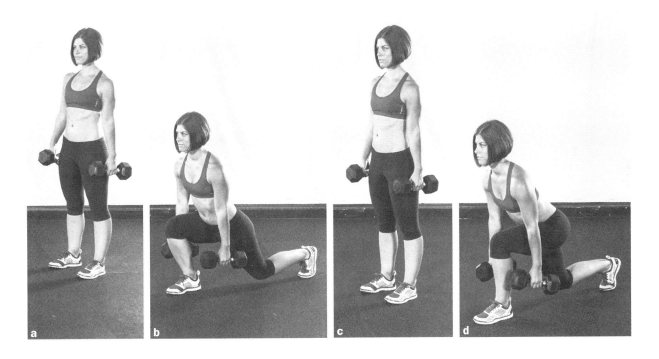

Dumbbell Anterior Lunge

Setup

Stand tall while holding a dumbbell in each hand by your sides with your feet hip-width apart (see figure a).

Action

Step forward with one leg, keeping your front knee bent 15 to 20 degrees and your back knee straight or slightly bent. As your front foot hits the ground, lean forward by hinging at your hips and allowing your rear heel to come off of the ground (see figure b). Your torso should be no lower than parallel to the floor and your back should be straight. Reverse the motion by stepping backward so that your feet are together again and you return to an upright position. Now perform the same motion, stepping forward with the other leg.

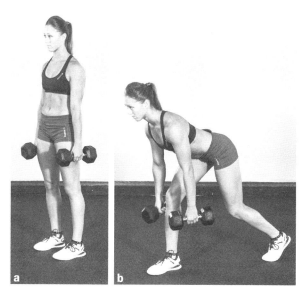

Coaching Tips

- Do not let the dumbbells touch the floor at any point.
- Do not allow your back to round out at the bottom of each lunge.
- Establish good rhythm and timing by performing the step and the hip hinge simultaneously and by reversing the motion in the same smooth, coordinated manner.

Bench Step-Up

Setup

Stand with your feet hip-width apart while facing a weight bench and holding a dumbbell in each hand by your hips. Place your right foot on top of the bench (see figure a).

Action

Step up by straightening your right knee (see figure b). Once you're on top of the bench, allow your left foot to gently contact the bench to help maintain your balance, then reverse the motion by stepping down with your left foot. Bring your right foot down to the floor and place your left leg on top of the bench to repeat with the other leg. Essentially, you're stepping up and stepping down with the same leg, then switching the working leg (i.e., the stepping leg) on the ground—not when you're on top of the bench.

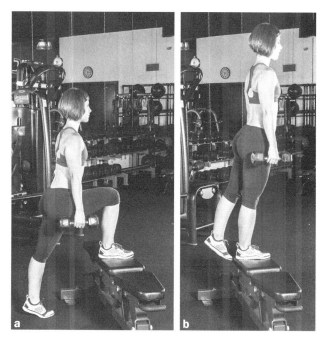

Coaching Tips

- Lean your torso slightly forward throughout the exercise to keep most of your weight on the front leg and make the exercise more knee friendly.
- Perform the exercise in a smooth, controlled fashion; avoid jerking your torso forward to complete each rep.
- You can also perform this exercise using only body weight by placing your hands on your hips.

Weight-Sled Push

Setup

You'll need a weight sled with upright handles to perform this exercise. Stand with a sled in front of you and your feet in a split stance. Hold the sled poles with your hands toward the top and position your body at about a 45-degree angle (see figure *a*).

Action

Drive your legs into the ground and push the sled by taking long strides (see figures *b* and *c*).

Coaching Tips

- Do not round your back or allow your head to sag toward the ground at any time; keep your torso and arms straight throughout.
- Do not run with the sled or take short, choppy steps. Use a weight heavy enough to force you to lean in and move in a deliberate manner. Take long strides, pushing hard from your legs and driving your feet diagonally into the ground with each step.

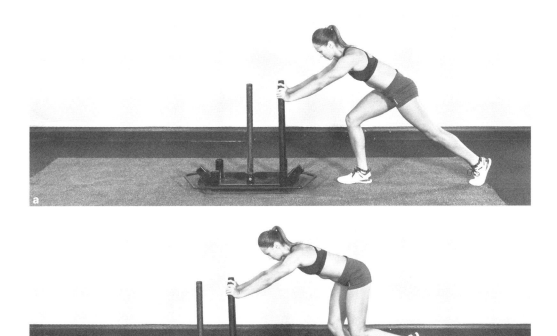

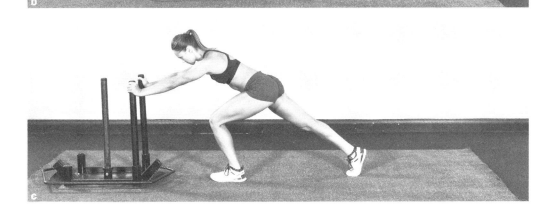

Weight-Sled Forward Pull

Setup

You'll need a weight sled with strap handles to perform this exercise. Stand with the sled about 2 yards behind you while holding the strap handles in each of your hands by your hips. Position your body at about a 45-degree angle with one leg in front of the other and keep your arms in line with your torso (see figure a).

Action

Drive your legs into the ground and move forward by stepping one leg after the other and taking long strides (see figures b and c).

Coaching Tips

- Do not round your back or allow your head to sag toward the ground at any time; keep your torso and arms straight throughout.

- Do not allow your arms to get pulled behind your torso; your arms should remain against your sides throughout.

- Do not run with the sled or take short, choppy steps. Use a weight heavy enough to force you to lean in and move in a deliberate manner. Take long strides, pushing hard from your legs and driving your feet diagonally into the ground with each step.

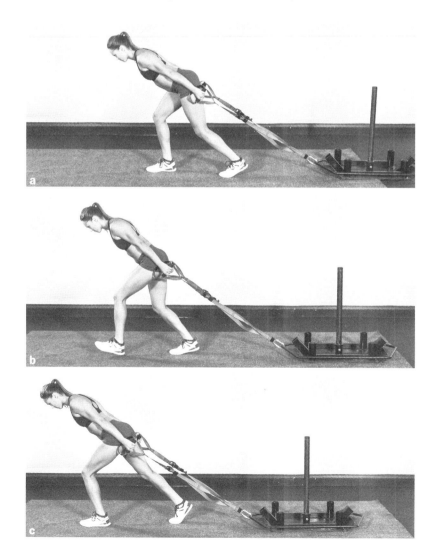

Weight-Sled Backward Pull

Setup

You'll need a weight sled with strap handles to perform this exercise. Stand with the sled about 2 yards in front of you while holding the strap handles in your hands with your arms straight at hip height. Assume a partial squat position so your thighs are at roughly a 45-degree angle to the floor (see figure *a*).

Action

Drive your legs into the ground and move backward by stepping one leg after the other (see figure *b*).

Coaching Tips

- Do not round your upper back at any time; keep your torso and arms straight throughout.
- Use a weight load that's neither light enough for you to run with nor heavy enough that you have to lean your body backward at a 45-degree angle. Instead, find a load at which you can move the sled in a smooth, deliberate manner with each step.

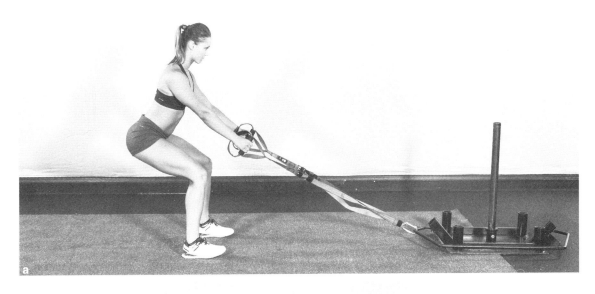

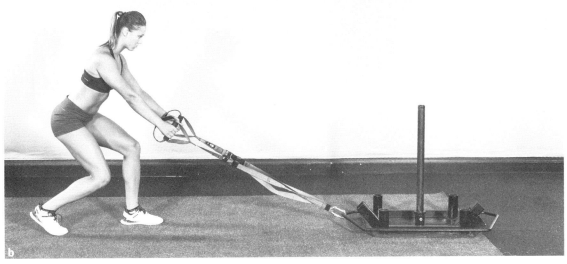

Weight-Sled Lateral Pull

Setup

You'll need a weight sled with strap handles to perform this exercise. With your feet hip-width apart, stand in an athletic position perpendicular to the sled, which is positioned about 2 yards to your left. With your knees slightly bent, hold both strap handles in your left hand with your left arm extended toward the sled at about belly-button height. Shift your weight onto your left leg by picking your right foot slightly off the ground (see figure a).

Action

Drive your left leg into the ground and move laterally to your right by stepping your right leg out to your side while simultaneously shifting your weight over to your right leg (see figure b). Then step your left leg back underneath your left hip to reset the starting position before performing the next rep (see figure c). Perform all reps moving in the same direction before turning around and moving toward your right.

Coaching Tips

- Keep your torso and arms straight throughout.

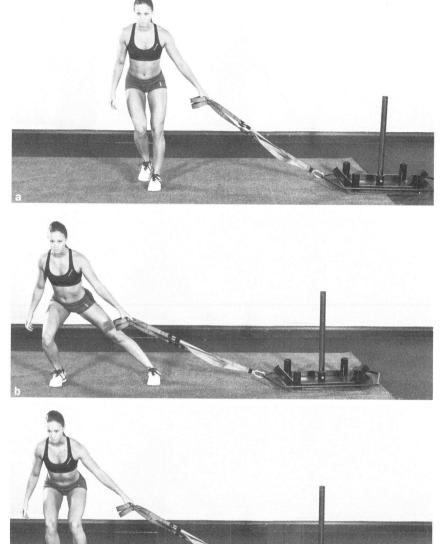

- Use a weight load that's not light enough for you to run laterally with it. Find a load with which you can maintain a consistent body angle while moving the sled in a smooth, deliberate manner with each step.

Isolation Exercises

These are single-joint movements that focus on individual muscle groups. These exercise applications consist primarily of classic bodybuilding exercises that target either the glutes, hamstrings, quadriceps, or calf musculature.

One-Leg Dumbbell Bench Hip Thrust

Setup
Sit on the floor with your shoulders elevated on a weight bench or chair and your head and shoulders resting on the bench. Position the left arm out to the side across the bench or on your left hip; with the right hand hold a dumbbell in front of your right hip. Position your legs so that your knees are bent about 90 degrees and your feet are directly below your knees. Keeping your right knee bent 90 degrees, lift your left knee above your hip and lift your hips so that your body makes a straight line from knee to nose (see figure a).

Action
Keeping your left leg lifted, lower your hips toward the floor until you either lightly contact the floor or can't go any deeper (see figure b). Drive your hips back up to the top position, thus completing the rep.

Coaching Tips
- Push through your heel on each repetition; do not lift the heel off of the ground at the top.
- Position the dumbbell over your hip in a manner that feels comfortable to you.
- Pause for one or two seconds at the top of each repetition.
- Extend from your hips, not your lower back.
- You can also perform this exercise using only body weight.

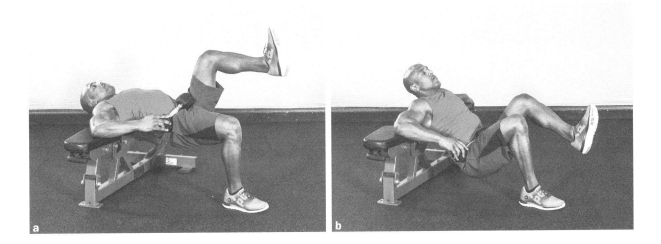

Hip Thrust Hamstring Curl Combo

Setup

Position between two weight benches. Your shoulders are elevated and your head and shoulders are resting on one bench. Open your arms to the sides with your palms facing up. Position your legs on top of another bench so that your knees are bent about 90 degrees and your ankles are flexed. Keep your toes up so that only your heels contact the bench (see figure a).

Action

Drive your hips up until your hips form a straight line with your torso (see figure b). Lower your hips toward the floor until you either lightly contact the floor or can't go any deeper, thus completing the rep.

Coaching Tips

- Pause for one or two seconds at the top of each repetition.
- Extend from your hips, not your lower back.
- You can add load to this exercise by holding a weighted bar across your hips, preferably one of the padded bars commonly used in group exercise classes.

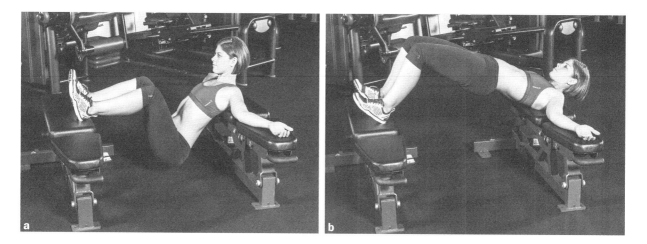

One-Leg Hip-Thrust Hamstring-Curl Combination

Setup

Position between two weight benches. Your shoulders are elevated on one bench with your shoulders resting on the bench. Open your arms to the sides with your palms facing up. Position your legs on top of another bench so that your knees are bent about 90 degrees and your ankles are flexed. Keep your toes up so that only your heels contact the bench. Keep your right knee bent 90 degrees and lift it above your hip (see figure a).

Action

Keeping your right leg lifted, drive your hips up until your hips form a straight line with your torso (see figure b). Lower your hips toward the floor until you either lightly contact the floor or can't go any deeper, thus completing the rep. Perform all reps on the same leg before switching sides.

Coaching Tips

- Pause for one or two seconds at the top of each repetition.
- Extend from your hips, not your lower back.

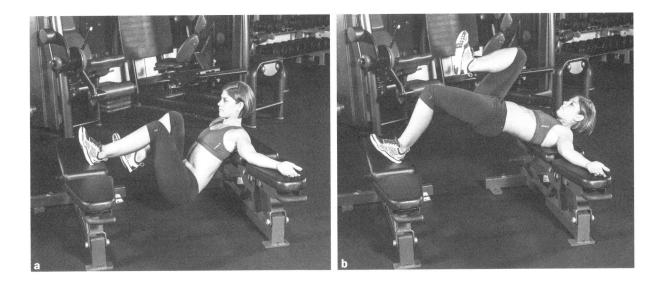

One-Leg Hip Lift

Setup

Lie on your back with your legs together, your knees bent 15 degrees, and your feet resting on top of a weight bench or chair. Raise one leg off of the bench or chair, flexing your hip and knee slightly beyond a 90-degree angle. Hold a weight plate at your shin of the flexed leg with both hands (see figure *a*).

Action

Holding your one leg flexed, raise your hips straight up as high as you can while keeping a slight bend in your knee (see figure *b*). Slowly reverse the motion, allowing your hips to lightly touch the floor. Complete all repetitions on one side before switching to the other leg.

Coaching Tips

- Do not overextend at your lower back at any time.
- Do not allow your hips to rotate during the exercise.
- You can also perform the exercise using only body weight.

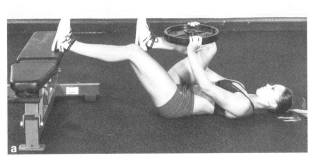
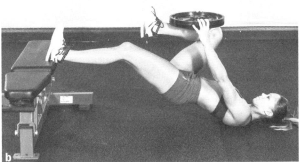

Lateral Mini-Band Shuffle

Setup

Place a mini-band around your legs just above your ankles. With your hands on your hips and your feet positioned hip-width apart, squat until your knees are bent roughly 45 degrees (see figure *a*).

Action

Take small lateral steps to your left, always maintaining tension in the band (see figures *b* and *c*), then sidestep back to your right in the same manner.

Coaching Tips

- Do not allow your torso to wobble from side to side; keep your spine and pelvis stable throughout the exercise.
- Do not allow your knees to give in to the band and drop toward the midline. Keep your knees in line with your feet throughout.

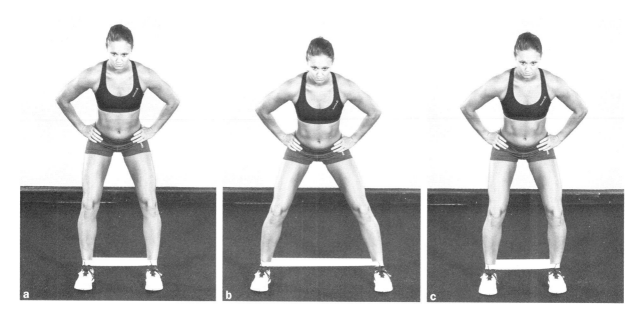

Low Lateral Mini-Band Shuffle

Setup

Place a mini-band around your legs just above your knees. With your hands on your hips and your feet positioned at hip-width apart, squat down until your thighs are just above parallel with the floor (see figure *a*).

Action

Take small steps laterally to your left, always maintaining tension on the band (see figures *b* and *c*). Then sidestep back to your right.

Coaching Tips

- Do not allow your torso to wobble from side to side. Keep your spine and pelvis stable throughout this exercise.
- Do not allow your knees to give into the band and drop toward the midline. Keep your knees in-line with your feet throughout.

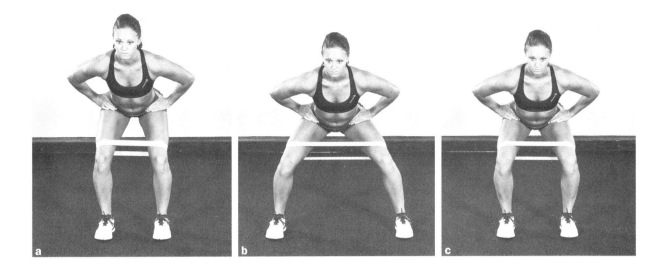

Supine Hip-Bridge March With Mini Band

Setup

Lie on your back with your legs hip-width apart, your knees slightly bent, and your feet resting on top of a weight bench or chair with a mini band around the tops of your feet. Raise your hips so that your torso forms a straight line (see figure a).

Action

Keep your hips elevated off of the ground so that your torso remains in a straight line. Flex one hip and bring your knee toward your head until your hip is bent just above a 90-degree angle (see figure b). Reverse the motion, placing your foot back on top of the bench or chair, then repeat with the other leg.

Coaching Tips

- Keep your ankles flexed by pulling your toes toward your nose throughout the exercise.
- Do not overextend at your lower back; hold your body in a straight line.
- Do not allow your hips to rotate at any time.

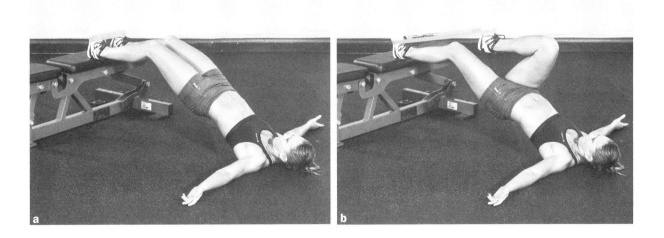

45-Degree Hip Extension

Setup

To perform this exercise, you will need a specially designed apparatus known as a 45-degree back extension. With your feet hip-width apart, rest your thighs against the pad, which is positioned below your hip bones, then cross your arms in front of your chest (see figure a).

Action

Hinge at your hips, keeping your back straight (see figure b). Reverse the motion by extending at your hips, without overarching your lower back, to pull yourself up so that your body forms a straight line from shoulders to hips to ankles.

Coaching Tips

- You can perform a unilateral version of this exercise by placing one leg over the ankle pad instead of underneath it.
- To make the exercise more difficult, hold a weight plate at your belly or chest.
- Although this exercise is commonly referred to as a 45-degree *back* extension, the motion should occur via *hip* extension—hence the name used here.

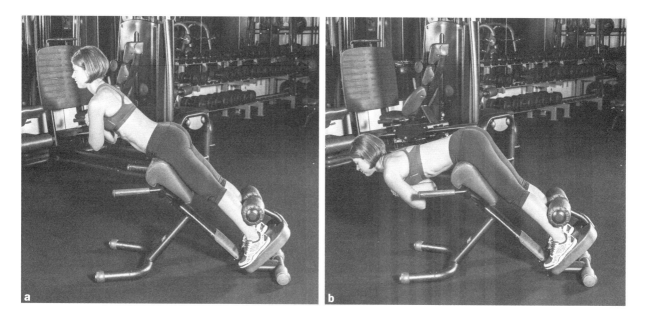

Nordic Hamstring Curl

Setup

This exercise requires either a partner or suitable gym equipment to securely lock your lower legs in place. Assume a tall kneeling position with your legs hip-width apart and your calves anchored (see figure a).

Action

Keeping your hips and back straight, slowly lower yourself toward the floor by extending at your knees (see figure b). At the point where you can no longer lower yourself in a controlled manner, allow your body to fall to the floor, using your hands to control your decent and landing in a position that resembles a kneeling push-up (see figure c). Use your hands to push back off of the floor and help you reverse the motion so that you return to the tall kneeling position (see figures d and e), thus completing the rep.

Coaching Tips

- Do not allow your hips to drift more than a few degrees behind you.
- Maintain a fairly straight line from your knees to your shoulders throughout.

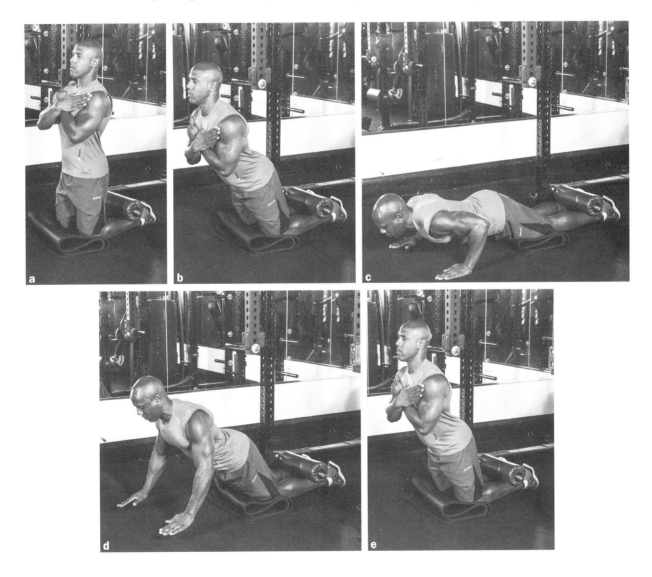

Stability-Ball Leg Curl

Setup

Lie on your back on the floor with your legs hip-width apart, your heels resting on top of a 22- to 26-inch (55- to 65-cm) stability ball, and your arms out to the sides for balance. Raise your hips off of the floor until your body forms a straight line (see figure *a*).

Action

Pull your heels toward your body while raising your hips toward the sky until your feet are underneath you (see figure *b*). Slowly reverse the motion and repeat without allowing your hips to rest on the floor.

Coaching Tips

- Do not overextend at your lower back at any time.
- Your body should form a straight line from your shoulders to your knees at the top of each rep.
- If your feet drift lower on the ball while performing a set, adjust foot position as needed.

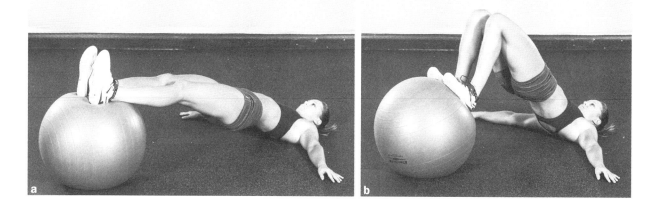

One-Leg Stability-Ball Leg Curl

Setup

Lie on your back on the floor with your legs hip-width apart, your heels resting on top of 22- to 26-inch (55- to 65-cm) stability ball, and your arms out to the sides for balance. Raise your hips off of the floor until your body forms a straight line, then raise one leg off of the ball, flexing your hip and knee slightly above a 90-degree angle (see figure *a*).

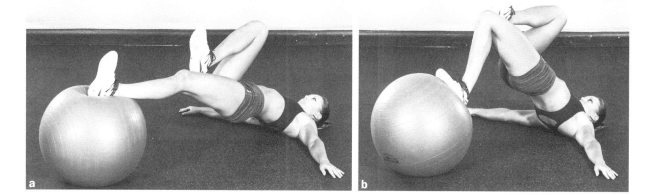

Action

Holding your one leg flexed, pull the ball toward your body with the heel of the foot that's on the ball while raising your hips toward the sky until your foot is underneath you (see figure *b*). Slowly reverse the motion and repeat without allowing your hips to rest on the floor. Complete all repetitions on one side before switching to the other leg.

Coaching Tips

- Do not overextend at your lower back at any time.
- Your body should form a straight line from your shoulders to your knee at the top of each rep.
- If your feet drift lower on the ball while performing a set, adjust foot position as needed.

Glute-Ham Roller Leg Curl

Setup

To perform this exercise, you'll need to use the glute ham roller device from Sorinex. Lie in a supine position on the floor with your legs hip-width apart and your heels resting in the center of the Sorinex glute-ham roller with your knees bent to 90-degrees and your arms out to the sides. Raise your hips up off the floor until your shoulders, hips, and knees form a straight line (see figure *a*).

Action

Slowly extend your legs until your knees are almost fully straight without allowing your glutes to rest on the floor (see figure *b*). Reverse the motion by pulling your heels toward your body while simultaneously raising your hips up toward the sky until your feet are once again underneath your hips.

Coaching Tips

- Be sure not to over-extend at your lower back at any time.
- You can also perform a single-leg version of this exercise, which is very challenging, by keeping one hip flexed to 90-degrees in the same manner as shown above in the one-leg stability-ball leg curl.

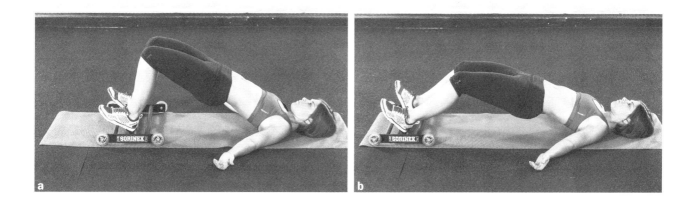

Machine Seated Hamstring Curl

Setup

To perform this exercise, use a seated hamstring-curl (aka leg-curl) machine. Sit tall and position the pad you'll be pushing at the bottom of your calves. Position your legs hip-width apart and the backs of your knees in contact with the seat pad (see figure *a*).

Action

Holding onto the handles, pull your calves against the pad by bending your knees to curl your legs underneath you as far as the machine will allow (see figure *b*). Slowly reverse the motion under control to complete the rep.

Coaching Tips

- Do not allow the portion of the weight stack that you're moving to rest on the other portion of the stack; rather, allow it to just gently touch the rest of the stack at the end of each rep.
- Perform each rep with deliberate control.

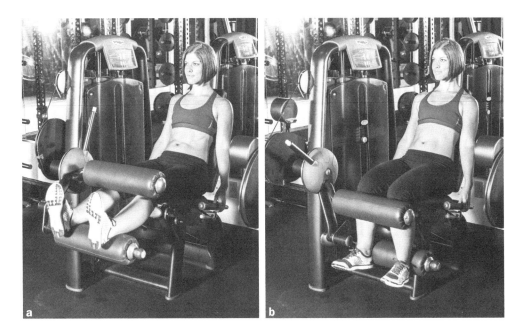

Machine Leg Extension

Setup

To perform this exercise, you'll need to use the machine that's commonly known as the leg extension machine. Sit tall with the pad you'll be extending your legs against at roughly low-shin level with your legs hip-width apart and the backs of your knees in contact with the seat pad (see figure *a*).

Action

Holding onto the handles, push your shins into the pad, and extend your legs keeping your ankles dorsiflexed until just before your knees are fully straight (see figure *b*). Slowly reverse the motion to complete one rep.

Coaching Tips

- Do not allow the weight stack you're moving to rest back on the rest of the stack. Just allow it to gently touch the rest of the stack at the end of each rep.
- Perform each rep using deliberate control.

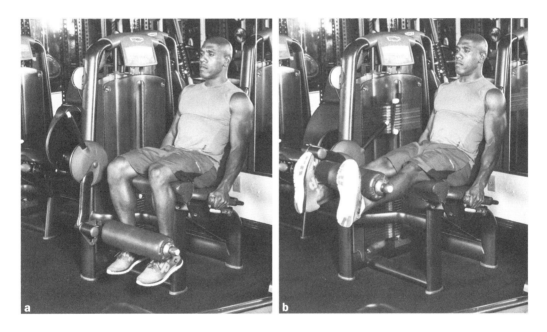

Barbell Calf Raise

Setup

Place small weight plates underneath the front portion of your feet. Stand tall with your feet hip-width apart and place a barbell across the tops of your shoulders behind your head (see figure *a*).

Action

Push your toes into the weight plates and lift your heels as high as you can off of the floor, thus ending up on the balls of your feet (see figure *b*). Slowly lower yourself until your heels touch the floor to complete the rep.

Coaching Tips

- Do not bounce; perform each rep with deliberate control.
- Control the lowering (eccentric) portion of each rep by allowing your heels to touch the floor gently—not to fully rest on the floor—until all reps have been completed.

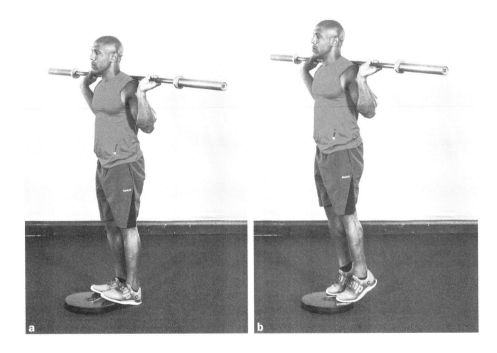

The next chapter introduces you to the Core 4 training formula and provides you with plenty of effective exercises for improving core strength and performance. It also clarifies some myths and misconceptions related to this popular topic.

7

Core

Just about everyone interested in training uses the term *core*, but most are unaware that it was coined some 30 years ago to describe the muscles that make up the center of the body and control the head, neck, ribs, spine, and pelvis (1). In other words, your core isn't just your abs and lower back; rather, it consists of all the muscles in your torso, including your chest, shoulders, lats, midback, glutes, lower back, abs, and obliques.

Of course, you can find plenty of work for your pecs and shoulders in chapter 4 (Upper Body—Pushing), for your lats and midback musculature in chapter 5 (Upper Body—Pulling), and for your glutes and low-back muscles in chapter 6 (Lower Body). Therefore, the exercises presented in this chapter focus on helping you maximize the strength of your abdominals and obliques; they also help you improve your rotational strength and power.

The Core 4

As the name implies, the Core 4 are four categories of exercise that strengthen your abdominals, obliques, lower back, and hips:

- Anterior (front) core exercises
- Lateral core exercises
- Rotational core exercises
- Posterior (back) core exercises

Your core-training routine must hit each of these categories in order to be comprehensive. A well-rounded routine covers the major types of movement performed by your torso and coordinates the muscles that make those movements possible.

The importance of approaching the core in this manner is highlighted by the persistent but false belief that squats and deadlifts provide sufficient stimulus for the anterior and lateral core musculature. Although research has shown that barbell back squats and conventional barbell deadlifts are great core exercises, the question to ask is this: Which aspect of the core?

The research demonstrates that exercises like squats and deadlifts effectively activate the posterior core muscles (i.e., back extensors, lumbar stabilizers). However, it does *not* show them to activate the *anterior* core muscles (i.e., abdominals, obliques) better than exercises focused on the anterior aspect of the core (2 and 3). Indeed, this reality should be obvious because squats and deadlifts drive the torso forward into flexion, which necessitates constant work by the back extensors to resist that force and maintain spinal alignment.

So, squats and deadlifts may not provide sufficient stimulus to train the anterior and lateral core aspects; nonetheless, lower-body strength does play a vital role in producing and improving maximal rotational power. Put simply, a strong lower body and core create a powerful linkage that increases rotational power. And rotational power, in turn, plays a big role in sport—for example, in batting, golfing, punching, and throwing, to name just a few key actions. A throw, punch, or swing depends not only on the strength of the arm but also on how well you can unleash combined power through rotary action in your hips, trunk, and arm (or arms). In short, if you want to improve your rotational power, you've got to improve not only your upper-body strength, but also your lower-body strength and your core strength. And that is exactly what the functional-spectrum training workout programs presented in this book enable you to do.

Total-Body Power Exercises

These explosive exercises require you to summate force by coordinating all of the muscles in your body that emphasize rotation. A few of these exercises are also included in other chapters because they are double-duty tools.

Medicine-Ball Horizontal Punch Throw

Setup

Stand roughly perpendicular to a solid wall with your feet shoulder-width apart and your knees slightly bent. Position your front foot (the one closest to the wall) at about a 45-degree angle and point your back foot straight ahead. With your torso upright, hold a medicine ball weighing 6.5 to 11 pounds (3 to 5 kg) between your hands at your chest with your elbows pointed outward (see figure a).

Action

Explosively rotate your hips and shoulders simultaneously toward the wall while extending your rear arm to throw the ball horizontally as if throwing a punch (see figure b). Allow the ball to bounce back to you, then reset your position for the next repetition. Perform all reps on one side before facing the other direction and performing the exercise on the opposite side.

Coaching Tips

- Allow your back foot to rotate toward the wall as you throw.
- Begin each throw with most of your weight shifted away from the wall; finish each throw with most of your weight on the leg closest to the wall with your rear heel off of the ground.
- Throw the ball at the wall as hard as you can.
- Keep your rear elbow parallel to the floor before each throw.
- If using a rubber, air-filled ball, which has a lot of bounce, stand far enough from the wall so that you don't feel rushed in catching the ball on the rebound after each throw. Specifically, stand far enough from the wall that the ball bounces at least once before it gets to you after each throw.
- If using a Dynamax-type medicine ball, which has limited bounce, you can stand much closer to the wall than if using a rubber medicine ball. Again, stand at a distance from the wall that allows the ball to bounce or roll back to you after each throw without forcing you to feel rushed.

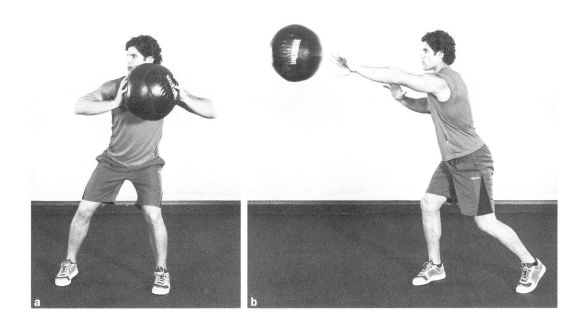

Medicine-Ball Shot-Put Throw

Setup

Stand roughly perpendicular to a solid wall with your feet shoulder-width apart and your knees slightly bent. Position your front foot (the one closest to the wall) at about a 45-degree angle point your back foot straight ahead. With your torso upright, hold a medicine ball weighing 6.5 to 11 pounds (3 to 5 kg) between your hands at your chest with your elbows pointed outward (see figure *a*).

Action

Explosively rotate your hips and shoulders simultaneously toward the wall while extending both your legs and your rear arm to throw the ball upward at a 45-degree angle in a shot-put type of action (see figure *b*). Allow the ball to bounce back to you, then reset your position for the next repetition. Perform all reps on one side before facing the other direction and performing the exercise on the opposite side.

Coaching Tips

- On every throw, your feet should leave the ground, and you should land facing the wall due to the rotation of your body.
- If using a Dynamax-type medicine ball, which has limited bounce, you can stand much closer to the wall than if using a rubber medicine ball. Stand at a distance from the wall that allows the ball to bounce back to you after each throw without forcing you to feel rushed.
- If using a sand-filled, non-bounce medicine ball, you can throw the ball into open space as far as possible at a 45-degree angle. Then walk to where it lands and throw it back to where you started.

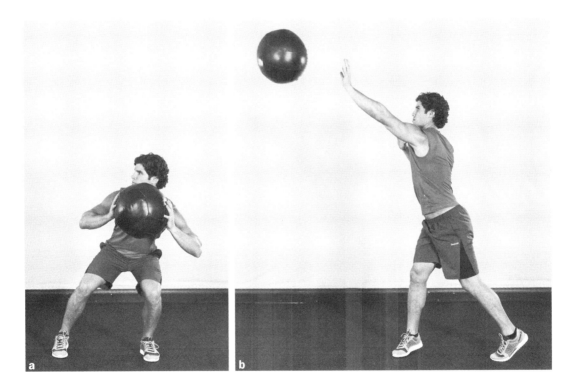

Medicine-Ball Side-Scoop Horizontal Throw

Setup

Stand perpendicular to a solid wall at your right side with your feet shoulder-width apart and your knees slightly bent. Hold a medicine ball weighing 6.5 to 11 pounds (3 to 5 kg) with both hands by your left hip and shift your weight to your left leg while hinging forward slightly at your hips. Lift your right heel off of the ground, allowing your right foot to rotate slightly and point toward your left side (see figure a).

Action

Explosively shift your hips toward your right while turning your hips and shoulders to throw the ball horizontally, using both hands in a scooplike motion (see figure b). Perform all reps on one side before switching sides.

Coaching Tips

- Keep your back in good alignment when setting up each throw.
- Keep your elbows slightly bent throughout.
- As you throw, lift your back heel off of the ground and rotate in the same direction as you're throwing by pivoting on the ball of your foot.
- If using a Dynamax-type medicine ball, which has limited bounce, you can stand much closer to the wall than if using a rubber medicine ball. Stand at a distance from the wall that allows the ball to bounce back to you after each throw without forcing you to feel rushed.

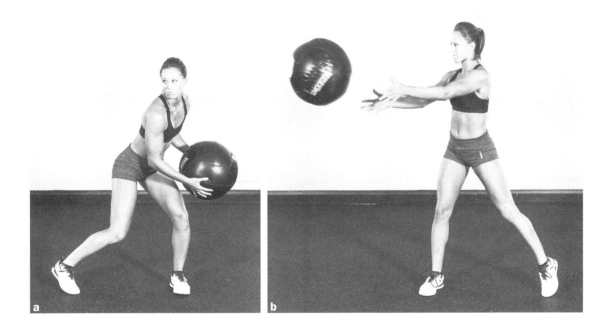

Medicine-Ball Side-Scoop Diagonal Throw

Setup

Stand perpendicular to a solid wall at your right side with your feet shoulder-width apart and your knees slightly bent. Hold a medicine ball weighing 6.5 to 11 pounds (3 to 5 kg) with both hands by your left hip and shift your weight to your left leg while hinging forward slightly at your hips (see figure a).

Action

Explosively shift your hips toward your right while turning your hips and shoulders to throw the ball horizontally with both hands in a scooplike motion (see figure b). Aim for a target on the wall that's roughly at your torso height. Alternate sides on each throw. Perform 8 to 10 reps.

Coaching Tips

- On each throw, simultaneously extend your legs and rotate your torso; in addition, keep your elbows slightly bent throughout.
- On each throw, your feet should leave the ground, and you should land facing the wall due to the rotation of your body.
- If using a Dynamax-type medicine ball, which has limited bounce, you can stand much closer to the wall than if using a rubber medicine ball. Stand at a distance from the wall that allows the ball to bounce back to you after each throw without forcing you to feel rushed.
- If using a sand-filled, non-bounce medicine ball, you can throw the ball into open space as far as possible at a 45-degree angle (as shown). Then walk to where it lands and throw it back to where you started.

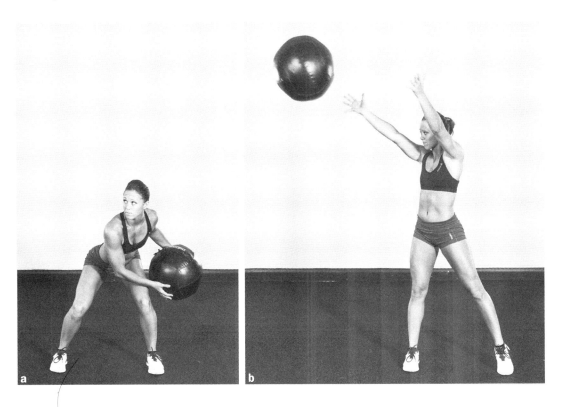

Medicine-Ball Front-Scoop Horizontal Throw

Setup

Stand facing the wall with your feet roughly shoulder-width apart and put most of your weight on your left leg. Rotate your shoulders toward your left side, placing a medicine ball weighing 6.5 to 11 pounds (3 to 5 kg) outside of your left thigh. Your right heel should be off of the ground, and your right foot should be rotated and pointed toward your left side (see figure a).

Action

Explosively throw the ball horizontally at the wall by unwinding your body back to the center position. Throw the ball in a scooplike fashion, in the same way you performed the side-scoop horizontal throw (see figure b). Stand at a distance from the wall that enables you to catch the ball before it bounces. You can either perform all reps on one side before switching or alternate sides with each repetition.

Coaching Tips

- Do not just throw the ball with your arms; rather, use your legs, hips, and torso to create rotational power.
- Keep your back in good alignment when setting up each throw.
- Keep your elbows slightly bent throughout.
- If using a Dynamax-type medicine ball, which has limited bounce, you can stand much closer to the wall than if using a rubber medicine ball.

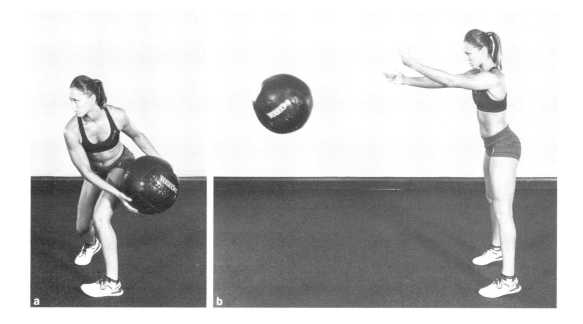

Medicine-Ball Downward-Chop Throw

Setup

Stand perpendicular to a wall on your right side with your feet slightly farther than shoulder-width apart. Hold a medicine ball weighing 6.5 to 11 pounds (3 to 5 kg) with both hands diagonally above your left shoulder and most of your weight shifted toward your left side (see figure a).

Action

Explosively shift your weight toward your left while turning your hips and shoulders to throw the ball downward at a 45-degree trajectory. Throw with both hands in a chopping fashion and aim at a point on the ground just in front of the wall (see figure b). Allow the ball to bounce off of the wall and hit the ground before you catch it and reset your position for the next repetition. Perform all reps on the same side before switching sides.

Coaching Tips

- To set up before each throw, reach your arms high enough to create a slight stretch in the front of your torso.
- Keep your elbows slightly bent throughout.
- As you throw, lift your back heel off of the ground and rotate in the same direction as you're throwing by pivoting on the ball of your foot.
- If using a Dynamax-type medicine ball, which has limited bounce, you can stand much closer to the wall than if using a rubber medicine ball.

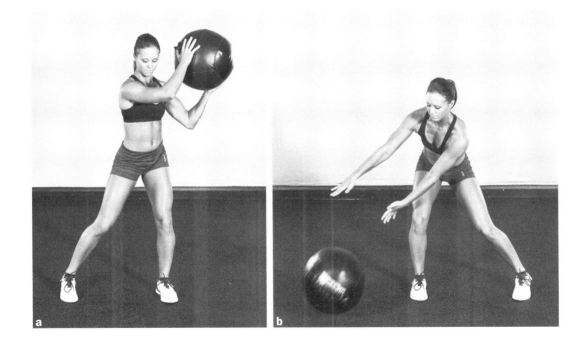

Cross-Body Exercises

The core musculature is engaged by all of the cross-body applications presented in chapters 4, 5, and 6 for upper-body pushing, upper-body pulling, and lower-body exercise. Even so, those exercises emphasize the pushing, pulling, or lower-body actions. In contrast, the following cross-body exercises emphasize the torso musculature required to perform rotation or to resist both rotation and lateral flexion.

Dumbbell Plank Row

Setup

Holding a dumbbell in each hand, assume a push-up position with your feet roughly shoulder-width apart (see figure a).

Action

From the top of the push-up position, pick up the dumbbell in your left hand and row it into your body (see figure b). Slowly lower it to the floor and repeat the action with your right hand. Continue to alternate hands until you've completed the indicated number of reps.

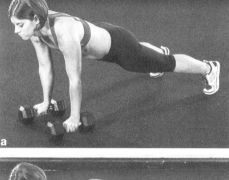

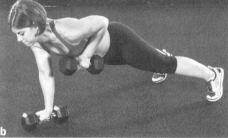

Coaching Tips

- Keep your head and hips from sagging toward the floor.
- Do not allow your body to shift from side to side as you perform each row.
- Do not allow your hips to rotate as you perform each row.
- Perform each row in a controlled manner by slowly lowering the dumbbell to the floor on each rep.
- To ensure that the dumbbells do not roll, place your hands directly underneath your shoulders.

One-Arm Dumbbell Farmer's Walk

Setup

Stand tall and hold a heavy dumbbell on the left side of your body by your left hip.

Action

Walk up and down the length of a room, keeping the dumbbell by your hip and maintaining your strong, upright posture (see figure). Then switch hands and repeat while holding a dumbbell on the other side.

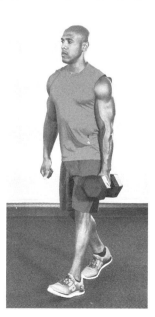

Coaching Tips

- This exercise is a great tool for improving your grip strength, which, along with core strength, can be a limiting factor in your ability to carry weight.
- If grip becomes a limiting factor in performing this exercise, you can carry the dumbbell in front of your shoulder.

Low-to-High Cable Chop

Setup

Stand perpendicular to a cable column on your left side. With both hands, hold each end of a rope handle, which is attached to the lowest position, with your arms extended toward the cable's origin. Position your feet slightly farther than shoulder-width apart.

Action

Squat and shift most of your weight to your left leg while your arms reach at a downward angle toward the origin of the cable (see figure a). Stand up while shifting your weight toward your right leg and driving the cable diagonally upward across your body. Finish at the top with your arms above your head on your right side (see figure b). Reverse the motion to return to the starting position, then repeat. Perform all reps on the same side before switching sides.

Coaching Tips

- Keep your torso fairly perpendicular to the cable column; do not rotate your torso away from the cable column more than a few degrees as you reach the top of the range of motion (doing so greatly reduces the rotational tension on your torso muscles.

- Keep your spine in a neutral position throughout the exercise; in the bottom position, set your hips back.

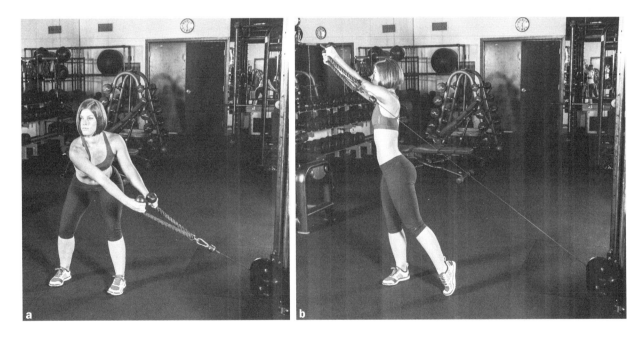

High-to-Low Cable Chop

Setup

Stand perpendicular to a cable column on your left side with the cable attached in the highest position. Hold a rope handle with both hands with your arms extended toward the cable's origin. Position your feet slightly father than shoulder-width apart.

Action

With your arms above your head on your left side and most of your weight shifted onto your left leg (see figure *a*), drive the cable diagonally downward across your body as you shift your weight to your right leg (see figure *b*). Once the cable touches your arm, slowly reverse the motion to complete the rep.

Coaching Tips

- Keep your torso fairly perpendicular to the cable column; do not rotate your torso away from the cable column more than a few degrees as you reach the bottom of the range of motion (doing so greatly reduces the rotational tension on your torso muscles.

- Keep your spine in a fairly neutral position throughout the exercise; in the bottom position, set your hips back slightly.

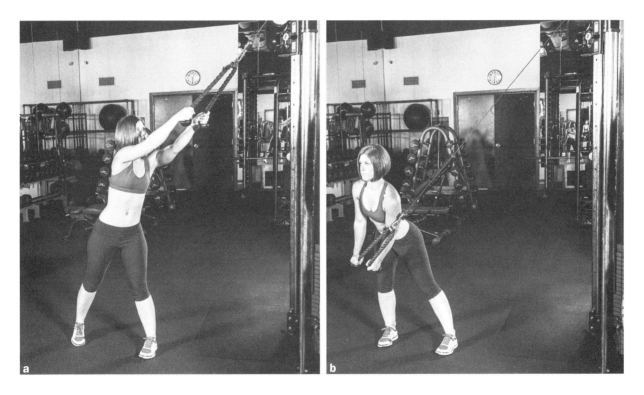

Plate Chop

Setup

Squat and rotate your hips and torso while holding a weight plate weighing 10 to 45 pounds (4.5 to 20 kg) outside your left knee (see figure *a*).

Action

Stand up as you rotate to your right side and drive the plate across your body in a diagonal pattern, finishing with it above your head (see figure *b*). Reverse the motion by driving the plate back down across your body on the same diagonal path you used to lift it. Perform all reps to one side, then repeat the exercise to the other side.

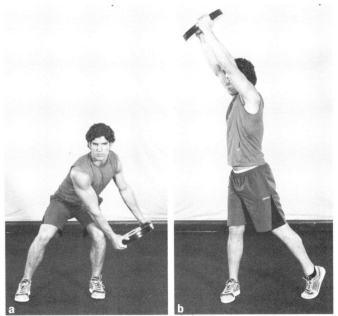

Coaching Tips

- Perform this exercise in a smooth and rhythmic fashion, coordinating your upper body and lower body during both the lifting and the lowering phase of each repetition.

- Keep your spine in a fairly neutral position throughout the exercise; in the bottom position, set your hips back slightly.

Cable or Band Tight Rotation

Setup

Stand with your feet shoulder-width apart, your knees slightly bent, and the handle(s) of a cable or resistance band on your left side at shoulder level. The cable or band should be attached to a stable structure or inside a doorjamb (many resistance bands come with such an attachment). Hold the handle(s) on your left side with your elbows slightly bent (see figure *a*).

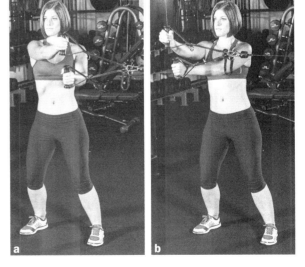

Action

Pull the handle(s) across your body to the right until both arms are just outside your right shoulder (see figure *b*). Move your arms horizontally in the opposite direction (toward the origin of the cable) until they reach a position just outside your left shoulder. The range of motion in this exercise is small—roughly the same as the width of your shoulders. Perform all reps on one side before switching to the other side.

Coaching Tips

- Stand tall throughout.

- Allow minimal rotation at your hips, which should move in the same direction and at the same speed as your shoulders.

Cable or Band Anti-Rotation Press

Setup

Kneel perpendicular to a cable handle or band that's attached at shoulder height to a stable structure or inside a doorjamb (many resistance bands come with such an attachment). With your knees roughly shoulder-width apart hold the handle with both hands at the center of your chest (see figure a).

Action

Reach your arms straight out in front of you at shoulder height without allowing your torso to rotate toward the origin of the cable or band (see figure b). Then slowly reverse the action and bring your hands back to the center of your chest. Perform all reps on one side before switching to the other side.

Coaching Tips

- Stay tall throughout.
- Do not allow your arms to drop below chest height as you reach.

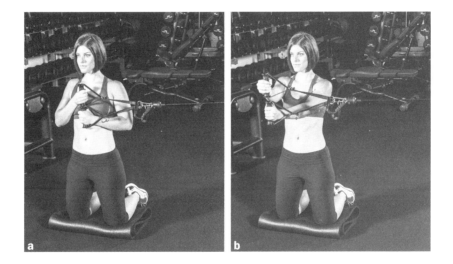

One-Arm Plank

Setup

Begin in a push-up position with your hands shoulder-width apart and your feet a few inches farther than shoulder-width apart.

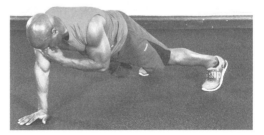

Action

Lift one arm off of the ground and place it on your chest without allowing your shoulders or hips to rotate or your head or belly to sag toward the floor (see figure). Pause for several seconds before switching hands.

Coaching Tips

- You can choose to perform this exercise from the elbows; if so, place a pad, pillow, or folded towel under your elbows for protection.
- To make the exercise more difficult, raise the lifted arm out to the side instead of across your chest.
- To make the exercise easier, start with your hands closer than shoulder-width apart, which shortens the lever arm.

Angled Barbell Tight Rainbow

Setup

Place one end of a barbell in a corner or into a landmine device. Hold the other end with both hands while standing tall with your feet roughly shoulder-width apart.

Action

Move the barbell from side to side in a rainbow-like arc from one shoulder to the other (see figures *a* and *b*).

Coaching Tips

- Maintain a straight spine.
- Avoid any rotation at your torso; as you move the barbell from side to side, your torso should remain facing the barbell's anchored end.
- Maintain a slight bend in your elbows throughout.
- The movement of the barbell should come from your shoulders, not your elbows.

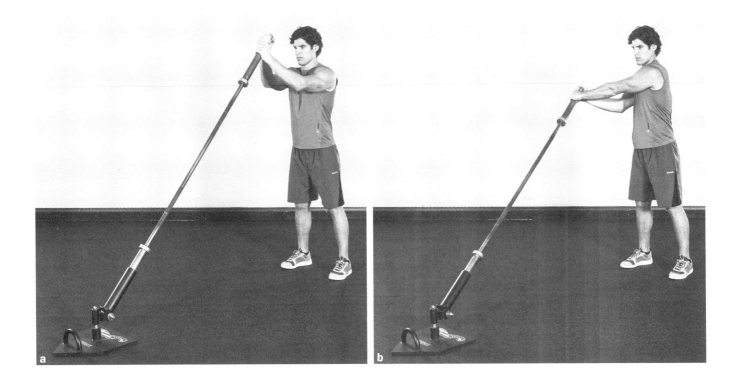

Compound Core Training

One principle of good weight training is to emphasize compound (multijoint) exercises but supplement them with isolation (single-joint) exercises. As you've already learned, the functional-spectrum training system takes this weight-training principle a step further by also incorporating cross-body exercises.

This approach is atypical but well founded. Many of the most common abdominal exercises are isolation oriented; in fact, the compound-movement principle is rarely applied in abdominal training. However, if we recall the original definition of the term core, given at the start of this chapter, research finds the greatest activation of abdominal and lumbar muscles during exercises that also require deltoid and gluteal recruitment (4). This finding establishes a principle of core training—that, as with every other muscle group, a comprehensive core-training routine should emphasize integrated, compound exercises and supplement them with isolation moves. That's exactly what the functional-spectrum training system delivers for core training. And you can now appreciate a key fact: All of the cross-body exercises provided in the pushing, pulling, and lower-body chapters also serve as fantastic core-training exercises because they elicit crisscross force production between the shoulder and the opposite hip through the torso.

Compound Exercises

These front and lateral core (i.e., abdominal and oblique) exercises integrate the shoulders and hips.

Stability-Ball Knee Tuck

Setup

Hold yourself in a push-up position with your hands directly underneath your shoulders and your feet and shins resting on top of a (55 to 65 cm size) stability ball (see figure a). Keep your legs hip-width apart.

Action

Pull your knees in to your chest (see figure b). Reverse the motion and repeat.

Coaching Tips

- Do not allow your head or lower back to sag toward the floor.
- Perform the exercise smoothly with deliberate control.

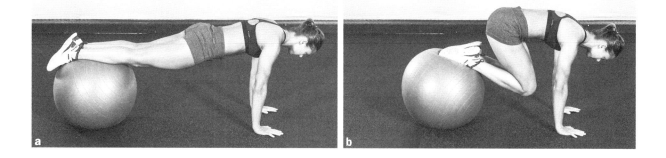

Stability-Ball Rollout

Setup

Kneel on the floor with your knees hip-width apart, your arms straight, and your palms shoulder-width apart on a stability (about 55 to 65 cm size) (see figure a).

Action

Drive the ball away from you by extending your arms overhead as if diving into a pool. Push the ball out as far as you can without allowing your head or lower back to sag toward the floor (see figure b). Once you've gone as far as you can, or your arms are completely up overhead in a straight line with your torso, reverse the motion and pull the ball back to the starting position.

Coaching Tips

- To make this exercise easier, simply begin with your forearms resting on top of the ball and perform the rest of the exercise as described.
- Do not flex at your hips at any time.

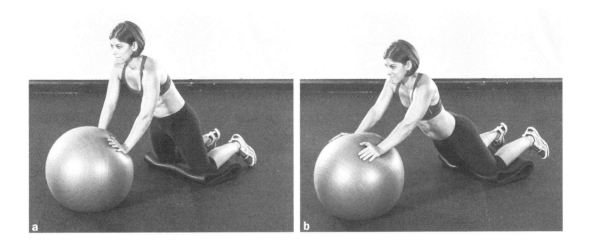

Stability-Ball Pike

Setup

Assume a push-up position with your hands directly underneath your shoulders and your feet and shins hip-width apart on top of a fitness ball (about 55 to 65 cm size) (see figure *a*).

Action

Use your abs to raise your hips toward the sky while keeping your legs fairly straight. Raise your hips until just before they reach above your shoulders (see figure *b*). Slowly lower to the starting position with your body straight.

Coaching Tips

- To make the exercise easier, start with the ball closer to your belly button.
- Do not allow your hips or head to sag toward the floor as you extend your hips back into the starting position.

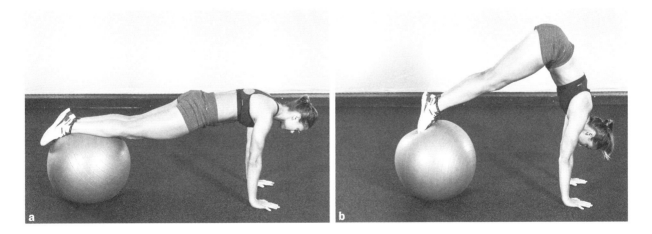

Stability-Ball Pike Rollout

Setup

This exercise combines the ball pike and the ball rollout into one comprehensive abdominal exercise. Hold yourself in a push-up position with your hands directly underneath your shoulders and your feet hip-width apart on top of a (55 to 65 cm size) ball (see figure a).

Action

Keep your legs straight and push your hips toward the ceiling while keeping your back fairly flat (see figures b and c). After straightening your hips and coming back to the starting position, push your body backward on the ball until your arms are fully extended in front of you and your legs are fully extended behind you. Reverse the motion, then repeat.

Coaching Tips

- To make the exercise easier, start with the ball closer to your belly button.
- Do not allow your hips or head to sag toward the floor as you extend your arms into the rollback portion of the exercise.
- When performing the pike portion of the exercise, raise your hips until just before they reach above your shoulders

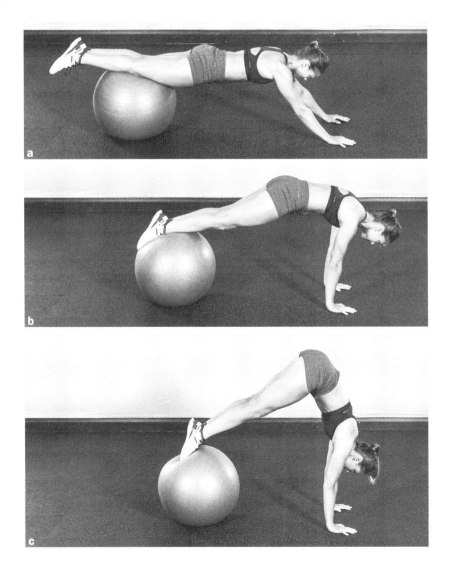

Stability-Ball Stir-the-Pot

Setup

Place both forearms on top of a fitness ball and assume a plank position with your body in a straight line and your feet just farther than shoulder-width apart (see figure a). Contract your glutes and posteriorly rotate your pelvis by bringing your front hip bones toward your head and your tailbone toward your feet. In other words, if you imagine your pelvis as a bucket of water, the posterior pelvic tilt would tip the bucket so that water would spill out of your back, whereas an anterior pelvic tilt would make water spill out from the front.

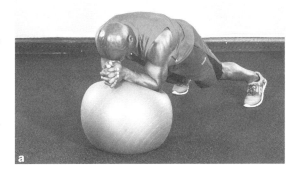

Action

Move your arms in small ovals (see figure b). Alternate between clockwise ovals and counterclockwise ovals without allowing your head or hips to sag toward the floor.

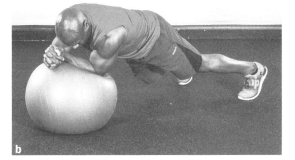

Coaching Tips

- Keep your body in a straight line throughout; do not allow your hips or head to sag toward the floor.
- Your arms should not move in circles so much as in ovals, going farther longways than to the sides, so that you don't fall off of the ball to either side.
- Squeeze your glutes tightly each time that you reach your arms out.
- Reach your arms as far as you can without feeling discomfort in your lower back.

Mini-Band Plank March

Setup

Assume a push-up position with a mini-band around your feet with legs hip-width apart and your wrists directly underneath your shoulders (see figure a).

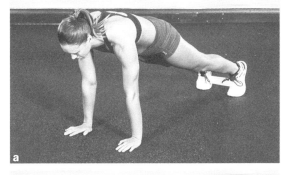

Action

Keeping your body in a straight line, flex one hip and bring your knee toward your head until your hip is bent just above a 90-degree angle without allowing your toes to touch the floor (see figure b). Reverse the motion by placing your foot back to the start position, then repeat the same motion on the other leg.

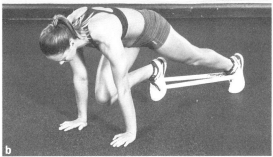

Coaching Tips

- Be sure to keep your ankles flexed by pulling your toes toward your nose throughout this exercise.
- Be sure not to round out your back as you flex your hip and pull your knee in.
- Do not allow your hips to rotate at any time.

Arm Walkout

Setup

Assume a kneeling position with your hands flat on the floor just above your shoulders and your arms straight under your shoulders (see figure a). Your torso should form a fairly straight line from your head to your knees. You may also need to place a pad, pillow, or folded towel under your knees for comfort.

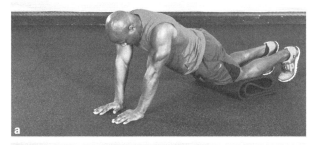

Action

Walk your arms out in front of you as far as possible without allowing your lower back to extend beyond the starting position (see figures b and c). Reverse the motion, walking your hands back so that they end up just in front of your shoulders.

Coaching Tips

- Keep your body in a straight line throughout; do not allow your hips or head to sag toward the floor.

- Squeeze your glutes tightly each time that you walk your hands out to the long position.

- Walk your arms out only as far as you can without feeling discomfort in your lower back.

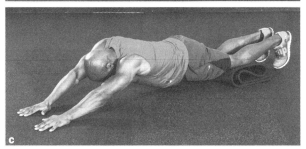

Medicine-Ball Walkout

Setup

Assume a kneeling position with your hands on the top of a rubber or sand-filled medicine ball just above your shoulders and your arms straight (see figure a). Your torso should form a fairly straight line from your head to your knees. You may also need to place a pad, pillow, or folded towel under your knees for comfort.

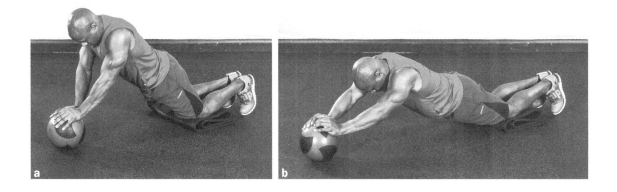

Action

Roll the ball out in front of you by walking with your arms in hand-over-hand fashion as far as possible without allowing your lower back to extend beyond the starting position (see figure b). Reverse the motion, rolling the ball back toward you by walking your hands back so that they end up just in front of your shoulders.

Coaching Tips

- Keep your body in a straight line throughout; do not allow your hips or head to sag toward the floor.
- Squeeze your glutes tightly each time that you walk your hands out to the long position.
- Walk your arms out only as far as you can without feeling discomfort in your lower back.
- If using a rubber medicine ball (the kind found at most gyms), choose one that is fully inflated and large enough—at least 8 pounds (3.5 kg)—to accommodate both of your hands.
- If using a sand-filled ball, you can make the exercise harder by using a heavier ball.

Suspension Ab Fallout

Setup

Facing away from the anchor point of a suspension trainer, grab the handles and lean your weight forward in a push-up position with your arms shoulder-width apart (see figure a).

Action

Without bending your elbows, reach your arms above your head as if diving into a pool (see figure b). Pull your arms back in to complete the rep.

Coaching Tips

- Do not allow your hips to sag toward the floor.
- To increase the difficulty, start the exercise from a more severe forward lean, which brings your body closer to the floor.

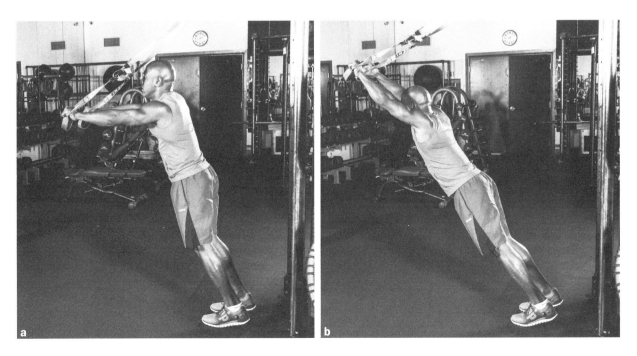

Ab Snail

Setup

You'll need a surface on which you can slide your feet; alternatively, you can place your heels on a paper plate or on furniture sliders. Sit on the floor with your legs outstretched and your hands supporting you, just behind your hips, with your fingers pointed backward (see figure a).

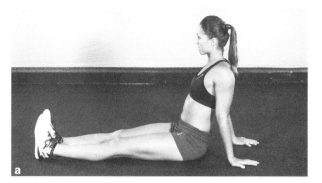

Action

Push against the ground with your hands and raise your hips (see figure b). Pull your hips through your hands as far as possible (see figure c), then slowly lower them to the floor. Place your hands back behind you and repeat the sequence, moving along the floor with each repetition.

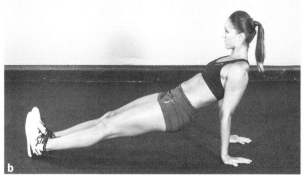

Coaching Tips

- Do not reach your arms too far behind you to begin each rep. Place your hands just a few inches behind your hips.
- Once you've pulled your hips through your arms as far as you can, pause for one or two seconds before lowering your hips and resetting your hands to start the next rep.
- Lift your hips as high as possible as you pull them through your arms.

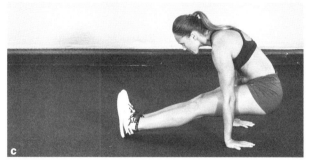

Side Elbow Plank

Setup

Lying on your side, place your right forearm on the floor, with the elbow directly underneath your shoulder, and your feet split apart with one in front of the other or stacked on top of each other. Place your left hand on your left hip.

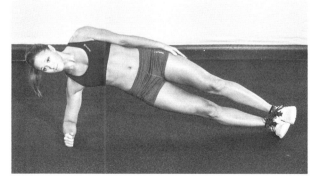

Action

Raise your hips off the ground (see figure). Maintain this position for indicated given number of seconds. Repeat on the other side.

Coaching Tips

- Keep a straight line in your entire body, from your nose to your belly button to the middle of your legs.
- Use a pad or a rolled towel underneath your elbow for comfort.

Isolation Exercises

These are movements that focus on individual muscle groups. These exercise applications consist primarily of traditional bodybuilding movements, along with a few not-so-traditional exercises that target the abdominal and oblique musculature.

Stability-Ball Plate Crunch

Setup
Lie down with a fitness ball in the arch of your lower back and hold a weight plate directly above your chest with your arms outstretched (see figure a).

Action
Perform a crunch, reaching the weight plate toward the sky (see figure b). Slowly reverse the motion, allowing your abdominal muscles to stretch over the ball.

Coaching Tips
- Do not let the ball roll at any point.
- Do not sit all the way up (with your torso perpendicular to the floor); doing so removes the tension from the abs.
- Do not allow your neck to hyperextend in the bottom position; keep your neck in a fairly neutral position throughout.
- Pause for one or two seconds at the top of each rep.

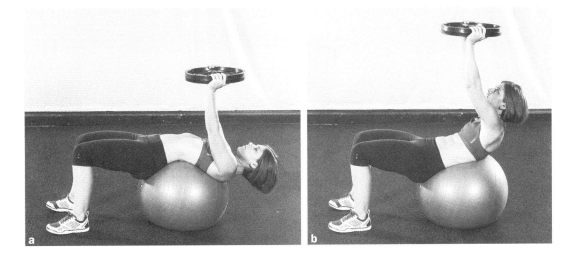

Reverse Crunch

Setup
Lie on your back on the floor with your knees bent and your hips flexed into your belly. With your elbows slightly bent, hold a dumbbell, kettlebell, or medicine ball that is resting on the floor behind your head (see figure a).

Action
In a smooth, controlled fashion, perform a reverse crunch by rolling your lower back up off of the floor and bringing your knees toward your chin (see figure b). Slowly reverse this motion, allowing your back to lower toward the floor one vertebra at a time.

> continued

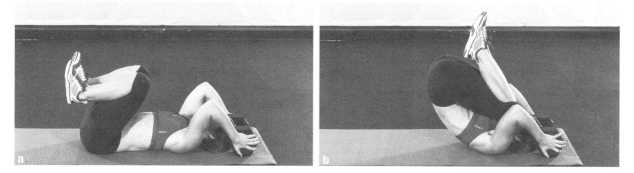

Coaching Tips

- Do not use momentum or jerk your body.
- Do not allow your legs to extend or your head to lift off of the ground at any point.
- Use a dumbbell, kettlebell, or medicine ball that is just heavy enough to prevent you from lifting it off of the ground. As your abdominal strength improves, you'll require less of an anchor, which means you'll be able to use a *lighter* dumbbell, kettlebell, or medicine ball without lifting it off of the floor.

Leg Lowering With Band

Setup

Lie on your back on the floor with your knees bent, your hips flexed above 90 degrees, and your arms outstretched in front of your torso, just below shoulder level. In each hand, hold the handle of a resistance band attached about 12 inches off of the floor to a stable structure or inside a doorjamb behind you (see figure *a*).

Action

Maintaining tension against the band with your arms, slowly lower your legs toward the floor. Keep your knees bent and do not allow your lower back to come off of the floor (see figure *b*). Once your heels lightly touch the floor, reverse the motion and bring your knees back above your hips.

Coaching Tips

- To make this exercise more challenging, simply extend your legs farther as you lower them toward the floor—the farther you straighten your legs, the harder the exercise; the closer your heels are to your hips, the easier the exercise.
- Do not allow your lower back to lose contact with the floor at any point.

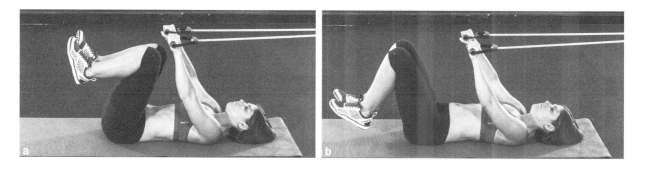

Now that you've seen the wide variety of exercises used in the functional-spectrum training system, it's time to show you the warm-up sequences and cool-down methods that you'll use to get more out of the workout programs presented later in the book.

8

Warm-Up and Cool-Down

A dynamic warm-up is a transition stage from normal activity to more athletic activity. A cool down is just the opposite—a transition stage from athletic activity to more normal activity. This chapter covers the warm-up protocols and cool-down techniques that you should use to bookend your functional-spectrum training workouts.

Warm-Up

Just as there are general and specific exercises in the functional-spectrum training system, there are also general and specific warm-ups. Specific warm-ups serve essentially as "build-up" sets because they are simply lighter, less intense versions of whatever exercises you're getting ready to perform; they are used to build up gradually to your working intensity. For example, if you're going to run sprints, you first do some light runs, building up your speed with each round. If you're going to perform a heavy lift, you first do a few lighter sets of that lift in order to build up to your working weight.

The warm-up sequences presented here are general warm-ups because they involve a few general athletic movements and coordination exercises. They not only get your heart rate up but also prepare your entire body for the more athletic functional-spectrum training workouts that follow. These warm-up sequences also include exercises that help you maintain and increase your overall joint mobility, which can improve joint health. Joints are designed primarily to function in their mid-range of motion, but they also need activity using their full range of motion in order to stay healthy and maintain their current range. As the saying goes, "If you don't use it, you lose it."

The mobility exercises included in the following warm-up sequences complement your training for size, strength, and speed (i.e., power). Specifically, they require your joints to move into their end range of motion, whereas the strength-training principles applied in this book avoid end-range joint actions in order to maximize safety in handling heavy loads. The mobility exercises presented here also help you improve in other areas: squatting deeper, deadlifting with a straighter back, and performing lifts with more comfort and less restriction.

As you can see, these warm-up sequences do far more than just boost your body temperature. They're also used in the functional-spectrum training system to increase the variety of activity in your workouts. In addition, they help you develop a more well-rounded body that's not just stronger and better looking but also more mobile—benefits that the typical warm-up on the treadmill or bike simply can't match.

The functional-spectrum training system uses three types of warm-up protocol: in-place, large-space, and medicine-ball. These protocols give you warm-up options to prepare yourself to perform the functional-spectrum workout programs provided in the chapters that follow. Although one of these warm-up protocols is suggested for each workout program, all of the protocols can be used interchangeably to add variety to your training and to fit your training environment. In addition, though there's already plenty of variety in these sequences, you can also mix and match specific exercises to create your own warm-up sequences.

Each of the following warm-up sequences can—and should—be completed in no more than seven minutes once you become proficient at them. Initially, however, they may take a bit longer as you learn how to perform them.

In-Place Warm-Ups

As the name implies, these sequences can be done anywhere because they require little space and only one piece of equipment: a mat. Select one of the following sequences to add variety to your training or to enable you to warm up when space is limited.

In-Place Warm-Up 1

This sequence includes the following exercises:

One-leg hip bridge	1 set × 10–15 reps each side
One-arm quadruped hip circle	1 set × 10–12 reps clockwise each side 1 set × 10–12 reps counterclockwise each side
Slow-motion mountain climber	1 set × 6 or 7 reps each leg
Lateral yoga-plex	1 set × 3–5 reps each side
Shoulder Y	1 set × 12–15 reps
Seal jack	1 set × 20–25 reps

1. One-Leg Hip Bridge

Setup

Lie on your back with your legs hip-width apart and your knees bent about 90 degrees. Keeping your right knee bent 90 degrees, lift it above your hip (see figure a).

Action

Lift your hips so that your body makes a straight line from knee to nose (see figure b). Keeping your right leg lifted, lower your hips toward the floor to complete the rep. Do 10 to 15 reps on each side; perform all reps on one side before switching sides.

Coaching Tips

- Keep your base foot flat on the ground throughout the exercise.
- Do not bounce; keep your motion smooth and your range controlled, finishing each rep at the top with your hips elevated as far as possible without overextending at your lower back.

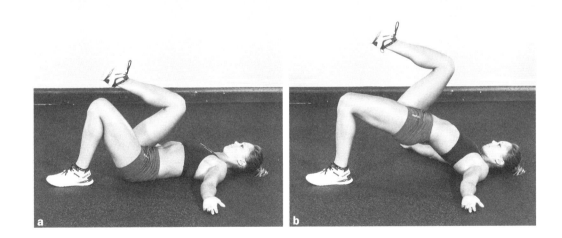

> continued

2. One-Arm Quadruped Hip Circle

Setup

Begin on all fours with your knees underneath your hips and your wrists underneath your shoulders. Keeping your back straight, lift your right hand off of the floor and place it on your left shoulder (see figure *a*).

Action

Keeping your left knee bent roughly 90 degrees, rotate clockwise at your left hip using the largest range of motion you can while maintaining a flat back (see figures *b* and *c*). Once you've performed 10 to 12 clockwise rotations, reverse direction and perform 10 to 12 counterclockwise rotations. Then switch sides by placing your left hand on your right shoulder and rotating at your right hip.

Coaching Tips

- Keep your back fairly flat and straight throughout to ensure that the rotation comes from your hip, not your spine.
- Keep your neck straight; do not allow your head to sag toward the floor.

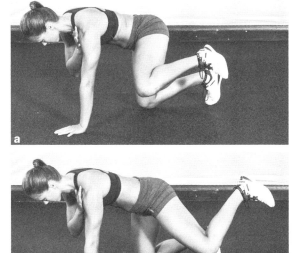

3. Slow-Motion Mountain Climber

Setup

Start at the top of a push-up with your feet hip-width apart and your wrists directly below your shoulders (see figure *a*).

Action

Pick up your right foot and slowly bring your right knee toward your right shoulder as far as possible (see figure *b*). Hold for two seconds, then return to the starting position. Alternate legs until you've done 12 to 14 total reps (6 or 7 per leg).

Coaching Tips

- Do not allow your head or hips to sag toward the floor; keep your body in a straight line throughout.
- Your toes should not touch the floor when you bring your knee toward your shoulder.

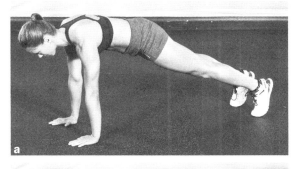

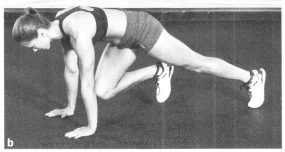

4. Lateral Yoga-Plex

Setup

Begin in a push-up position with your wrists underneath your shoulders and your feet positioned roughly 6 inches (15 cm) farther to each side than shoulder-width apart (see figure *a*).

Action

Step your left foot roughly 6 inches (15 cm) to the outside of your left arm so that your torso now forms a straight line with your right leg. Rotate your torso to the right as you reach your right arm toward the ceiling (see figures *b* and *c*). Reverse the motion and perform the same action by stepping up with your right leg and reaching with your left arm. Perform 3 to 5 reps per side; alternating legs each time.

Coaching Tips

- Each time you step one foot to roughly the outside of your hands, that foot should stay flat on the floor. If you're unable to place your foot flat next to your hand when you step forward, you can make the exercise easier by elevating your hands on a platform (e.g., aerobic step).

- Do not pause for more than a second at any point; maintain a constant flow.

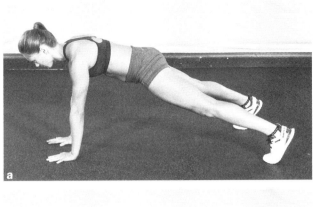

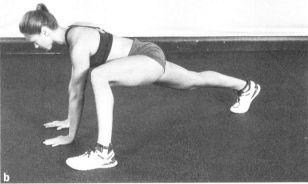

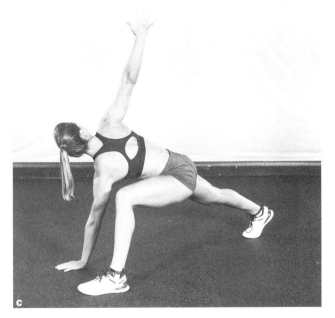

> continued

5. Shoulder Y

Setup

Standing with your feet hip-width apart, bend slightly at your knees and hinge at your hips to lower your torso until it's roughly parallel to the floor; let your arms hang from your shoulders (see figure *a*).

Action

Raise your arms out to shoulder height by keeping your arms fairly straight at a 45-degree angle to form a Y; point your thumbs toward the sky (see figure *b*). Slowly lower your arms back down; perform 12 to 15 reps.

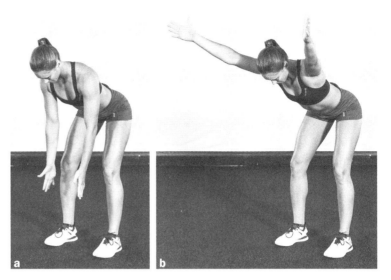

Coaching Tips

- Do not swing your arms up.
- Pause for a second or two at the top of each rep.
- The hip and back positioning of this exercise are virtually the same as for a Romanian deadlift; do not allow your back to round out at any point.

6. Seal Jack

Setup

Stand with your feet together and your arms extended in front of you at shoulder level with your hands together (see figure *a*).

Action

As you open your arms horizontally to the side, jump up just enough to spread your feet wide (see figure *b*). Without pausing, quickly reverse the movement. Perform 20 to 25 reps.

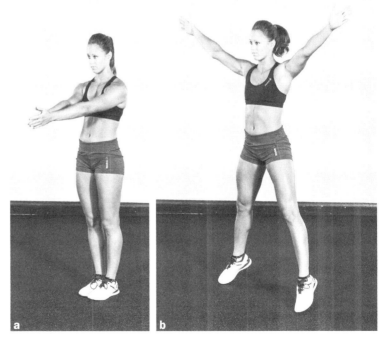

Coaching Tips

- Be as light on your feet as possible.
- Minimize the time that your feet are in contact with the ground.
- Perform the exercise in a smooth, coordinated fashion, opening and closing your legs and arms simultaneously.

In-Place Warm-Up 2

This sequence includes the following exercises:

Arm crossover	1 set × 6–8 reps each side
Side-lying hip adduction and internal rotation	1 set × 10–12 reps each side
Quadruped T-spine rotation	1 set × 6–8 reps each side
Superdog	1 set × 12–15 reps each side
Shoulder L	1 set × 12–15 reps
In-place high-knee skip	1 set × 20–25 reps each leg

1. Arm Crossover

Setup

Lie on your right side with your knees and hips bent just above 90 degrees and straighten both arms in front of you with your palms facing each other (see figure *a*).

Action

While keeping your right arm and both legs in position, rotate your torso to the left as far as you can until your left hand and upper back are flat on the floor (see figure *b*). Hold for one or two seconds, then return to the starting position. Perform 6 to 8 reps on each side. Do all reps on one side before switching sides.

Coaching Tips

- Rotate as far as you can without forcing anything.
- If you're unable to get remotely close to touching the floor with the shoulder you're rotating, perform this exercise with a small medicine ball or rolled towel between your knees to allow for greater range of motion.

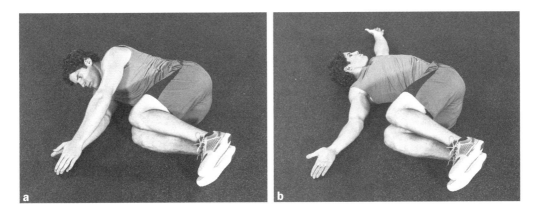

2. Side-Lying Hip Adduction and Internal Rotation

Setup

Lie on your right side with your head resting on your right arm (your bottom arm), which is extended across the floor at roughly a 45-degree angle above you. Keep your right leg (your bottom leg) straight and in line with your torso. Bend your left leg (your top leg) and bring it up until your foot is flat on the floor in front of your bottom knee. Grab your left ankle with your left (top) hand (see figure *a*).

> continued

Action

Keeping your knee straight and your ankle flexed, lift your right leg off of the ground as you internally rotate it so that your toes point toward the ceiling (see figure *b*). Slowly reverse the motion, allowing your leg to return to the floor. Perform 10 to 12 reps on each side. Do all reps on one side before switching sides.

Coaching Tips

- Lift and rotate your bottom leg as much as possible without allowing your hip to flex; your bottom leg should stay fairly in line with your torso throughout.

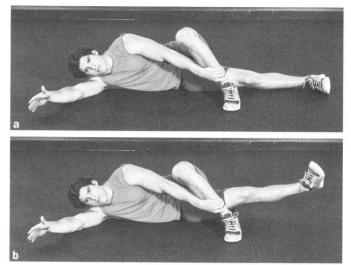

- Do not allow your torso to roll at any point; keep your shoulders and hips perpendicular to the floor.

3. Quadruped T-Spine Rotation

Setup

Begin on all fours with your arms shoulder-width apart and your hands on the floor just above your head. Spread your knees wide and sit back on your hips. Place your left hand on the back of your head.

Action

Rotate your upper back and your left arm upward as far as you can go, so that your left elbow now points toward the ceiling (see figure *a*). Slowly reverse the motion by rotating your upper back downward and bringing your left elbow down toward the elbow of your right (bracing) arm (see figure *b*). That's one rep. Perform 6 to 8 reps on each side before switching sides.

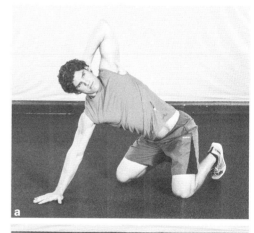

Coaching Tips

- Each time you rotate your elevated arm toward the ceiling, go only as far as is comfortable, without forcing anything.

- Move in a slow, controlled manner, pausing for one second at the top position on each rep.

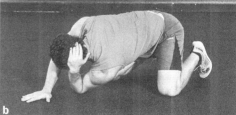

4. Superdog

Setup

Kneel and place your elbows on the floor. Slide your left hand forward and stretch your right leg behind you until your arm and leg are both straight (see figure *a*).

Action

Raise your left arm and your right leg as high as you can, forming a straight line from your fingertips to your toes without allowing your rear end to lift more than a few degrees (see figure *b*). Hold for one second, then return to the starting position. That's one rep; do 12 to 15 reps on each side. Perform all reps on one side before switching sides.

Coaching Tips

- Place a pad or rolled towel underneath your bent knee for comfort.
- Do not allow your hips to lift or your torso to shift forward as you perform this exercise.

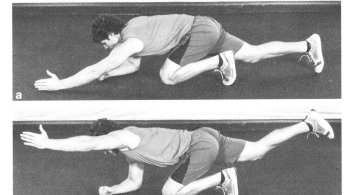

5. Shoulder L

Setup

Stand with your feet hip-width apart and bend at your hips, lowering your torso until it's roughly parallel to the floor. Raise your arms out to the sides to shoulder height, bending your elbows 90 degrees so that your hands point down toward the ground (see figure a).

Action

Without moving your elbows, rotate your arms up as far as you can bring your hands toward the ceiling (see figure b). Slowly reverse the motion to return to the starting position. That's one rep; perform 12 to 15 reps.

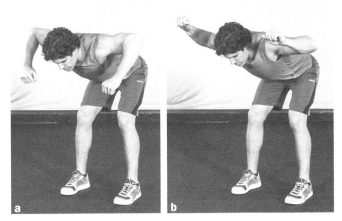

Coaching Tips

- Pause for a second or two at the top of each rep.
- The hip and back positioning of this exercise are virtually the same as for a Romanian deadlift; do not allow your back to round out at any point.

6. In-Place High-Knee Skip

Setup

Stand tall with your feet hip-width apart and your elbows bent roughly 90 degrees.

Action

Lift your left knee to a point just above your hip while also lifting your right arm and moving your left arm back (see figure). Quickly reverse your arm positions as you drive your left leg down to the ground and elevate your right knee. Much like jumping rope, skipping requires a double-foot strike pattern, or right-right hops followed by left-left hops. Perform 20 to 25 reps per leg.

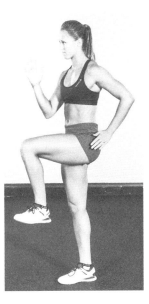

Coaching Tips

- This is not running in place; to skip in place, you must coordinate your arm pumping with your double-foot strikes.
- Keep your torso upright throughout.

In-Place Warm-Up 3

This sequence includes the following exercises:

Crab bridge with overhead reach	1 set × 6–8 reps each side
Dynamic pigeon	1 set × 6–8 reps each side
Yoga-plex	1 set × 4–6 reps each side
Half-kneeling knee lift	1 set × 4–6 reps each side
Zombie lateral lunge	1 set × 4–6 reps each side
Shoulder T	1 set × 12–15 reps
Crossover jack	1 set × 20–25 reps

1. Crab Bridge With Overhead Reach

Setup

Sit on the floor with your legs bent 90 degrees, your feet flat on the floor, and your hands flat on the floor just behind your shoulders with your fingers pointed behind you (see figure *a*).

Action

Use your feet and hands to push into the ground and raise your hips so that your torso assumes a tabletop-like position. As you raise your hips, reach one arm overhead and across your body (see figure *b*). Slowly reverse the motion to complete the rep. Alternate arms with each rep; perform 6 to 8 reps on each side

Coaching Tips

- Push through your heels and keep your feet flat each time that you raise your hips.
- You wrists should be underneath your shoulders at the top of each bridge.

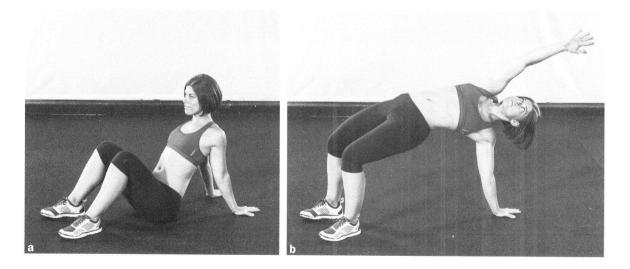

2. Dynamic Pigeon

Setup

This is a dynamic version of a yoga position known as pigeon pose. Get on all fours with your hands underneath your shoulders and your knees under your hips.

Action

Extend your left leg straight at a 45-degree angle across your right leg (see figure *a*). Shift your hips backward as you drive your left leg back at a 45-degree angle as far as you can without lifting your hands off of the floor (see figure *b*). Reverse the motion, bringing your left knee back down underneath your left hip. After brining the left knee back, extend your right leg behind you at a 45-degree angle to perform the same action. Alternate legs and perform 6 to 8 reps with each leg.

Coaching Tips

- Keep your shoulders parallel to the floor throughout.
- As you shift your hips backward, allow your arms to extend fully without allowing your hands to lift off of the floor.
- Perform each rep in a smooth, controlled manner without pausing at any time.

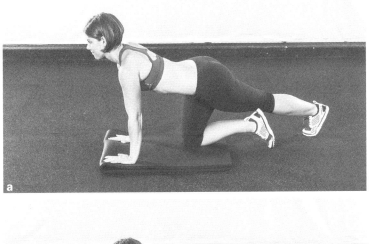

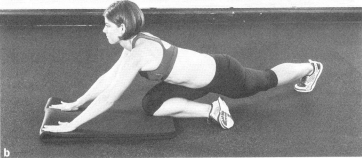

> *continued*

3. Yoga-Plex

Setup

Begin in a push-up position with your wrists underneath your shoulders and your feet hip-width apart (see figure *a*).

Action

Step your left foot up to your left hand while simultaneously lifting your left hand off the floor and reaching your left arm directly above you to form a straight line with your torso and right leg (see figure *b* and *c*). With your left foot flat on the floor, rotate your torso to the left as you reach your left arm toward the ceiling using a circular (clockwise) motion at your shoulder (see figure *d*). Continue the arm circle motion until your left arm comes back down to where your left foot is (see figure *e*). Step your left foot back and place your left hand back down to resume the starting position (see figure *f*). Repeat on the other side by stepping up with your right foot and making a circular (clockwise) motion at your right shoulder. Continue to alternate sides; Perform 4 to 6 reps on each side.

Coaching Tips

- Maintain a constant flow; do not pause for more than one second at any point.
- If you're unable to place your foot flat when it comes next to your hand on the forward step, you can make the exercise easier by elevating your hands on a platform (e.g., aerobic step).

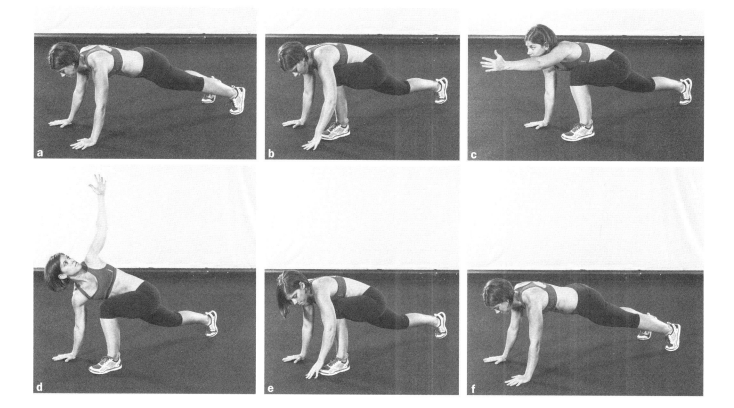

4. Half-Kneeling Knee Lift

Setup

Using a mat or rolled towel for comfort, assume a half-kneeling position on the floor with your torso straight and both knees bent 90 degrees. Interlace your fingers behind your head with your elbows pointed outward (see figure *a*).

Action

Keeping your torso straight, flex your hip and lift your front foot off of the ground; keep your knee bent 90 degrees (see figure *b*). Lower your foot back to the floor and repeat. Perform 4 to 6 reps on each side.

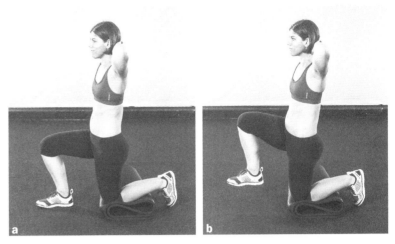

Coaching Tips

- Do not allow your torso to bend forward or lean backward; your torso should remain in line with your down knee throughout.
- Lift your knee as high as possible on each repetition.
- Each rep should take only one or two seconds because it can be difficult to balance when your front foot is lifted.

5. Zombie Lateral Lunge

Setup

Stand with your feet hip-width apart and your arms straight in front of you at shoulder height (see figure *a*).

Action

Step to one side and lower into a side lunge (see figure *b*). Your arms remain outstretched to the front. Step back to the middle and repeat on the other side. Continue to alternate sides; perform 4 to 6 reps on each side.

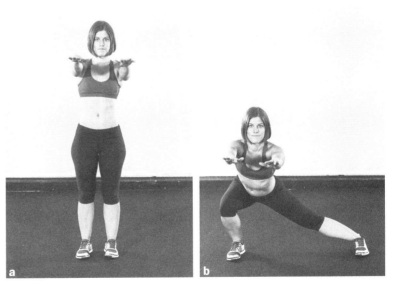

Coaching Tips

- Maintain good rhythm and timing, both when stepping and when reversing the action; the movement should not look choppy.
- Keep your training leg straight and both of your feet flat as you step laterally.

> continued

6. Shoulder T

Setup

Stand with your feet hip-width apart and bend at your hips, lowering your torso until it's roughly parallel to the floor; let your arms hang from your shoulders (see figure *a*).

Action

With a slight bend in your elbows and your thumbs pointed out to the sides, lift your arms out to the sides until they're parallel to the floor so that they form a T with your torso (see figure *b*). Slowly reverse the motion to complete the rep. Perform 12 to 15 reps.

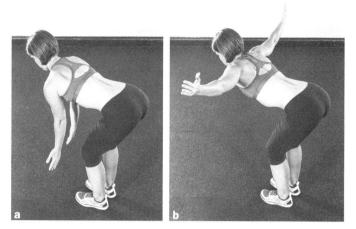

Coaching Tips

- Pause for one or two seconds at the top of each rep.
- The hip and back positioning of this exercise are virtually the same as for a Romanian deadlift; do not allow your back to round out at any point.

7. Crossover Jack

Setup

Stand with your feet slightly wider than hip-width apart and your arms straight out to your sides at shoulder level (see figure *a*).

Action

Simultaneously cross your arms in front of your chest and jump up just enough to cross one leg in front of the other (see figure *b*). Without pausing, quickly reverse the motion and return to the starting position. Repeat, crossing your other leg in front and crossing your opposite arm on top. Continue to switch your front leg and top arm on each rep; perform 20 to 25 total reps.

Coaching Tips

- Be as light on your feet as possible.
- Minimize the time that your feet are in contact with the ground.
- Perform the exercise in a smooth, coordinated fashion, moving your legs and arms simultaneously when opening and closing.

In-Place Warm-Up 4

This sequence includes the following exercises:

T-roll push-up	1 set × 4–6 reps each side
Arm circle	1 set × 10–12 reps clockwise 1 set × 10–12 reps counterclockwise
Rotational arm swing	1 set × 6–8 reps each side
Single-leg hip circle	1 set × 10–12 reps clockwise set × 10–12 reps counterclockwise
Zombie squat with reach-through	1 set × 6–8 reps each side
Jumping jack	1 set × 20–25 reps

1. T-Roll Push-Up

Setup

Assume a plank position with your hands just outside your shoulders and your feet shoulder-width apart (see figure a).

Action

Perform a push-up (see figure b). At the top position, rotate your entire body 90 degrees so you're positioned sideways to the ground, move your hips and shoulders at the same rate, and then reach your top arm toward the sky (see figure c). Roll back to the starting position and repeat on the other side. Perform 4 to 6 reps on each side.

Coaching Tips

- If it is difficult for you to perform a few push-ups, simply eliminate the push-up component of the exercise and perform only the T-roll while remaining in the starting plank position. Do not allow your head or hips to sag toward the floor.

- Rotate your hips and shoulders together and at the same rate each time that you go in and out of the T-roll.

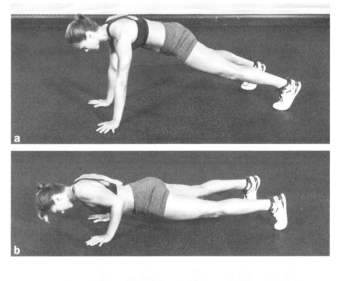

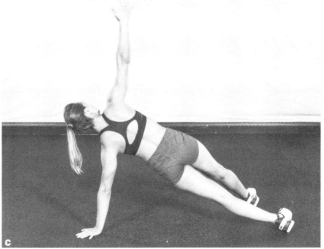

> continued

2. Arm Circle

Setup

Stand tall with your arms reaching above your head and your feet hip-width apart.

Action

Keeping your arms straight, swing your arms dynamically to make circles (see figure). Perform 10 to 12 clockwise rotations and 10 to 12 counterclockwise rotations.

Coaching Tips

- Make the biggest circles you can without any discomfort.
- The action should be smooth and rhythmic.
- Although your arms are straight, do no lock-out your elbows.

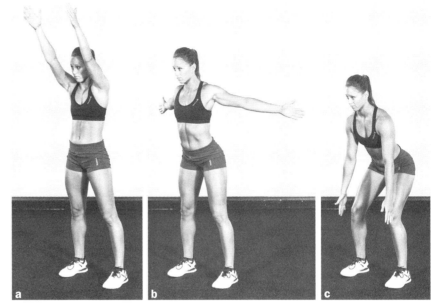

3. Rotational Arm Swing

Setup

Stand tall with your feet hip-width apart and reach your arms straight out in front of your shoulders (see figure *a*).

Action

Quickly rotate your torso to one side, driving both your left hip and your left arm behind you while allowing your other foot to rotate freely by elevating your heel and turning on the ball of your foot (see figure *b*). Return to the starting position and repeat the same motion to the other side. Make your motions fast and dynamic. Perform 6 to 8 reps on each side.

Coaching Tips

- To better allow your hips to rotate, raise your heel off of the ground as you turn.
- Rotate your hips and shoulder simultaneously, moving them at the same rate.

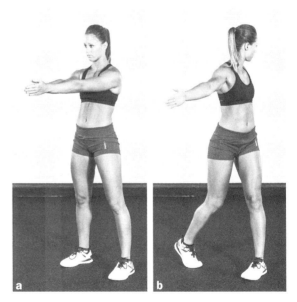

4. Single-Leg Hip Circle

Setup

Stand tall balancing on your right leg with your left knee bent around 90-degrees and your fingers interlaced behind your head and your elbows pointed out to the sides.

Action

While keeping your left knee bent, rotate at your left hip and move your left leg clockwise as far as you can for 10 to 12 rotations and then counterclockwise for 10 to 12 rotations (see figures a-c). Then switch legs and repeat.

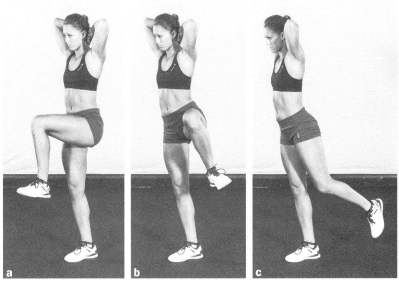

Coaching Tips

- Make the biggest circles you can without any discomfort.
- The action should be smooth and rhythmic.
- Try to keep your torso straight and your shoulders level with the ground throughout.

5. Zombie Squat With Reach-Through

Setup

Stand with your feet slightly farther than shoulder-width apart and your toes pointed slightly outward. Reach your arms through your legs, keeping your knees slightly bent (see figure a).

Action

As you bring your torso upright, simultaneously bend your hips and drop them into a squat. Finish with your arms outstretched in

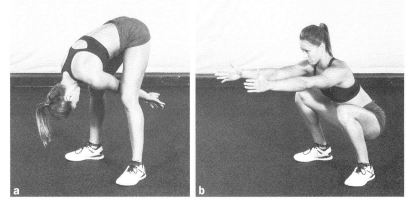

front of you at shoulder level (see figure b). Reverse to return to the starting position. Perform 6 to 8 reps.

Coaching Tips

- Squat as deep as you can on each rep.
- Keep your heels flat on the floor and do not allow your knees to drop toward the midline as you squat.
- For a slightly more advanced variation, perform the exercise in the same manner but place your arms overhead, in line with your torso, each time you drop into the squat.

> continued

6. *Jumping Jack*

Setup

Stand with your feet together and your hands at your sides (see figure *a*).

Action

As you raise your arms above your head, jump up just enough to spread your feet wide (see figure *b*). Without pausing, quickly reverse the movement. Perform 20 to 25 reps.

Coaching Tips

- Be as light on your feet as possible.
- Minimize the time that your feet are in contact with the ground.
- Perform the exercise in a smooth, coordinated fashion, moving your legs and arms simultaneously when opening or closing.

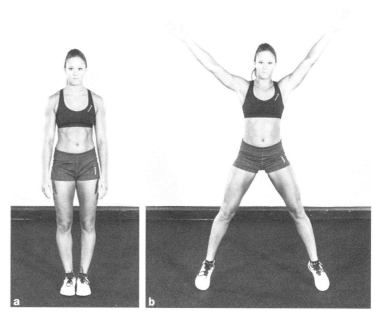

Large-Space Warm-Ups

The following warm-up sequences don't call for any special equipment, but they do require at least 20 yards of space for locomotion exercises. Use one of these sequences for training variety or for sessions when you have plenty of space to move around in.

Large-Space Warm-Up 1

This sequence includes the following exercises:

Traveling knee hug	1 set × 15–20 yards
Reverse lunge with posterior reach	1 set × 15–20 yards
Lateral hip shift with shuffle	1 set × 15–20 yards each direction
Arm-circle skip	1 set × 15–20 yards each direction
Lateral shuffle with arm crossover	1 set × 15–20 yards each direction
Carioca	1 set × 15–20 yards each direction
Alligator crawl	1 set × 15–20 yards

1. Traveling Knee Hug

Setup

Stand tall with your feet hip-width apart and your hands by your sides.

Action

Take a step forward with your left foot and lift your right knee above your hips. Grab your leg just below the knee and lightly hug your leg into your body as you lift your knee a bit more (see figure). Place your right leg down on the floor, stepping forward with it. Repeat on the other leg. Perform in alternating fashion for 15 to 20 yards.

Coaching Tips

- Walk three small-stride steps between one knee hug and the next; since three is an odd number, you'll alternate legs with each knee hug.
- Keep your torso upright throughout.
- Bring your knee up to your arms rather than reaching your arms down to grab your leg.

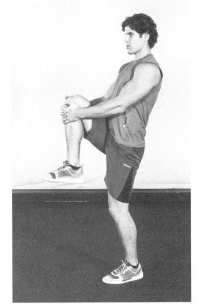

2. Reverse Lunge With Posterior Reach

Setup

Stand tall with your feet together and your arms by your sides.

Action

Step backward with one leg, dropping into a lunge while reaching your arms overhead and leaning your torso slightly backward (see figure a). Stand back up tall while bringing your front leg backward to meet your back leg and stepping backward with the front leg from the previous rep (see figures b and c). Perform for 15 to 20 total yards.

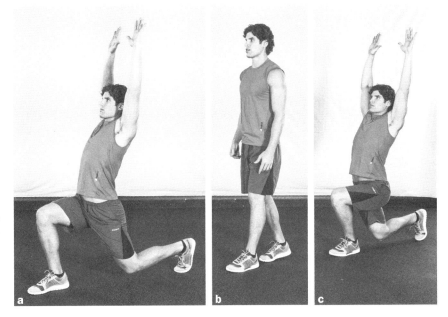

Coaching Tips

- Walk three small-stride steps between one lunge and the next; since three is an odd number, you'll alternate legs with each lunge.
- Do not overstretch when leaning backward; reach your arms and extend backward only slightly—just enough to get a stretch without forcing yourself into discomfort.

> continued

3. Lateral Hip Shift With Shuffle

Setup

Stand with your feet about 4 feet (1.2 m) apart, your feet pointed forward, and your arms extended in front of you at shoulder level.

Action

Shift your hips toward your right side and lower your hips (see figure a). Then, while staying low, shift your weight to your left (see figure b). Once all of your weight is on your left, shuffle to your right by explosively pushing your left foot into the ground and take a sideways step (to the right) with your left leg and then quickly take a sideways step to the right with your right leg while allowing your feet to slightly leave the ground (see figure c). Return to the original stance and repeat by continuing to move to your right in this manner for 15 to 20 yards. Then reverse the motion and travel 15 to 20 yards in the opposite direction.

Coaching Tips

- The sequence is shift, shift, shuffle.
- If you're moving down the room to your right, start each rep by shifting your hips to the right.
- Your feet should remain parallel with one another, with the toes facing forward, as you shift and shuffle.
- Stay light on your feet on each shuffle.

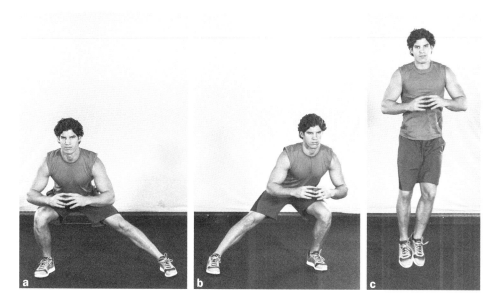

4. Arm-Circle Skip

Setup

Stay tall with your feet hip-width part and your arms above your head. Lift your right knee to a point just above your hip.

Action

Skip forward while making forward circles with both arms (see figures *a-d*). As with jumping rope, skipping requires a double-foot strike pattern, or right-right hops followed by left-left hops. Once you've traveled 15 to 20 yards, skip backward while making backward arm circles for another 15 to 20 yards.

Coaching Tips

- Coordinate your arm circles with your double-foot strikes.
- Keep your torso upright throughout.

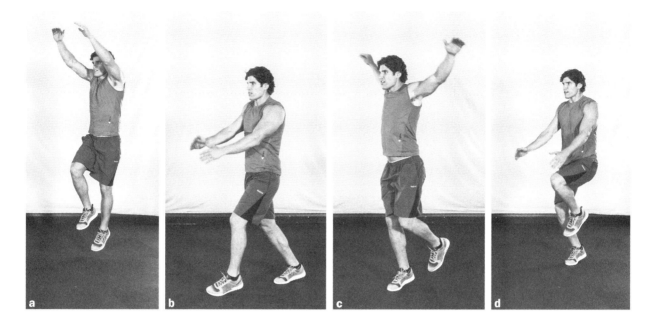

5. Lateral Shuffle With Arm Crossover

Setup

Stand tall with your knees slightly bent and your arms crossed in front of your torso with your elbows slightly bent (see figure *a*).

Action

Shuffle to your right by shifting your weight onto your left foot and explosively pushing your left foot into the ground and take a sideways step (to the right) with your left leg and then quickly take a sideways step to the right with your right leg while allowing your feet to slightly leave the ground. Continue to move to your right in this manner; picking up your right foot and placing it to the right while pushing your left foot into the ground to generate force and momentum for the sideways movement. Meanwhile, cross your arms and open them out to your sides (see figures *b-d*). Reverse direction by shuffling left, back to the starting point. Move 15 to 20 yards in each direction.

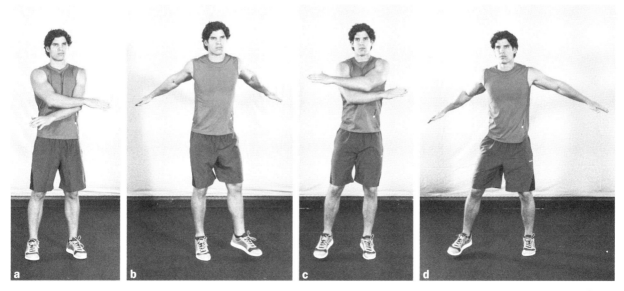

> *continued*

Coaching Tips

- Your feet should remain fairly parallel to one another, with the toes facing forward, as you shuffle.
- Stay light on your feet.
- Coordinate your arm swings with your strides in a smooth, rhythmic fashion.

6. Carioca

Setup

Start in an athletic ready position with your feet a little farther than hip-distance apart and your knees soft.

Action

Use your left foot to push off, crossing it in front of your right foot and transferring your weight onto it (see figure *a*). Move your right foot to the side until you're back to your starting stance (see figure *b*). Now cross your left foot over and move your right foot to the side (see figure *c*). Continue moving to your right, crossing your left foot behind

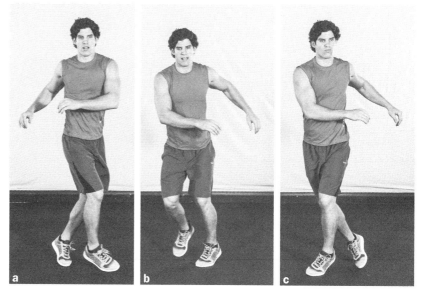

and then in front, until you have traveled 15 to 20 yards. Then reverse direction and travel another 15 to 20 yards.

Coaching Tips

- Face the same direction in traveling both ways.
- Stay light on your feet.
- Allow your hips to rotate as you keep your shoulders facing fairly straight ahead.

7. Alligator Crawl

Setup

Assume a push-up position with your feet shoulder-width apart and your hands underneath your shoulders. Bend your elbows slightly and lower your chest slightly toward the ground.

Action

Reach forward with your right arm as you bring your left knee to your left elbow (see figure *a*). Then perform a mirror-image movement by reaching your left arm out in front, extending your left leg, and bringing your right knee to your right elbow (see figures *b* and *c*). Continue this alternating crawling action until you've traveled 15 to 20 yards.

Coaching Tips

- Allow your trailing leg to fully extend on each step.
- Your hips should shift and roll a bit toward the side of your extended arm.

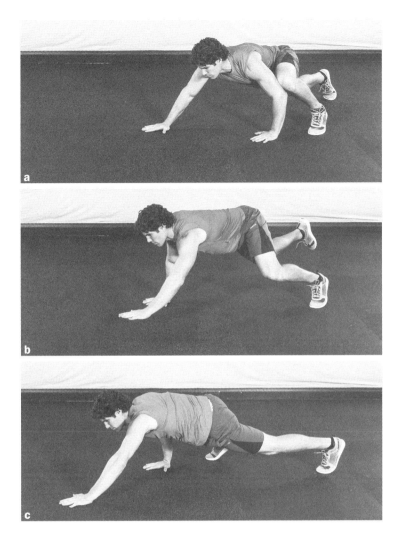

Large-Space Warm-Up 2

This sequence includes the following exercises:

High kick	1 set × 15–20 yards
Backward long-stride run	1 set × 15–20 yards
Forward traveling lunge with twist	1 set × 15–20 yards
Backward one-leg Romanian deadlift with floor touch	1 set × 15–20 yards
Traveling crossover lunge	1 set × 15–20 yards each direction
Hip-opener skip	1 set × 15–20 yards each direction
Low lateral shuffle	1 set × 15–20 yards each direction
Spider crawl	1 set × 10 yards each direction

> *continued*

1. High Kick

Setup

Stand tall with your feet hip-width apart and your arms by your sides.

Action

Begin walking forward as you kick your right leg up toward the sky, keeping your knee slightly bent; simultaneously, reach your left arm out in front of you at shoulder level (see figure *a*). Continue walking forward, alternating legs and using the opposite-side arm with each kick (see figures *b* and *c*). Continue in this alternating manner for 15 to 20 yards.

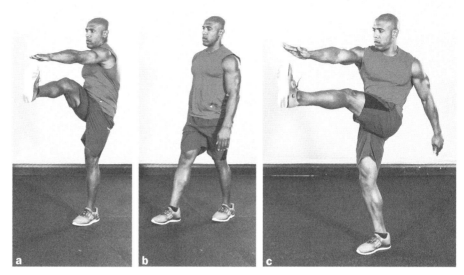

Coaching Tips

- Walk three small-stride steps between one high kick and the next; since three is an odd number, you end up alternating legs with each kick.
- Keep your torso upright throughout.
- Keep your ankle flexed as you kick.

2. Backward Long-Stride Run

Setup

Face away from the area into which you'll be running. Assume an athletic ready position with your feet hip-width apart, your knees bent, and your hips slightly flexed.

Action

Taking long strides, run backward for 15 to 20 yards while pumping your arms (see figures *a-c*).

Coaching Tips

- Run in a smooth, athletic manner and coordinate your arm pumping with your stride.
- Take the longest strides you can without losing rhythm or feeling out of control.

3. Forward Traveling Lunge With Twist

Setup

Stand tall with your feet hip-width apart, your fingers hooked in front of your chest, and your elbows pointed out to your sides (see figure *a*).

Action

Take a large step forward and drop your body so that your back knee lightly touches the floor. As you step, rotate your torso to the same side as your stepping leg (see figure *b*). Stand back up tall while bringing your rear leg forward to meet your front leg and returning your torso to a forward-facing position (see figure *c*). Repeat by stepping forward with the opposite leg (the one that was behind you on the last rep) and rotating toward that side (see figure *d*). Repeat in alternating fashion as you move down the room for 15 to 20 yards.

Coaching Tips

- At the bottom of each lunge, it is okay to use a slight forward torso lean—with a straight spine—instead of an upright torso to make the exercise a bit easier on your knees (the slight forward lean helps recruit your glutes).

- When rotating, you can use the arm on the same side as your forward leg to slightly pull your torso.

- Walk three small-stride steps between one lunge and the next; since three is an odd number, you end up alternating legs with each lunge.

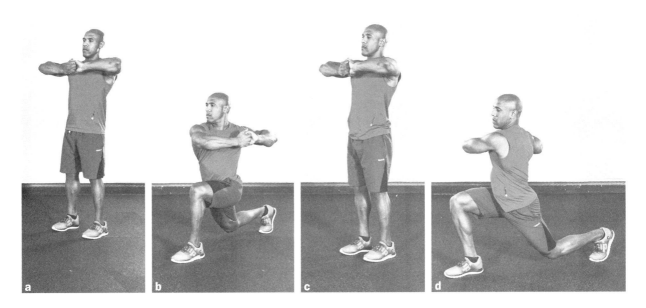

4. Backward One-Leg Romanian Deadlift With Floor Reach

Setup

Stand tall with your feet hip-width apart and your arms by your sides (see figure *a*).

Action

Hinge at your hip and lift one leg while bending forward toward the floor, keeping your weight-bearing knee bent at a 15- to 20-degree angle. As you hinge, allow your non-weight-bearing leg to elevate so that it remains in a fairly straight line with your torso (see figure *b*). Once the tips of your fingers touch the floor, or once you can't go down any farther, stand back up tall, place your non-weight-bearing leg on the ground behind you, and walk backward three steps. Repeat the sequence while balancing on your other leg. Alternate legs as you move backward down the room for 15 to 20 yards.

> *continued*

Coaching Tips

- Outwalk three small-stride steps between one lunge and the next; since three is an odd number, you end up alternating legs with each lunge.

- Keep your back (non-weight-bearing) foot pointed down toward the floor as you hinge at your hip and reach your arms down.

- Your back leg should rise as your torso lowers, thus creating a motion like that of a seesaw.

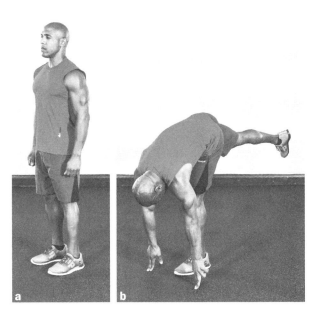

5. Traveling Crossover Lunge

Setup

Stand in a staggered stance with your left leg in front of your right leg and your arms straight in front of you (see figure *a*).

Action

Step your left leg in and across your right leg and lower your right knee toward the floor (see figures *b* and *c*). Push off with your left foot to stand as you step your right leg laterally and repeat the lunge (see figure *d*). Continue this action to move to your right across the floor. Then switch your stance and reverse direction by leading with your right leg across your left leg. Move 15 to 20 yards in each direction.

Coaching Tips

- Size your steps properly (not too big) so that you can get in and out of the lunge with deliberate control.

- Keep your front foot flat on the floor as you drop into each lunge.

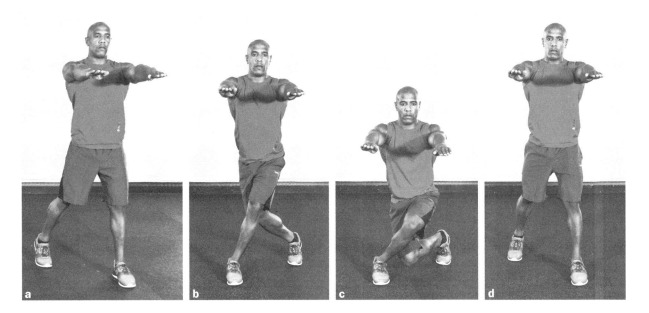

6. Hip-Opener Skip

Setup

Stand tall with your feet hip-width apart and your elbows bent roughly 90 degrees.

Action

As in rope jumping, skipping requires a double-foot strike pattern, or right-right hops followed by left-left hops. In doing so, lift your left knee out to the side just above your hip (see figure *a*). Drive your left leg toward the midline of your body, rotating your hips as if you're closing a gate (see figure *b*). Quickly drive your left leg down to the ground while elevating your right knee out to the side above your right hip. Continue this action forward with your legs following an out-to-in pattern. Once you've traveled 15 to 20 yards, reverse the action by moving backward, with your legs following an in-to-out pattern, for another 15 to 20 yards.

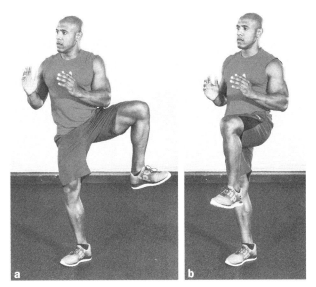

Coaching Tips

- Remain light on your feet.
- Keep your torso upright throughout.

7. Low Lateral Shuffle

Setup

Assume an athletic ready position with your feet hip-width apart, your knees bent, your weight back, and your hips flexed.

Action

Shuffle to your right by shifting your weight onto your left foot and explosively pushing your left foot into the ground. Take a sideways step (to the right)

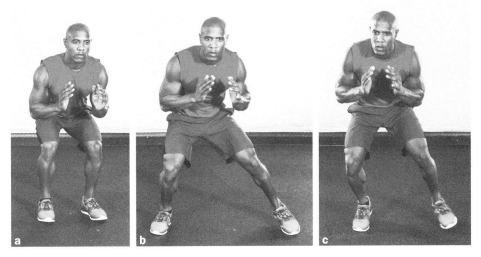

with your left leg and then quickly take a sideways step to the right with your right leg while allowing your feet to slightly leave the ground (see figures *a-c*). Continue to move to your right in this manner; picking up your right foot and placing it to the right while pushing your left foot into the ground to generate force and momentum for the sideways movement. Then reverse direction and shuffle back to the starting point. Move 15 to 20 yards to the right and 15 to 20 yards back to the left.

Coaching Tips

- Your feet should remain parallel to one another with the toes facing forward.
- Stay as light on your feet as possible.
- Do not allow the insides of your feet to touch as you shuffle.

> continued

8. Spider Crawl

Setup

Assume a push-up position with your feet together and your hands just farther than shoulder-width apart (see figure *a*).

Action

Move laterally to your right by stepping your right leg out to the side and crossing your left hand over your right (see figures *b* and *c*). Continue moving to the right for 10 yards by moving your legs apart and then together while stepping your arms apart and then crossed. Reverse the motion to move in the opposite direction for another 10 yards.

Coaching Tips

- Cross your hands but not your legs as you move laterally.
- Don't let your body—from your hips to your head—sag toward the floor.
- Do not lift your rear end any higher than your shoulders.

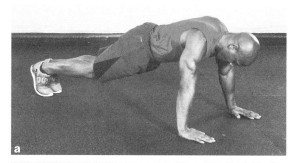

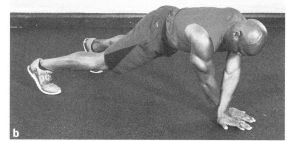

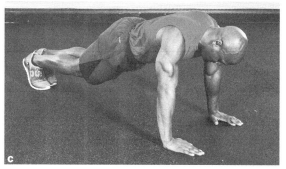

Medicine-Ball Warm-Ups

The following warm-up sequences use a medicine ball weighing about 4.5 to 6.5 pounds (2 to 3 kg). Because they're designed to keep you in place, they require little space. Select one of these sequences to add variety to your training or to use when space is limited.

Medicine-Ball Warm-Up 1

This sequence includes the following exercises:

Perform 2 rounds with 30 sec. of rest between rounds.	
Medicine-ball rotation	15–20 reps each side
Medicine-ball diagonal chop	10–12 reps each side
Medicine-ball lateral ribbon lunge	6–8 reps each side
Medicine-ball prisoner squat swing combo (behind the head)	10–12 reps

1. Medicine-Ball Rotation

Setup

Stand tall while holding the medicine ball at chest height with your feet slightly wider than shoulder-width apart and your arms extended in front of you (see figure *a*).

Action

Rotate your torso to the right side while raising your left heel off of the ground and rotating on the ball of your foot as you turn (see figure *b*). Quickly reverse the motion and repeat on the other side. Continue moving dynamically until you've performed 15 to 20 reps on each side.

Coaching Tips

- Do not pause at any time during this exercise; move fast while using deliberate control.
- Your nonrotating foot should point fairly straight ahead on each rep.
- Rotate your hips and shoulders together, at the same rate, while looking straight ahead.

2. Medicine-Ball Diagonal Chop

Setup

Stand with your feet hip-width apart. Slightly bend at the knees and rotate your hips and torso to the left by pivoting on the ball of your right foot while holding the medicine ball outside of your left knee (see figure *a*).

Action

Stand up as you rotate your torso to the right side while raising your left heel off of the ground and driving the medicine ball across your body, finishing with it outside of your right shoulder and above eye level (see figure *b*). Quickly reverse the action, driving the ball down at the same angle until you return to the starting position. Perform all reps on this side, then repeat on the other side.

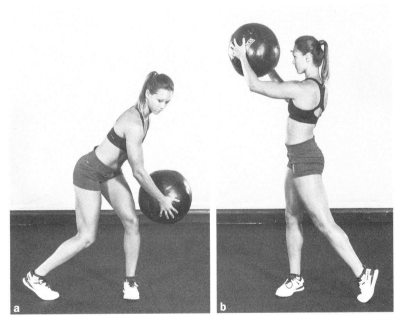

Coaching Tips

- Perform this exercise in a smooth, rhythmic fashion, coordinating your upper body and lower body in the lifting and lowering phases of each repetition.
- Keep your elbows slightly bent throughout.
- Shift your weight to the same side as the ball.

> *continued*

3. Medicine-Ball Lateral Ribbon Lunge

Setup

Stand with your feet positioned about a yard (or a little more) apart. Keeping your left leg straight and both feet flat on the floor, shift your weight onto your right leg while slightly bending your right knee and sitting back at your hips, while holding the ball in front of your right shin (see figure a and the inset).

Action

Push your left foot into the ground and step your right foot towards the midline of your body and place it down so your feet are now hip width apart. As you step in, simultaneously swing the ball in circular motion to the left (see figure b). Continue swinging the ball until it's overhead (see figure c). Repeat by stepping out laterally with your left leg as you swing the ball out to your left shin, then reverse the motion, once again finishing with the ball overhead. Continue to alternate side; perform 6 to 8 reps on each side.

Coaching Tips

- This exercise involves moving the ball in a ribbon-shaped pattern, with the round portion of the loop occurring as you swing the ball overhead; the "X" of the ribbon occurring each time you swing the ball across your torso; and each end of the ribbon ending at the bottom of each lunge.
- Do not allow your back to round out at the bottom of each lunge.
- Keep your feet flat on the floor throughout.
- Perform the exercise smoothly with good rhythm and timing in your arm movement and stepping.

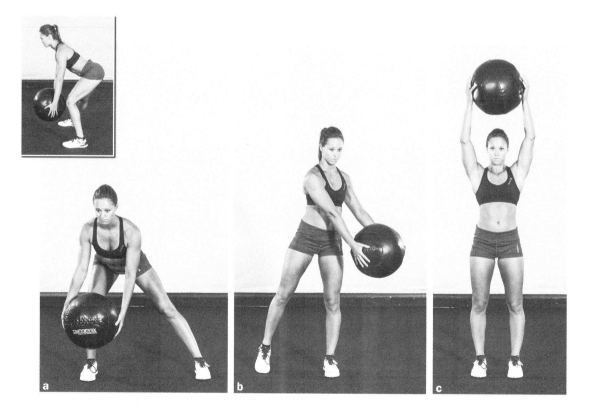

4. Medicine-Ball Prisoner Squat Swing Combo

Setup

Stand tall with your feet shoulder-width apart and your toes turned out about 10 degrees. Hold the medicine ball behind your head with your elbows pointing out to the sides.

Action

Perform a squat by bending your knees and sitting back at your hips (see figure *a*); go as low as you can. As you rise out of the squat, lift the ball from behind your head and perform a swing by driving it between your legs as if hiking a football (see figures *b* and *c*). Hinge forward at your hips, keeping your knees bent at roughly a 15- to 20-degree angle. Reverse the motion by swinging the ball back up and replacing it behind your head to complete one rep. Perform 10 to 12 reps.

Coaching Tips

- As you squat, do not allow your heels to come off of the ground or your knees to come together toward the midline of your body.
- Do not allow your back to round out at any point.

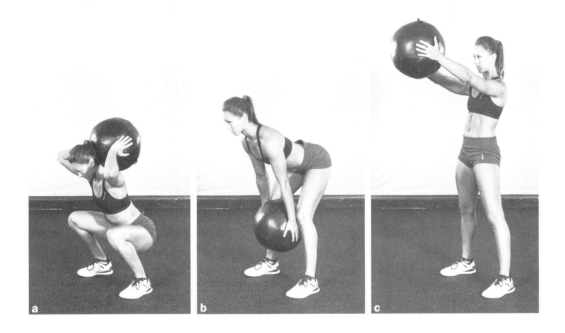

Medicine-Ball Warm-Up 2

This sequence includes the following exercises:

Perform 2 rounds with 30 secs. of rest between rounds.	
Medicine-ball swing	12–14 reps
Medicine-ball U swing	6–8 reps each side
Medicine-ball reverse lunge with twist	6–8 reps each side
Medicine-ball hip-shift squat	6–8 reps each side

> continued

1. Medicine-Ball Swing

Setup

With your feet roughly hip-width apart, hold a medicine ball with both hands with your arms straight and in front of your body.

Action

Hinge forward at your hips, keeping your knees bent at roughly a 15- to 20-degree angle. Drive the medicine ball between your legs as if hiking a football (see figure *a*). Once your forearms come into contact with your thighs, quickly reverse the motion by simultaneously driving your hips forward and swinging the medicine ball upward (see figure *b*). Finish with the ball at eye-level, then reverse the motion to complete one rep. Perform 12 to 14 reps.

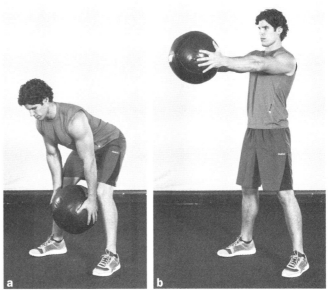

Coaching Tips

- Perform this exercise in a smooth, rhythmic fashion, coordinating your upper body and lower body in the lifting and lowering phases of each repetition.
- Do not allow your back to round out at the bottom of each rep.
- Perform the exercise in dynamic fashion without pausing at any point.

2. Medicine-Ball U Swing

Setup

Assume an athletic stance with your feet shoulder-width apart and your hips and knees bent while holding the medicine ball between your legs (see figure *a*).

Action

Keeping your arms straight, drive the medicine ball upward as you rotate your hips and shoulders to the right and extend your legs as you pivot on the ball of your left foot (see figure *b*). Quickly reverse the motion by swinging the ball back down to the middle of your legs, then continue to swing it in a U-shaped fashion and finish with it on your left side. Perform 6 to 8 reps on each side.

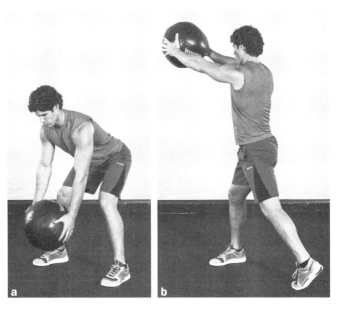

Coaching Tips

- Perform this exercise in a smooth, rhythmic fashion, coordinating your upper body and lower body in the lifting and lowering phases of each repetition.
- Do not allow your back to round out at the bottom of each rep.
- Perform this exercise in a dynamic fashion without pausing at any point.
- To better allow your hips to rotate, raise the heel (of your trailing leg) off of the ground as you turn and pivot your foot in the same direction you're swinging the ball.

3. Medicine-Ball Reverse Lunge With Twist

Setup

Stand with your feet hip-width apart and hold the medicine ball at your chest (see figure a).

Action

Step backward with your right foot and drop your body so that your knee lightly touches the floor as you rotate your torso to the left (see figure b). Reverse the movement by coming out of the lunge and bringing your right foot forward so that you are back to the starting position with your torso facing forward. Perform the same movement with the other leg while turning to the other side. Continue to alternate sides; perform 6 to 8 reps on each side.

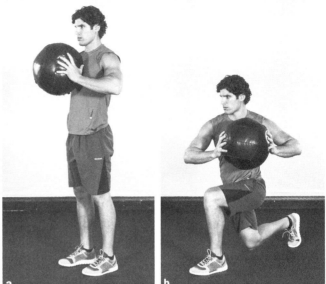

Coaching Tips

- Perform this exercise in a smooth, rhythmic fashion, coordinating your upper body and lower body in the lifting and lowering phases of each repetition.

- Keep your head facing forward throughout; in other words, your shoulders rotate, but your head does not. This technique keeps you from getting dizzy and helps maintain range of motion in your neck.

4. Medicine-Ball Hip-Shift Squat

Setup

Stand with your feet hip-width apart and hold the medicine ball at your chest (see figure a).

Action

Bend your knees and sit your hips back roughly 45 degrees to your left as you reach the medicine ball out at shoulder level 45 degrees to the right (see figure b). Reverse the motion and return to the middle. Repeat on the other side. Perform 6 to 8 reps on each side (12 to 16 total reps).

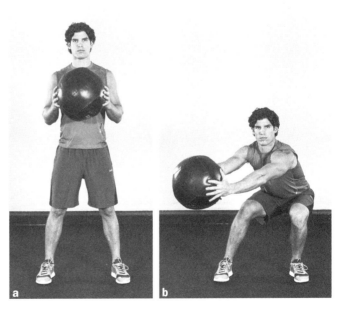

Coaching Tips

- As you stand up out of each squat, pull the ball back in to your chest.

- Use a range of motion that you can perform with good control and without discomfort.

- Focus not on squat depth but on shifting your hips.

> continued

Cool-Down

The functional-spectrum training system uses self-massage techniques as cool-down activities to help you feel looser and more relaxed after intense strength and conditioning training, such as the workouts provided in the following chapters. Self-massage can be performed with a foam roller, a rubber medicine ball, or (for smaller, more targeted areas) a tennis ball.

Because self-massage can improve joint flexibility and range of motion, some people use it at the beginning of a workout as a "pre-warm-up" before moving into a dynamic warm-up. This approach is fine if you prefer it. The recommendation here, however, is to use self-massage at the end of your workouts because, as a form of massage, it relaxes you and therefore helps you transition from intense activity to more normal activity. In contrast, the warm-up sequences provided in this chapter not only enhance your working range of motion but also get your body and mind ready for action.

Before addressing self-massage for specific areas of the body, here are a few guidelines to hold in mind:

- Roll the length of the muscle group you're massaging (up and down) 15 to 20 times; if you prefer to think in terms of time, roll each area for 30 to 40 seconds.

- Start by placing the ball or roller in the middle of the area you're going to massage and work out from there.

- Tenderness (mild discomfort) is okay, but avoid painful spots.

- Apply only an amount of pressure that allows you to remain relaxed and maintain a normal breathing rate.

- Do not roll an injured or inflamed area (e.g., one suffering from tendonitis).

You certainly don't have to roll every single body area addressed in the following sections after every workout. After any given workout, simply pick a few areas that you feel need to be targeted. In addition, if you think self-massage would help you feel better in an area of your body that isn't mentioned in this chapter, simply place a tennis ball on that spot and go to town. Just keep in mind the guidelines in the preceding list—especially the one about avoiding inflamed areas, because rolling on them could increase the irritation.

Self-Massage: Feet

Setup

Place most of your weight on your right leg with a tennis ball underneath the center of your left foot.

Action

Roll the ball up and down the length of the bottom of your foot (see figure). Perform 15 to 20 rolls on each foot. Finish all rolls on one foot before switching to the other.

Coaching Tips

- Hold onto something for added balance if needed.
- To increase massage pressure, place more weight on the tennis ball.

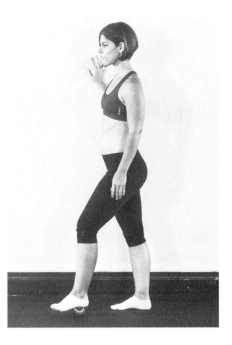

Self-Massage: Calves

Setup

Sit with your legs outstretched and your right leg crossed over your left leg with a foam roller underneath the center of your left calf.

Action

Slightly lift your hips off of the ground and use your arms to move your left calf over the roller; use your top (right) leg to add some pressure (see figure). Perform 15 to 20 rolls on each side and finish all rolls on one calf before switching to the other.

Coaching Tips

- Begin with the roller underneath the center of your calf.
- To reduce the massage pressure, uncross your legs and place both calves on the roller.

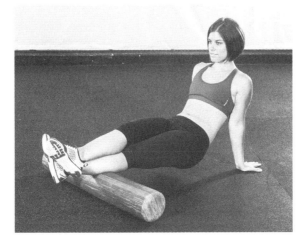

Self-Massage: Midback

Setup

Lie on your back on a foam roller positioned underneath your midback and cross your arms on top of your chest.

Action

With your hips lifted slightly off of the ground, use your legs to move the roller up and down your midback, or thoracic spine (see figure). Perform 15 to 20 rolls.

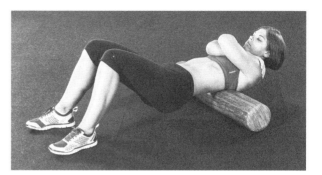

Coaching Tips

- Roll from the bottom of your ribs to just below your shoulder level.
- If you need additional neck support, interlace your fingers behind your head and keep your elbows pointed toward the ceiling.

Self-Massage: Lats

Setup

Lie on your left side with your left latissimus dorsi resting on the roller with the roller positioned a few inches below your armpit and your left arm outstretched above you with your left palm turned toward the sky. Bend your right knee slightly and place your right foot on the floor in-front of your left knee (see figure).

Action

Using your right leg to move you, roll up and down the muscle from few inches below your armpit to the bottom of your rib cage. Perform 15 to 20 rolls on each side. Finish all rolls on one side before switching to the other.

Coaching Tips

- Keep your torso fairly perpendicular to the floor as you roll.
- You can place your top hand on the floor in front of your torso (below the roller) for additional stability or to reduce the massage pressure.

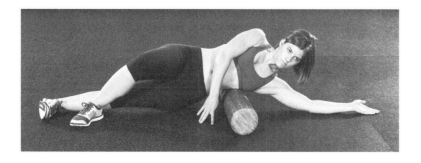

Self-Massage: Quads

Setup

Assume a prone position on your elbows with the center of your left thigh resting on top of the roller and your right knee bent away from your body.

Action

Use your arms to move your whole body, including your left thigh, up and down the roller (see figure). Perform 15 to 20 rolls on each side; finish all rolls on one side before switching to the other.

Coaching Tips

- Do not allow your belly to sag toward the floor at any point.
- To reduce the massage pressure, place more weight on your arms.

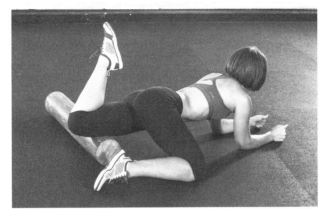

Self-Massage: Glutes

Setup

Sit on top of a foam roller or a medicine ball positioned underneath your left glute with your left hand on the floor behind you. Cross your left leg over your right leg (see figure).

Action

Roll across your entire left gluteal region. Once you've finished all rolls on the left side, switch sides, cross your legs the opposite way, and roll on the right glute. Perform 15 to 20 rolls on each side.

Coaching Tips

- To reduce the massage pressure, place more weight on your arms.
- If using a medicine ball, you can roll in a circular motion and focus on more targeted areas.

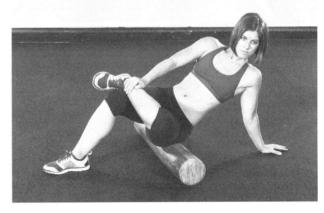

Self-Massage: Pectorals and Biceps

Setup

From a kneeling position with your legs spread, rest your right shoulder on top of a well-inflated rubber medicine ball. Position your right arm outstretched to the side and your left hand on the floor to provide light support.

Action

Roll the ball horizontally across your right arm, from your biceps to your right pectoral area (see figure). After completing all rolls on your right side, switch to your left side; perform 15 to 20 rolls on each side.

Coaching Tips

- Keep your weight leaning into the ball.
- To reduce the massage pressure, shift some of your weight back onto your hips.
- Do not press into the ground with the arm on the side that you're massaging; instead, use your opposite arm (on the nonrolling side) for support.

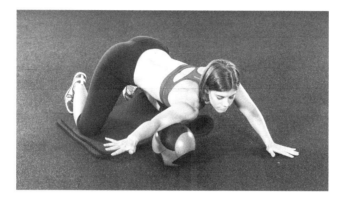

Now, let's dig into workout programming, beginning with programs that help you build the solid training foundation to safely and effectively use the functional-spectrum training system.

PART III

Workout Programs

9

Foundational Programming

As the title indicates, this chapter enables you to lay the foundation for the functional-spectrum workout programs presented in chapters 10, 11, and 12. Specifically, chapter 10 is dedicated to programs that emphasize performance improvement, chapter 11 to programs that emphasize muscle building, and chapter 12 to workouts that address both performance and muscle without emphasizing one over the other. So, whatever your goal—maximizing muscle, performance, or both—the workout programs provided in this book have plenty to offer you.

Regardless of which program you use, each workout includes exercise applications for each of the three S's of the functional-spectrum training system: speed, strength, and size. The exercise applications for each of these categories are demanding and therefore *not* designed to be used without first building a solid training foundation. In other words, training smart means using smart progression to build a training foundation by gradually increasing the intensity of your workouts to ensure that you continually improve (i.e., progress) with much less risk of injury or overtraining.

That's where the workout programs provided in this chapter come in. They help you build a training foundation to ensure that your body is ready to safely perform the more intense workouts using the three S's. So, regardless of which of the three following chapters you use, it is smartest and safest to start with the progressive workout programs provided in this chapter.

Foundational Workout Program Guidelines

Each of the four workout programs provided in this chapter is broken into phases of gradually increasing intensity. Each training phase builds the foundation needed to more safely and effectively perform the next phase. This progressive method of training gives you the foundation needed to get the most out of performing functional-spectrum workout programs, which, as you've learned, involve a mixture of fitness demands.

Each phase of the training presented here consists of two workouts: workout A and workout B. You alternate workouts and perform them for a combined total of two, three, or four times per week—but no more than two days in a row, to allow for sufficient recovery since these are total-body workouts. Once you've performed each workout six times with the indicated set-and-rep progression, you're ready to move on to the next phase of training. For guidance in the setup of each phase, see table 9.1.

TABLE 9.1 **Weekly Training Frequency Chart**

Training frequency	Phase length	Weekly setup examples
2 × per week	6 weeks	**Example 1** Monday (A), Thursday (B) **Example 2** Tuesday (A), Saturday (B)
3 × per week	4 weeks	**Example 1** Week 1: Monday (A), Wednesday (B), Friday (A) Week 2: Monday (B), Wednesday (A), Friday (B) **Example 2** Week 1: Tuesday (A), Thursday (B), Saturday (A) Week 2: Tuesday (B), Thursday (A), Saturday (B)
4 × per week	3 weeks	**Example 1** Monday (A), Tuesday (B), Thursday (A), Friday or Saturday (B) **Example 2** Tuesday (A), Wednesday (B), Friday (A), Saturday or Sunday (B)

Foundational Workout Programs

The following programs develop your training foundation. Use them to ensure that your body is ready to safely and effectively perform the functional-spectrum workout programs provided in the next three chapters. The workouts are divided into four phases: break-in, muscle base, strength base, and power base. Begin with the appropriate phase for your current training level based on the descriptions accompanying the phase presentations.

First, a few key points regarding these workouts:

- Perform exercises categorized as *a* and *b* in pairs. Perform all indicated sets and reps for a given pair before moving on to the next exercise or pair.

- If necessary, rest a bit longer than indicated between sets in order to complete the designated number of reps with good control. This program emphasizes movement quality over quantity!

- Focus on the technique of each exercise and use deliberate control on each rep.

- Before you begin your workout, perform one of the dynamic warm-up sequences of your choice (provided in chapter 8).

- To help you personalize these workouts to best fit you, refer to chapter 12.

Break-In Workout Program

If you're just starting out, or if it's been a while since you've done any strength training, I suggest that you perform the break-in workout program. If, on the other hand, you've been regularly using moderate levels of resistance training, you can begin with the next phase (muscle base), which is presented in the next section.

The main goal of this phase, as its name suggests, is to familiarize your body with the demands of performing basic exercises—primarily, to help your brain learn how to engage your muscles more efficiently as you progress through the early stages of the program. These neural adaptations often bring rapid strength improvements during this phase. However, even though neural adaptations are primarily responsible for increased strength in the early phases of training, research has also found that changes in muscle size are detectable within the first three or four weeks of resistance training (1, 2).

Your primary focus in this training phase is not to reach full exercise fatigue but to improve your exercise technique and your muscle awareness when performing the exercises. With this goal in mind, use a weight load that challenges you enough for the entire set but allows you to maintain good control and creates only mild muscle fatigue at the end of each set. In other words, choose a weight for each set that allows you to complete all indicated reps while still being capable of performing a few more (two or three) before you reach muscular failure.

TABLE 9.2 **Break-In Program: Workout A**

Exercise sets*	Page	Day 1	Day 2	Day 3	Day 4	Day 5	Day 6
1a. Reverse lunge	35	2 × 8 each side	2 × 9 each side	2 × 10 each side	2 × 12 each side	3 × 8 each side	3 × 10 each side
1b. One-arm cable row	114	2 × 10 each side	2 × 12 each side	2 × 14 each side	3 × 10 each side	3 × 12 each side	3 × 14 or 15 each side
2a. Barbell Romanian deadlift	156	2 × 10	2 × 12	2 × 14	3 × 10	3 × 12	3 × 14 or 15
2b. Heavy-band step and press	96	2 × 18	2 × 20	2 × 22	2 × 24	3 × 22	3 × 24
3a. Shoulder Y	218	2 × 10	2 × 12	2 × 14 or 15	3 × 10	3 × 12	3 × 14 or 15
3b. Cable triceps rope extension	101	2 × 10	2 × 12	2 × 14 or 15	3 × 10	3 × 12	3 × 14 or 15
4a. One-leg dumbbell bench hip thrust	177	2 × 10–12 each side	2 × 12–14 each side	2 × 15 each side	3 × 10–12 each side	3 × 12–14 each side	3 × 14 or 15 each side
4b. Stability-ball rollout	204	2 × 8–10 reps	2 × 8–10 reps	2 × 11 or 12 reps	3 × 11 or 12 reps	3 × 13–15 reps	3 × 13–15 reps

*Rest 60 to 90 seconds between paired sets.

TABLE 9.3 **Break-In Program: Workout B**

Exercise sets*	Page	Day 1	Day 2	Day 3	Day 4	Day 5	Day 6
1a. Dumbbell anterior lunge	172	2 × 8 each side	2 × 9 each side	2 × 10 each side	2 × 12 each side	3 × 8 each side	3 × 10 each side
1b. Push-up**	92	2 × 8–10	2 × 10–12	2 × 12–15	2 × 15	3 × 15	3 × 15–20
2a. Goblet squat	164	2 × 10	2 × 12	2 × 14	3 × 10	3 × 12	3 × 14 or 15
2b. Lat pull-down	121	2 × 10	2 × 12	2 × 14	3 × 10	3 × 12	3 × 14 or 15
3a. Shoulder T	226	2 × 10	2 × 12	2 × 14 or 15	3 × 10	3 × 12	3 × 14 or 15
3b. Dumbbell biceps curl	136	2 × 8	2 × 9	2 × 10	3 × 8	3 × 9	3 × 10
4a. Stability-ball leg curl	184	2 × 8–10	2 × 10–12	2 × 12–15	2 × 15	3 × 15	3 × 15–20
4b. Side elbow plank	210	2 × 10 sec. each side	2 × 12 sec. each side	2 × 14 or 15 sec. each side	2 × 14 or 15 sec. each side	3 × 15–17 sec. each side	3 × 17–20 sec. each side

*Rest for 60 to 90 seconds between paired sets.

**If needed, place your hands or feet on a bench to adjust the push-up to your ability level in order to perform the indicated number of reps.

Muscle-Base Workout Program

If you've finished the break-in program, or if you've been regularly using a moderate level of resistance training, then you're ready to use the muscle-base training program. If you've been regularly performing fairly intense resistance training, then you can begin with the strength-base workout program provided in the following section.

The primary goal of this phase is to add a fatigue element to your training. Doing so familiarizes your body with reaching muscular failure and achieving a muscle "pump" in order to focus on adding muscle tissue and increasing connective-tissue strength. So, unlike the break-in phase, this phase calls for you to use a weight load that allows you to achieve the indicated number of reps in each set—but no more.

In other words, at the end of each set, you should not be able to perform any more reps than indicated while maintaining proper control and technique. This approach is referred to as taking each set to "technical failure" because your muscle fatigue prevents you from maintaining proper technique. Be sure to maintain control in the eccentric (lowering) portion of each rep.

TABLE 9.4 **Muscle-Base Program: Workout A**

Exercise sets*	Page	Day 1	Day 2	Day 3	Day 4	Day 5	Day 6
1a. One-leg offset traveling lunge	154	3 × 7 each side	3 × 8 each side	3 × 9 each side	3 × 10 or 11 each side	3 × 11 or 12 each side	4 × 8–10 each side
1b. One-arm dumbbell bench row	114	3 × 8 each side	3 × 9 each side	3 × 10 each side	3 × 11 or 12 each side	3 × 12 or 13 each side	4 × 8–10 each side
2a. Barbell back squat	159	3 × 8	3 × 9	3 × 10	3 × 11 or 12	3 × 12 or 13	4 × 8–10
2b. Dumbbell biceps curl	136	3 × 8	3 × 9	3 × 10	3 × 11 or 12	3 × 12 or 13	4 × 8–10
3a. Lat pull-down	121	3 × 8	3 × 9	3 × 10	3 × 11 or 12	3 × 12 or 13	4 × 8–10
3b. Bent-over dumbbell shoulder fly	130	3 × 10	3 × 11	3 × 12	3 × 12–14	3 × 15	4 × 10–12
4a. High-to-low cable chop	199	3 × 8 each side	3 × 9 each side	3 × 10 each side	3 × 11 or 12 each side	3 × 12 or 13 each side	4 × 10–12 each side
4b. Rope face pull	134	3 × 10	3 × 11 or 12	3 × 12	3 × 12–14	3 × 15	4 × 10–12

*Rest for 60 to 90 seconds between paired sets.

TABLE 9.5 **Muscle-Base Program: Workout B**

Exercise sets*	Page	Day 1	Day 2	Day 3	Day 4	Day 5	Day 6
1a. One-leg one-arm dumbbell Romanian deadlift	149	3 × 8 each side	3 × 9 each side	3 × 10 each side	3 × 11 or 12 each side	3 × 12 or 13 each side	4 × 8–10 each side
1b. Barbell bench press	87	3 × 8	3 × 9	3 × 10	3 × 11 or 12	3 × 12 or 13	4 × 8–10
2a. 45-degree hip extension	182	3 × 10	3 × 11	3 × 12	3 × 12–14	3 × 15	4 × 10–12
2b. Dumbbell rotational shoulder press	81	3 × 7 each side	3 × 8 each side	3 × 9 each side	3 × 10 each side	3 × 10 each side	4 × 6–8 each side
3a. Cable triceps rope extension	101	3 × 10	3 × 11 or 12	3 × 12	3 × 12–14	3 × 15	4 × 10–12
3b. Cable compound straight-arm pull-down	135	3 × 10	3 × 11 or 12	3 × 12	3 × 12–14	3 × 15	4 × 10–12
4a. Dumbbell side shoulder raise	99	3 × 10	3 × 11 or 12	3 × 12	3 × 12–14	3 × 15	4 × 10–12
4b. Ab snail	210	3 × 5	3 × 6	3 × 7	3 × 8	3 × 8	4 × 8

*Rest for 60 to 90 seconds between paired sets.

Strength-Base Workout Program

If you've finished the muscle-base program, or if you've been regularly using bodybuilding-style training methods (methods similar to those featured in the muscle-base program), then you're ready to use the strength-base program. The primary goal of this phase is to familiarize your body with lifting heavier loads in order to increase motor unit recruitment and force output (i.e., strength). Therefore, your focus in this phase is to perform the concentric portion (the lift) of each exercise with maximal force. Still, as in the previous phase, be sure to maintain control in the eccentric (lowering) portion of each rep.

Also, as in the previous phase, at the end of each set you should not be able to perform any more reps than indicated while maintaining proper control and technique.

TABLE 9.6   Strength-Base Program: Workout A

Exercise sets*	Page	Day 1	Day 2	Day 3	Day 4	Day 5	Day 6
1a. Elevated barbell reverse lunge	163	4 × 3 or 4 each side	4 × 4 or 5 each side	4 × 5 or 6 each side	4 × 5 or 6 each side	4 × 5 or 6 each side	5 × 3 or 4 each side
1b. Dumbbell plank row	197	3 × 5 each side	3 × 5 each side	3 × 6 each side	3 × 6 each side	3 × 7 each side	4 × 6 or 7 each side
2a. Lat pull-down	121	4 × 3 or 4	4 × 4 or 5	4 × 5 or 6	4 × 5 or 6	4 × 5 or 6	5 × 4 or 5
2b. One-leg knee-tap squat	166	3 × 6 each side	3 × 7 each side	3 × 8 each side	3 × 8–10 each side	3 × 8–10 each side	4 × 6–8 each side
3a. One-arm freestanding dumbbell row	112	4 × 3 or 4 each side	4 × 4 or 5 each side	4 × 5 or 6 each side	4 × 5 or 6 each side	4 × 5 or 6 each side	5 × 4 or 5 each side
3b. Barbell calf raise	188	3 × 8	3 × 9	3 × 10	3 × 11 or 12	3 × 12 or 13	4 × 8–10
4a. Cable compound straight-arm pull-down	135	3 × 10–12	3 × 12–14	3 × 12–14	3 × 15	4 × 10	4 × 10–12
4b. Cable biceps curl	137	3 × 10	3 × 11 or 12	3 × 12–14	3 × 15	4 × 10	4 × 10–12

*Rest for 90 seconds to 3 minutes between paired sets.

TABLE 9.7   Strength-Base Program: Workout B

Exercise sets*	Page	Day 1	Day 2	Day 3	Day 4	Day 5	Day 6
1a. Barbell sumo deadlift	157	4 × 3 or 4	4 × 4 or 5	4 × 5 or 6	4 × 5 or 6	4 × 5 or 6	5 × 4 or 5
1b. Arm walkout	208	3 × 5	3 × 6	3 × 7	3 × 8	3 × 8	4 × 8
2a. Dumbbell bench press	88	4 × 3 or 4	4 × 4 or 5	4 × 5 or 6	4 × 5 or 6	4 × 5 or 6	5 × 4 or 5
2b. One-leg hip lift	179	3 × 8 each side	3 × 9 each side	3 × 10 each side	3 × 11 or 12 each side	3 × 12 or 13 each side	4 × 8–10 each side
3a. Nordic hamstring curl	183	3 × 10–12	3 × 12–14	3 × 12–14	3 × 15	4 × 10	4 × 10–12
3b. One-arm dumbbell rotational push press	80	3 × 4 each side	3 × 4 each side	3 × 5 each side	3 × 5 each side	3 × 6 each side	4 × 5 or 6 each side
4a. Dumbbell front shoulder raise	99	3 × 10–12	3 × 12–14	3 × 12–14	3 × 15	4 × 10	4 × 10–12
4b. Suspension triceps skull crusher	101	3 × 10–12	3 × 12–14	3 × 12–14	3 × 15	4 × 10	4 × 10–12

*Rest for 90 seconds to 3 minutes between paired sets.

Power-Base Workout Program

If you've finished the strength-base program, or if you've been regularly lifting heavy loads, then you're ready to use the power-base training program. The primary goal of this phase is to familiarize your body with performing fast, explosive movements by improving your rate of force production (i.e., power). Remember: Power = strength × speed. Now that you've established muscular control in the break-in phase, added some new muscle and increased your connective-tissue strength in the muscle-base phase, and built on that foundation by increasing force production in the strength-base phase, you're ready to add the final component—improving the speed at which your muscles can produce force.

This workout program uses a training concept referred to as *contrast training*, which is easy to explain: Start with a set of heavy lifts (3 to 5 reps) and follow it immediately with an unloaded explosive exercise using the same movement pattern and roughly the same number of reps. Or, to make it even simpler: Perform loaded squats followed by body-weight jump squats; bench presses followed by clap push-ups; or pull-ups followed by medicine-ball rainbow slams.

Research has demonstrated that contrast training creates an effect known as *post-activation potentiation*, or PAP, in which a muscle's explosive capability is enhanced when it is forced to perform maximal or near-maximal contractions (3). Contrast training is used here, however, not just to increase your rate and quality of force development—thus potentially maximizing your explosive power for athletic performance—but also because it gives you a simple way to train strength and power simultaneously. In addition, the increased work volume can improve your overall work capacity, thus giving you an even more solid foundation to take on the functional-spectrum workout programs provided in the following chapters.

When using this workout program, perform the heavy-lift portion (i.e., the first exercise in each contrast pair) in the same manner as described in the strength-base phase. Perform the explosive portion (i.e., the second exercise in each contrast pair) as powerfully as you can.

It's important to note that not all paired sets in this workout program are contrast sets. When using the non-contrast training sets in this workout program, perform the exercises in the same manner as described in the muscle-base phase.

TABLE 9.8 **Power-Base Program: Workout A**

Exercise sets*	Page	Day 1	Day 2	Day 3	Day 4	Day 5	Day 6
1a. Broad jump	146	5 × 3	5 × 3	5 × 4	5 × 4	5 × 5	5 × 5
1b. Stability-ball pike rollout	206	4 × 6–10	4 × 6–10	4 × 10–12	4 × 10–12	4 × 12–15	4 × 12–15
2a. Elevated barbell reverse lunge	163	4 × 5 each side	4 × 5 each side	4 × 5 each side	5 × 5 each side	5 × 5 each side	5 × 5 each side
2b. Anterior-leaning lunge scissor jump	147	4 × 3 each side	4 × 4 each side	4 × 5 each side	5 × 4 or 5 each side	5 × 4 or 5 each side	5 × 4 or 5 each side
3a. Chin-up or lat pull-down (with underhand grip)	119, 121	4 × 2 or 3	4 × 2 or 3	4 × 3 or 4	5 × 2–4	5 × 2–5	5 × 4 or 5
3b. Medicine-ball rainbow slam	105	4 × 5 each side	4 × 5 each side	4 × 6 each side	5 × 6 each side	5 × 6 each side	5 × 6 each side
4. One-arm compound cable row**	116	3 × 10–12 each side	3 × 12–14 each side	3 × 15 each side	4 × 8–10 each side	4 × 10–12 each side	4 × 10–12 each side
5a. Low-to-high cable chop	198	3 × 10–12 each side	3 × 12–14 each side	3 × 15 each side	4 × 8–10 each side	4 × 10–12 each side	4 × 10–12 each side
5b. Rope face pull	134	3 × 10–12	3 × 12–14	3 × 15	4 × 8–10	4 × 10–12	4 × 10–12

*Rest for 90 seconds to 3 minutes between paired sets.

**Rest for 60 to 90 seconds between sets.

TABLE 9.9 **Power-Base Program: Workout B**

Exercise sets*	Page	Day 1	Day 2	Day 3	Day 4	Day 5	Day 6
1a. Dumbbell high pull	107	5 × 3	5 × 3	5 × 4	5 × 4	5 × 5	5 × 5
1b. Leg lowering with band	212	4 × 6–10	4 × 6–10	4 × 10–12	4 × 10–12	4 × 12–15	4 × 12–15
2a. Barbell hybrid dead-lift	158	4 × 3–5	4 × 3–5	4 × 3–5	5 × 2–4	5 × 3–5	5 × 3–5
2b. Deadlift jump with arm drive	145	4 × 5	4 × 5	4 × 6	5 × 6	5 × 6	5 × 6
3a. Barbell bench press	87	4 × 3–5	4 × 3–5	4 × 3–5	5 × 2–4	5 × 3–5	5 × 3–5
3b. Clap push-up	94	4 × 5	4 × 5	4 × 6	5 × 6	5 × 6	5 × 6
4. Angled bar-bell press**	82	3 × 10–12 each side	3 × 12–14 each side	3 × 15 each side	4 × 8–10 each side	4 × 10–12 each side	4 × 10–12 each side
5a. Machine seated ham-string curl	186	3 × 10–12	3 × 12–14	3 × 15	4 × 8–10	4 × 10–12	4 × 10–12
5b. Plate chop	200	3 × 6–8 each side	3 × 8–10 each side	3 × 8–10 each side	4 × 10–12 each side	3 × 12–14 each side	3 × 15 each side

*Rest for 90 seconds to 3 minutes between paired sets.

**Rest for 60 to 90 seconds between sets.

You now understand the importance of possessing a solid foundation in speed and power training, heavy strength training, and bodybuilding. You also know how to develop that foundation by using the systematic training progression provided in this chapter. Implementing this approach prepares you to take on the demands of the functional-spectrum training workouts provided in the next three chapters.

10

Performance Programming

In chapter 2, I introduced you to the three S's of the functional-spectrum training system: speed, strength, and size. Every functional-spectrum workout program provided in this book includes a mixture of exercise applications to train each of the three S's. However, the amount of time that you spend on each S can be manipulated to maximize your improvements in your targeted areas.

The workout programs featured in this chapter focus on maximizing improvement in athletic performance. Since movement speed (i.e., explosiveness) and strength are critical components of athletic performance, the programs presented here include more exercise applications in the speed component than do the programs presented in the following two chapters. The programs included in this chapter also prioritize cross-body exercise applications since the body's X-factor relationships are also such a big part of athletic movement.

Performance Workout Program Guidelines

Each of the five functional-spectrum performance training programs presented here consists of three workouts: workout A, workout B, and workout C. Workout A focuses on pulling exercises, workout B focuses on lower-body and core exercises, and workout C focuses on pushing exercises.

You alternate workouts and perform them three, four, or five times per week depending on your preference and training schedule—but no more than three days in a row, to maximize recovery and minimize the risk of overtraining. I recommend training at least three times per week for best results. Perform the workouts in each program six times before moving on to a new program. Table 10.1 guides you in setting up your training based on the number of times you train per week.

TABLE 10.1   **Weekly Training Frequency Guide**

Training frequency	Program length	Weekly setup examples
3 × per week	6 weeks	Monday (A), Wednesday (B), Friday (C)
4 × per week	4.5 weeks	Week 1: Monday (A), Tuesday (B), Thursday (C), Friday or Saturday (A) Week 2: B, C, A, B Week 3: C, A, B, C Week 4: A, B, C, A Week 5: B, C
5 × per week	3.5 weeks	Week 1: Monday (A), Tuesday (B), Wednesday (C), Friday (A), Saturday (B) Week 2: C, A, B, C, A Week 3: B, C, A, B, C Week 4: A, B, C

What Strength and Conditioning Can and Can't Do

A good strength and conditioning workout helps you improve physical qualities that are not addressed by simply playing and practicing your sport, thus giving you the physical fitness to do what you need to do when you practice.

Of course, improving your physical fitness doesn't make you a winner if you lack the skills required to play your sport. But strength and conditioning do give you the physical fitness to do what you already know how to do. A good football player who is strong and fast in multiple directions is better than a good football player who is slow and relatively weak.

Performance Workout Programs

The functional-spectrum training system not only allows you to train both your hustle (performance) and your muscle (strength and size) but also can be adjusted easily to emphasize a particular aspect of training. The programs presented here focus on improving overall athleticism and functional capacity.

Here are a few key points to remember when performing the exercises:

Speed Exercises

- Perform each rep as explosively as possible.
- If the exercise involves jumping, land as quietly as possible.
- If the workout calls for throwing a medicine ball (outside or against a solid wall) and your training environment prevents you from doing so; simply choose an alternative, non-medicine ball exercise option from the Total-Body Power Exercises section of chapters 4 through 7. Perform the alternative exercise for roughly the same amount of sets and reps that were recommended for the original exercise.

Strength Exercises

- While maintaining optimal technique, perform the concentric lifting portion of each rep as forcefully as you can; during the eccentric (lowering) portion, maintain good control.

- Use a weight load that allows you to perform the indicated number of reps in the fashion described in the preceding point. In each workout, you ensure improvement in strength either by adding weight and performing the same number of reps as in the preceding workout or by performing more reps with the same weight.

Size Exercises

- Focus on the working muscles in each exercise and maintain strict form without "cheating" by using additional movements or momentum.

- Perform the concentric lifting portion of each rep at a normal tempo and maintain control during the eccentric (lowering) portion.

- The set and rep numbers used for exercises in this section are undulated with three schemes. Regardless of the scheme you're on, use a weight load that leaves you unable to perform any more reps than indicated while maintaining proper control and technique.

Cardio Conditioning

- If the workout calls for a particular supramaximal interval training (SMIT), steady-state cardio, or metabolic conditioning protocol (MCP) that your training environment prevents you from performing, simply choose a comparable alternative exercise from chapter 3. Perform the alternative exercise for roughly the same amount of reps, rounds, or time that were recommended for the original exercise.

- Only workouts A and C of each program involve a cardio conditioning component.

Performance Workout Programs (Three to Five Days Per Week)

In the following programs, perform *a*, *b*, and *c* exercises as tri-sets and perform *a* and *b* exercises as paired sets. Perform all indicated sets and reps in a given tri-set or paired set before moving on to the next set. If necessary, rest a bit longer than indicated between sets in order to complete the designated number of reps with good control. This program emphasizes movement quality over quantity!

Before you begin each workout in the following programs, be sure to perform one of the dynamic warm-up sequences (of your choice) provided in chapter 8. To help you personalize these workouts to *best* fit you, refer to chapter 12.

TABLE 10.2 **Performance Program 1: Workout A—Pulling**

	Page	Days 1 and 4	Days 2 and 5	Days 3 and 6
SPEED				
1a. Medicine-ball step and overhead throw (3–4 kg or 6.5–9 lbs.)	104	5 × 8	5 × 8	5 × 8
1b. Medicine-ball front-scoop horizontal throw (3–4 kg)	195	5 × 5 with 90 sec. rest between paired sets	5 × 5 with 90 sec. rest between paired sets	5 × 5 with 90 sec. rest between paired sets
2. 30-yard shuttle	142	4 or 5 sets with 60–90 sec. rest between sets	4 or 5 sets with 60–90 sec. rest between sets	4 or 5 sets with 60–90 sec. rest between sets
STRENGTH				
3. One-arm cable row	114	4 × 4–6 each side with 60–90 sec. rest between sets	4 × 4–6 each side with 60–90 sec. rest between sets	4 × 4–6 each side with 60–90 sec. rest between sets
SIZE				
4. Wide-grip seated row	126	3 × 10–12 with 60–90 sec. rest between sets	2 × 15–20 with 60–90 sec. rest between sets	4 × 6–8 with 60–90 sec. rest between sets
5a. Suspension biceps curl	138	3 × 10–12	2 × 15–20	4 × 6–8
5b. Bent-over dumbbell shoulder fly	130	3 × 10–12 with 60–90 sec. rest between paired sets	2 × 15–20 with 60–90 sec. rest between paired sets	4 × 6–8 with 60–90 sec. rest between paired sets
CARDIO CONDITIONING		MCP*: bilateral farmer's-walk complex (page 57)—2 or 3 sets with 2 min. rest between sets	Steady-state cardio on elliptical trainer (page 29) or upright bike (page 30) for 25–35 min.	SMIT**: shuttle run (page 25)—200 yd. × 5 or 6 with 2 min. rest between sets

*MCP = metabolic conditioning protocol.

**SMIT = supramaximal interval training.

TABLE 10.3 Performance Program 1: Workout B—Lower Body and Core

	Page	Days 1 and 4	Days 2 and 5	Days 3 and 6
SPEED				
1. 25-yard dash	141	× 5 or 6 with 60 sec. rest between sets	× 5 or 6 with 60 sec. rest between sets	× 5 or 6 with 60 rest sec. between sets
2. Squat jump with arm drive	144	5 × 4 or 5 with 90 sec. rest between sets	5 × 4 or 5 with 90 sec. rest between sets	5 × 4 or 5 with 90 sec. rest between sets
STRENGTH				
3a. Trap-bar squat	164	5 × 1–5	5 × 1–5	5 × 1–5
3b. Ab snail	210	4 × 5–8 with 2 min. rest between paired sets	4 × 5–8 with 2 min. rest between paired sets	4 × 5–8 with 2 min. rest between paired sets
SIZE				
4. One-leg one-arm dumbbell Romanian deadlift	149	2 × 15–20 each side with 60 sec. rest between sets	4 × 6–8 each side with 60 sec. rest between sets	3 × 10–12 each side with 60 sec. rest between sets
5a. Dumbbell plank row	197	2 × 14 or 15 each side	4 × 6–8 each side	3 × 10–12 each side
5b. Bench step-up	172	2 × 15–20 each side with 90 sec. rest between paired sets	4 × 6–8 each side with 90 sec. rest between paired sets	3 × 10–12 each side with 90 sec. rest between paired sets
6a. Leg lowering with band*	212	2 × 15–20	4 × 6–8	3 × 10–12
6b. 45-degree hip extension	182	2 × 15–20 with 90 sec. rest between paired sets	4 × 6–8 with 90 sec. rest between paired sets	3 × 10–12 with 90 sec. rest between paired sets

*There is an inverse relation between the amount of reps indicated and the resistance load of band you use or how far you extend your legs. Extend your legs the farthest you can control on the days you perform 6 to 8 reps or use the heaviest band, and use the lightest band or don't extend your legs out as far on the days you perform 15 to 20 reps.

TABLE 10.4 **Performance Program 1: Workout C—Pushing**

	Page	Days 1 and 4	Days 2 and 5	Days 3 and 6
SPEED				
1a. Medicine-ball vertical squat push throw (3–4 kg or 6.5–9 lbs.)	73	5 × 4 or 5	5 × 4 or 5	5 × 4 or 5
1b. Medicine-ball side-scoop diagonal throw (3–5 kg or 6.5–11 lbs.)	194	4 × 3 or 4 each side with 90 sec. rest between paired sets	4 × 3 or 4 each side with 90 sec. rest between paired sets	4 × 3 or 4 each side with 90 sec. rest between paired sets
2. 180-Degree squat jump with cross-arm drive	144	4 × 2 or 3 each side with 90 sec. rest between sets	4 × 2 or 3 each side with 90 sec. rest between sets	4 × 2 or 3 each side with 90 sec. rest between sets
STRENGTH				
3. Angled barbell rotational push press	83	4 × 4 or 5 each side with 90 sec. rest between sets	4 × 4 or 5 each side with 90 sec. rest between sets	4 × 4 or 5 each side with 90 sec. rest between sets
SIZE				
4. Box crossover push-up	86	4 × max (–2)* with 90 sec. rest between sets	3 × max (–1)* with 90 sec. rest between sets	2 × max with 90 sec. rest between sets
5a. Cable triceps rope extension	101	4 × 6–8	3 × 10–12	2 × 15–20
5b. Cable compound straight-arm pull-down	135	4 × 6–8 with 90 sec. rest between paired sets	3 × 10–12 with 90 sec. rest between paired sets	2 × 15–20 with 90 sec. rest between paired sets
CARDIO CONDITIONING		SMIT**: rower (page 28)—4–6 sets of 45–60 sec. as fast as possible with 90 sec. to 2 min. rest between sets	MCP***: Six-min. body-weight complex (page 32)—2 or 3 sets with 2 min. rest between sets	Steady-state cardio on elliptical trainer (page 29) or upright bike (page 30) for 25–35 min.

*(–1) means to stop the set one rep before failure; (–2) means to stop two reps before failure.

**SMIT = supramaximal interval training.

***MCP = metabolic conditioning protocol.

TABLE 10.5　Performance Program 2: Workout A—Pulling

	Page	Days 1 and 4	Days 2 and 5	Days 3 and 6
SPEED				
1a. Medicine-ball rainbow slam (3–4 kg or 6.5–9 lbs.)	105	5 × 3 or 4 each side	5 × 3 or 4 each side	5 × 3 or 4 each side
1b. Medicine-ball side-scoop diagonal throw (3–5 kg or 6.5 to 11 lbs.)	194	4 × 3 or 4 each side with 90 sec. rest between paired sets	4 × 3 or 4 each side with 90 sec. rest between paired sets	4 × 3 or 4 each side with 90 sec. rest between paired sets
2. Lateral bound	148	4 × 3 or 4 each side	4 × 3 or 4 each side	4 × 3 or 4 each side
STRENGTH				
3. One-arm freestanding dumbbell row	112	4 × 2–4 each side with 90 sec. between sets	4 × 2–4 each side with 90 sec. rest between sets	4 × 2–4 each side with 90 sec. rest between sets
SIZE				
4. Seated row	125	3 × 10–12 with 60–90 sec. rest between sets	2 × 15–20 with 60–90 sec. rest between sets	4 × 6–8 with 60–90 sec. rest between sets
5a. Cable biceps curl	137	3 × 10–12	2 × 15–20	4 × 6–8
5b. Rope face pull	134	3 × 10–12 with 60 sec. rest between paired sets	2 × 15–20 with 60 scc. rest between paired sets	4 × 6–8 with 60 sec. rest between paired sets
CARDIO CONDITIONING		MCP*: boxing and kickboxing with heavy bag (page 30)—4–6 2 min. rounds with 60 sec. rest between rounds	Steady-state cardio: brisk walking outside or on treadmill (page 29)—25–35 min.	SMIT**: gasser (page 26)—1–3 sets with 3 or 4 min. rest between sets

*MCP = metabolic conditioning protocol.

**SMIT = supramaximal interval training.

TABLE 10.6   **Performance Program 2: Workout B—Lower Body and Core**

	Page	Days 1 and 4	Days 2 and 5	Days 3 and 6
SPEED				
1. 30-yard shuttle	142	× 5 or 6 with 60–90 sec. rest between sets	× 5 or 6 with 60–90 sec. rest between sets	× 5 or 6 with 60–90 sec. rest between sets
2. Broad jump	146	5 × 3 with 90 sec. rest between sets	5 × 3 with 90 sec. rest between sets	5 × 3 with 90 sec. rest between sets
STRENGTH				
3a. Barbell hybrid dead-lift	158	5 × 2–4	5 × 2–4	5 × 2–4
3b. One-arm plank	201	4 × 15–20 secs. each side with 2 min. rest between paired sets	4 × 15–20 secs. each side with 2 min. rest between paired sets	4 × 15–20 secs. each side with 2 min. rest between paired sets
SIZE				
4a. Lateral lunge with cross-body reach	152	2 × 14 or 15 each side	4 × 6–8 each side	3 × 10–12 each side
4b. Stability-ball plate crunch	211	2 × 15–20 with 60–90 sec. rest between paired sets	4 × 6–8 with 60–90 sec. rest between paired sets	3 × 10–12 with 60–90 sec. rest between paired sets
5. Elevated barbell reverse lunge	163	2 × 14 or 15 each side with 90 sec. rest between sets	4 × 6–8 each side with 90 sec. rest between sets	3 × 10–12 each side with 90 sec. rest between sets
6a. Stability-ball abdominal exercise indicated	204, 206, 205	Stability-ball knee tuck 2 × 15–20	Stability-ball pike rollout 4 × 6–8	Stability-ball pike 3 × 10–12
6b. One-leg hip lift	179	2 × 15–20 each side with 60–90 sec. rest between paired sets	4 × 6–8 each side with 60–90 sec. rest between paired sets	3 × 10–12 each side with 60–90 sec. rest between paired sets

TABLE 10.7 Performance Program 2: Workout C—Pushing

	Page	Days 1 and 4	Days 2 and 5	Days 3 and 6
SPEED				
1a. Medicine-ball downward-chop throw (3–4 kg or 6.5 to 9 lbs.)	196	4 × 5 or 6 each side	4 × 5 or 6 each side	4 × 5 or 6 each side
1b. Power skip	142	4 × 8–10 each leg with 2 min. rest between paired sets	4 × 8–10 each leg with 2 min. rest between paired sets	4 × 8–10 each leg with 2 min. rest between paired sets
2. Angled barbell press and catch	78	4 × 4 or 5 each side with 90 sec. rest between sets	4 × 4 or 5 each side with 90 sec. rest between sets	4 × 4 or 5 each side with 90 sec. rest between sets
STRENGTH				
3. One-arm dumbbell rotational push press	80	4 × 2–4 each side with 2 min. rest between sets	4 × 2–4 each side with 2 min. rest between sets	4 × 2–4 each side with 2 min. rest between sets
SIZE				
4. Standing cable chest press	95	4 × 6–8 with 60 sec. rest between sets	3 × 10–12 with 60 sec. rest between sets	2 × 15–20 with 60 sec. rest between sets
5a. Cable triceps rope extension	101	4 × 6–8	3 × 10–12	2 × 15–20
5b. Push-up	92	4 × max (–2)* with 60 sec. rest between paired sets	3 × max (–1)* with 60 sec. rest between paired sets	2 × max with 60 sec. rest between paired sets
CARDIO CONDITIONING		SMIT**: treadmill (page 28)—× 5–7 sets running at top speed for 15–30 sec. with 60 sec. rest between sets	MCP***: unilateral leg complex (page 34)—× 1 or 2 sets with 2 min. rest between sets	Steady-state cardio: brisk walking outside or on treadmill (page 29)—25–35 min.

*(–1) means to stop the set one rep before failure; (–2) means to stop two reps before failure.

**SMIT = supramaximal interval training.

***MCP = metabolic conditioning protocol.

TABLE 10.8 Performance Program 3: Workout A—Pulling

	Page	Days 1 and 4	Days 2 and 5	Days 3 and 6
SPEED				
1a. Medicine-ball step and overhead throw (3–4 kg or 6.5–9 lbs.)	104	5 × 6–8	5 × 6–8	5 × 6–8
1b. Medicine-ball side-scoop horizontal throw (3–5 kg or 6.5–11 lbs.)	193	4 × 4 or 5 each side	4 × 4 or 5 each side	4 × 4 or 5 each side
1c. Power skip	142	5 × 8–10 each leg with 2 min. rest between tri-sets	5 × 8–10 each leg with 2 min. rest between tri-sets	5 × 8–10 each leg with 2 min. rest between tri-sets
STRENGTH				
2. One-arm compound cable row	116	4 × 5 or 6 each side with 90 sec. rest between sets	4 × 5 or 6 each side with 90 sec. rest between sets	4 × 5 or 6 each side with 90 sec. rest between sets
SIZE				
3a. Cable compound straight-arm pull-down	135	3 × 10–12	2 × 15–20	4 × 6–8
3b. Suspension row	127	3 × 10–12	2 × 15–20	4 × 6–8
3c. Suspension biceps curl	138	3 × 10–12 with 60–90 sec. rest between tri-sets	2 × 15–20 with 60–90 sec. rest between tri-sets	4 × 6–8 with 60–90 sec. rest between tri-sets
CARDIO CONDITIONING		MCP*: Six-min. body-weight complex (page 32)—2 or 3 sets with 2 min. rest between sets	Steady-state cardio on elliptical trainer or upright bike (page 29-30)—25–35 min.	SMIT**: rower (page 28)—4–6 sets of 45–60 sec. as fast as possible with 90 sec. to 2 min. rest between sets

*MCP = metabolic conditioning protocol.

**SMIT = supramaximal interval training.

TABLE 10.9 **Performance Program 3: Workout B—Lower Body and Core**

	Page	Days 1 and 4	Days 2 and 5	Days 3 and 6
SPEED				
1. Broad jump	146	5 × 3 or 4 with 90 sec. rest between sets	5 × 3 or 4 with 90 sec. rest between sets	5 × 3 or 4 with 90 sec. rest between sets
2. Anterior-leaning lunge scissor jump	147	4 × 2 or 3 each side with 90 sec. rest between sets	4 × 2 or 3 each side with 90 sec. rest between sets	4 × 2 or 3 each side with 90 sec. rest between sets
STRENGTH				
3a. Barbell hybrid dead-lift	158	4 × 3–5	4 × 3–5	4 × 3–5
3b. Stability-ball stir-the-pot	207	3 × 4–8 each direction with 2 min. rest between paired sets	3 × 4–8 each direction with 2 min. rest between paired sets	3 × 4–8 each direction with 2 min. rest between paired sets
SIZE				
4a. Angled barbell cross-shoulder reverse lunge	155	2 × 14 or 15 each side	4 × 6–8 each side	3 × 10–12 each side
4b. Angled barbell tight rainbow	202	2 × 15–20 each side with 90 sec. rest between paired sets	4 × 6–8 each side with 90 sec. rest between paired sets	3 × 10–12 each side with 90 sec. rest between paired sets
5a. Bulgarian split squat and Romanian dead-lift combination	168	2 × 14 or 15 each side	4 × 6–8 each side	3 × 10–12 each side
5b. Reverse crunch*	211	2 × 15–20 with 90 sec. rest between paired sets	4 × 6–8 with 90 sec. rest between paired sets	3 × 10–12 with 90 sec. rest between paired sets
6. One-leg dumbbell bench hip thrust	177	2 × 15–20 each side with 60 sec. rest between sets	4 × 6–8 each side with 60 sec. rest between sets	3 × 10–12 each side with 60 sec. rest between sets

*There is an inverse relation between the amount of reps indicated and the weight you'll use as an anchor, as the heavier the anchor the easier the exercise becomes. Use the lightest dumbbell, kettlebell, or medicine ball as an anchor on the days you perform 6 to 8 reps, and use the heaviest anchor on the days you perform 15 to 20 reps.

TABLE 10.10 **Performance Program 3: Workout C—Pushing**

	Page	Days 1 and 4	Days 2 and 5	Days 3 and 6
SPEED				
1a. Medicine-ball step and push throw (3 or 4 kg or 6.5–9 lbs.)	77	5 × 4–6	5 × 4–6	5 × 4–6
1b. Medicine-ball side-scoop horizontal throw (3–5kg or 6.5–11 lbs.)	193	4 × 4 or 5 each side with 90 sec. rest between paired sets	4 × 4 or 5 each side with 90 sec. rest between paired sets	4 × 4 or 5 each side with 90 sec. rest between paired sets
2. 180-degree squat jump with cross-arm drive	144	4 × 2 or 3 each side with 90 sec. rest between sets	4 × 2 or 3 each side with 90 sec. rest between sets	4 × 2 or 3 each side with 90 sec. rest between sets
STRENGTH				
3. One-arm push-up or angled barbell press	85, 82	4 × 1–5 or 4 × 3–6 each side with 90 sec. rest between sets	4 × 1–5 or 4 × 3–6 each side with 90 sec. rest between sets	4 × 1–5 or 4 × 3–6 each side with 90 sec. rest between sets
SIZE				
4. Incline barbell bench press	88	4 × 6–8 with 60–90 sec. rest between sets	3 × 10–12 with 60–90 sec. rest between sets	2 × 15–20 with 60–90 sec. rest between sets
5. Dumbbell overhead press	90	4 × 6–8 with 60–90 sec. rest between sets	3 × 10–12 with 60–90 sec. rest between sets	2 × 15–20 with 60–90 sec. rest between sets
6. Close-grip push-up	95	4 × max (−2)* with 2 min. rest between sets	3 × max (−1)* with 2 min. rest between sets	2 × max with 2 min. rest between sets
CARDIO CONDITIONING		SMIT**: shuttle run (page 25)—250 yd. × 4 or 5 with 2.5 min. rest between sets	MCP***: unilateral farmer's-walk complex (page 59)—2 or 3 sets with 2 min. rest between sets	Steady-state cardio on elliptical trainer or upright bike (page 29-30)—25–35 min.

*(−1) means to stop the set one rep before failure; (−2) means to stop two reps before failure.

**SMIT = supramaximal interval training.

***MCP = metabolic conditioning protocol.

TABLE 10.11 Performance Program 4: Workout A—Pulling

	Page	Days 1 and 4	Days 2 and 5	Days 3 and 6
SPEED				
1a. Anterior-leaning lunge scissor jump	147	5 × 3–5 each leg	5 × 3–5 each leg	5 × 3–5 each leg
1b. Medicine-ball side-scoop horizontal throw (3–5 kg or 6.5–11 lbs.)	193	5 × 4 or 5 each side with 2 min. rest between paired sets	5 × 4 or 5 each side with 2 min. rest between paired sets	5 × 4 or 5 each side with 2 min. rest between paired sets
2. Rope slam or medicine-ball rainbow slam (3–4 kg or 6.5–9 lbs.)	111, 105	4 × 10–12 or 4 × 6–8 each side with 90 sec. rest between sets	4 × 10–12 or 4 × 6–8 each side with 90 sec. rest between sets	4 × 10–12 or 4 × 6–8 each side with 90 sec. rest between sets
STRENGTH				
3. One-arm freestanding dumbbell row	112	4 × 2–4 each side with 90 sec. rest between sets	4 × 2–4 each side with 90 sec. rest between sets	4 × 2–4 each side with 90 sec. rest between sets
SIZE				
4. Lat pull-down	121	3 × 10–12 with 90 sec. rest between sets	2 × 15–20 with 90 sec. rest between sets	4 × 6–8 with 90 sec. rest between sets
5a. Dumbbell biceps curl	136	3 × 10–12	2 × 15–20	4 × 6–8
5b. Bent-over dumbbell shoulder fly	130	3 × 10–12 with 60 sec. rest between paired sets	2 × 15–20 with 60 sec. rest between paired sets	4 × 6–8 with 60 sec. rest between paired sets
CARDIO CONDITIONING		MCP*: Four-minute rope complex—2 or 3 sets with 2–3 min. rest between sets (page 47)	Steady-state cardio: brisk walking outside or on treadmill—25–35 min. (page 29)	SMIT**: treadmill—5–7 sets running at top speed for 15–30 secs. with 60 sec. rest between sets (page 28)

*MCP = metabolic conditioning protocol.

**SMIT = supramaximal interval training.

TABLE 10.12 Performance Program 4: Workout B—Lower Body and Core

	Page	Days 1 and 4	Days 2 and 5	Days 3 and 6
SPEED				
1. 25-yard dash	141	5–7 sets with 60 sec. rest between sets	5–7 sets with 60 sec. rest between sets	5–7 sets with 60 sec. rest between sets
2. Deadlift jump with arm drive	145	5 × 3–5 with 90 sec. rest per set	5 × 3–5 with 60 sec. rest per set	5 × 3–5 with 60 sec. rest per set
STRENGTH				
3a. Barbell sumo dead-lift	157	4 or 5 × 2–4	4 or 5 × 2–4	4 or 5 × 2–4
3b. Stability-ball pike rollout	206	3 or 4 × 8–12 with 2 min. rest between paired sets	3 or 4 × 8–12 with 2 min. rest between paired sets	3 or 4 × 8–12 with 2 min. rest between paired sets
SIZE				
4a. One-leg 45-degree cable Romanian deadlift	150	2 × 15–20 each side	4 × 6–8 each side	3 × 10–12 each side
4b. Stability-ball plate crunch	211	2 × 15–20 with 60–90 sec. rest between paired sets	4 × 6–8 with 60–90 sec. rest between paired sets	3 × 10–12 with 60–90 sec. rest between paired sets
5. Dumbbell fighter's lunge	170	2 × 14 or 15 each side with 90 sec. rest per set	4 × 6–8 each side with 90 sec. rest per set	3 × 10–12 each side with 90 sec. rest per set
6a. One-arm dumbbell farmer's walk	197	3 × 45 sec. each side	3 × 45 secs each side	3 × 45 sec. each side
6b. Leg-curl exercise variation indicated	184, 184, 178	Stability-ball leg curl 2 × 15–20 with 60–90 sec. rest between paired sets	One-leg stability-ball leg curl 4 × 6–8 with 60–90 sec. rest between paired sets	Hip thrust hamstring curl combo 3 × 10–12 with 60–90 sec. rest between paired sets

TABLE 10.13 Performance Program 4: Workout C—Pushing

	Page	Days 1 and 4	Days 2 and 5	Days 3 and 6
SPEED				
1a. Medicine-ball shot-put throw (3 or 4 kg or 6.5–9 lbs.)	192	4 × 3 or 4 each side	4 × 3 or 4 each side	4 × 3 or 4 each side
1b. Medicine-ball front-scoop horizontal throw (3–5 kg or 6.5–11 lbs.)	195	4 × 5 or 6 each side with 90 sec. rest between paired sets	4 × 5 or 6 each side with 90 sec. rest between paired sets	4 × 5 or 6 each side with 90 sec. rest between paired sets
2. Lateral bound	148	4 × 3 or 4 each side with 90 sec. rest between sets	4 × 3 or 4 each side with 90 sec. rest between sets	4 × 3 or 4 each side with 90 sec. rest between sets
STRENGTH				
3. One-arm dumbbell rotational push press	80	5 × 2 or 3 each side with 90 sec. rest between sets	5 × 2 or 3 each side with 90 sec. rest between sets	5 × 2 or 3 each side with 90 sec. rest between sets
SIZE				
4. Push-up lock-off	86	4 × max (–2)* each side with 90 sec. rest between sets	3 × max (–1)* each side with 90 sec. rest between sets	2 × max each side with 90 sec. rest between sets
5a. Bent-over dumbbell shoulder fly	130	4 × 6–8	3 × 10–12	2 × 15–20
5b. Dumbbell triceps skull crusher	100	4 × 6–8 with 60 sec. rest between paired sets	3 × 10–12 with 60 sec. rest between paired sets	2 × 15–20 with 60 sec. rest between paired sets
CARDIO CONDITIONING		SMIT**: gasser—1–3 with 3 or 4 min. rest between sets (page 26)	MCP***: 20-20-10-10 leg complex—2 or 3 sets with 2 min. rest between sets (page 37)	Steady-state cardio: brisk walking outside or on treadmill—25–35 min. (page 29)

*(–1) means to stop the set one rep before failure; (–2) means to stop two reps before failure.

**SMIT = supramaximal interval training.

***MCP = metabolic conditioning protocol.

TABLE 10.14   Performance Program 5: Workout A—Pulling

	Page	Days 1 and 4	Days 2 and 5	Days 3 and 6
SPEED				
1a. Medicine-ball horizontal punch throw (3 or 4 kg or 6.5–9 lbs.)	75	5 × 3 or 4 each side	5 × 3 or 4 each side	5 × 3 or 4 each side
1b. Medicine-ball rainbow slam (3 or 4 kg)	105	5 × 4 or 5 each side with 2 min. rest between paired sets	5 × 4 or 5 each side with 2 min. rest between paired sets	5 × 4 or 5 each side with 2 min. rest between paired sets
2. Lateral bound	148	4 × 4–6 each side with 60 sec. rest between sets	4 × 4–6 each side with 60 sec. rest between sets	4 × 4–6 each side with 60 sec. rest between sets
STRENGTH				
3. One-arm cable row	114	4 × 4–6 each side with 90 sec. rest between sets	4 × 4–6 each side with 90 sec. rest between sets	4 × 4–6 each side with 90 sec. rest between sets
SIZE				
4. Suspension row	127	3 × 10–12 with 60–90 sec. rest between sets	2 × 15–20 with 60–90 sec. rest between sets	4 × 6–8 with 60–90 sec. rest between sets
5. Cable compound straight-arm pull-down	135	3 × 10–12 with 60–90 sec. rest between sets	2 × 15–20 with 60–90 sec. rest between sets	4 × 6–8 with 60–90 sec. rest between sets
6. Suspension biceps curl	138	3 × 10–12 with 60–90 sec. rest between sets	2 × 15–20 with 60–90 sec. rest between sets	4 × 6–8 with 60–90 sec. rest between sets
CARDIO CONDITIONING		MCP*: weight-plate push—4–6 sets × 40–50 yds. with 90 sec. rest between sets (page 50)	Steady-state cardio on elliptical trainer or upright bike—25–35 min. (page 29-30)	SMIT**: shuttle run—2 or 3 × 300 yd. with 3 min. rest between sets (page 25)

*MCP = metabolic conditioning protocol.

**SMIT = supramaximal interval training.

TABLE 10.15 Performance Program 5: Workout B—Lower Body and Core

	Page	Days 1 and 4	Days 2 and 5	Days 3 and 6
SPEED				
1. Squat jump with arm drive	144	5 × 4 or 5 with 90 sec. rest between sets	5 × 4 or 5 with 90 sec. rest between sets	5 × 4 or 5 with 90 sec. rest between sets
2. Lateral power shuffle	143	4 × 5 or 6 each direction with 90 sec. rest between sets	4 × 5 or 6 each direction with 90 sec. rest between sets	4 × 5 or 6 each direction with 90 sec. rest between sets
STRENGTH				
3a. Barbell hybrid deadlift	158	5 × 2–4	5 × 2–4	5 × 2–4
3b. Leg lowering with band*	212	4 × 8–15 with 2 min. rest between paired sets	4 × 8–15 with 2 min. rest between paired sets	4 × 8–15 with 2 min. rest between paired sets
SIZE				
4a. One-leg offset traveling lunge	154	2 × 15–20 each side	4 × 6–8 each side	3 × 10–12 each side
4b. Rollout exercise variation indicated	204, 208, 208	Stability-ball rollout 2 × 15–20 with 60–90 sec. rest between paired sets	Medicine-ball walkout 4 × 6–8 with 60–90 sec. rest between paired sets	Arm walkout 3 × 10–12 with 60–90 sec. rest between paired sets
5a. Dumbbell anterior lunge	172	2 × 15–20 each side	4 × 6–8 each side	3 × 10–12 each side
5b. High-to-low cable chop	199	2 × 14 or 15 each side with 60–90 sec. rest between paired sets	4 × 6–8 each side with 60–90 sec. rest between paired sets	3 × 10–12 each side with 60–90 sec. rest between paired sets
6. Leg-curl exercise variation indicated	184, 178, 178	Stability-ball leg curl 2 × 15–20 with 60–90 sec. rest between sets	One-leg hip thrust hamstring curl combo 4 × 6–8 with 60–90 sec. rest between sets	Hip thrust hamstring curl combo 3 × 10–12 with 60–90 sec. rest between sets

*Use a heavier band or extend your legs farther as you lower them toward the floor.

TABLE 10.16 Performance Program 5: Workout C—Pushing

	Page	Days 1 and 4	Days 2 and 5	Days 3 and 6
SPEED				
1a. Power skip	142	5 × 8–10 each leg	5 × 8–10 each leg	5 × 8–10 each leg
1b. Medicine-ball side-scoop horizontal throw (3–5 kg or 6.5–11 lbs.)	193	5 × 5 or 6 each side with 2 min. rest between paired sets	5 × 5 or 6 each side with 2 min. rest between paired sets	5 × 5 or 6 each side with 2 min. rest between paired sets
2. One-arm dumbbell rotational push press	80	4 × 2 or 3 each side with 90 sec. rest between sets	4 × 2 or 3 each side with 90 sec. rest between sets	4 × 2 or 3 each side with 90 sec. rest between sets
STRENGTH				
3. Angled barbell press	82	4 × 2–5 each side with 90 sec. rest between sets	4 × 2–5 each side with 90 sec. rest between sets	4 × 2–5 each side with 90 sec. rest between sets
SIZE				
4. Close-grip push-up	95	4 × max (–2)* with 2 min. rest between sets	3 × max (–1)* with 2 min. rest between sets	2 × max with 2 min. rest between sets
5a. Dumbbell side shoulder raise	99	4 × 6–8	3 × 10–12	2 × 15–20
5b. Suspension triceps skull crusher	101	4 × 6–8 with 60–90 sec. rest between paired sets	3 × 10–12 with 60–90 sec. rest between paired sets	2 × 15–20 with 60–90 sec. rest between paired sets
CARDIO CONDITIONING		SMIT**: rower—4–6 sets of 45–60 sec. as fast as possible with 90 sec. to 2 min. rest between sets (page 28)	MCP***: boxing and kickboxing with heavy bag—3–5 3-min. rounds with 90 sec. rest between rounds (page 30)	Steady-state cardio on elliptical trainer or upright bike—25–35 min. (page 29-30)

*(–2) means to stop the set two reps before failure and (–1) means to stop the set one rep before failure.

**SMIT = supramaximal interval training.

***MCP = metabolic conditioning protocol.

Performance Workout Programs (Two Days Per Week)

Although I recommend training at least three times per week, you can still get positive results if your schedule allows only two training days per week. Designed to meet that need, the following programs are alternative versions of the programs provided in the preceding sections of the chapter.

Each of the following three programs consists of two workouts: workout A and workout B. Workout A focuses on pulling and pushing exercises, and workout B focuses on lower-body and core exercises. Perform the workouts in each program six times before moving on to a new program. In other words, if you're training twice per week, use the same program for six weeks before switching to the next program and performing that one for another six weeks, and so on.

In each of the following programs, workout B (lower body and core) is almost identical to the corresponding workout in the preceding sections, with the exception of an additional exercise application in the speed category. On the other hand, the version of workout A used in these programs is a combination of the corresponding workout A and workout C in the preceding sections. Therefore, although they feature exercises also found in the preceding sections, each workout A presented here involves performing several more exercises.

TABLE 10.17 **Two-Day Performance Program 1: Workout A—Pulling and Pushing**

	Page	Days 1 and 4	Days 2 and 5	Days 3 and 6
SPEED				
1a. Medicine-ball step and overhead throw (3 or 4 kg or 6.5–9 lbs.)	104	5 × 8	5 × 8	5 × 8
1b. Medicine-ball front-scoop horizontal throw (3–5 kg or 6.5–11 lbs.)	195	5 × 5 each side with 90 sec. rest between paired sets	5 × 5 each side with 90 sec. rest between paired sets	5 × 5 each side with 90 sec. rest between paired sets
2. 30-yard shuttle	142	4 or 5 sets with 45–60 sec. rest between sets	4 or 5 sets with 45–60 sec. rest between sets	4 or 5 sets with 45–60 sec. rest between sets
3. 180-Degree squat jump with cross-arm drive	144	4 × 2 or 3 each side with 90 sec. rest between sets	4 × 2 or 3 each side with 90 sec. rest between sets	4 × 2 or 3 each side with 90 sec. rest between sets
STRENGTH				
4a. One-arm cable row	114	4 × 4–6 each side	4 × 4–6 each side	4 × 4–6 each side
4b. Angled barbell rotational push press	83	4 × 4 or 5 each side with 2 min. rest between paired sets	4 × 4 or 5 each side with 2 min. rest between paired sets	4 × 4 or 5 each side with 2 min. rest between paired sets
SIZE				
5a. Wide-grip seated row	126	3 × 10–12	2 × 15–20	4 × 6–8
5b. Box crossover push-up	86	3 × max (−1)* with 60–90 sec. rest between paired sets	2 × max with 60–90 sec. rest between paired sets	4 × max (−2)* with 60–90 sec. rest between paired sets
6a. Suspension biceps curl	138	3 × 10–12	2 × 15–20	4 × 6–8
6b. Cable triceps rope extension	101	3 × 10–12 with 60–90 sec. rest between paired sets	2 × 15–20 with 60–90 sec. rest between paired sets	4 × 6–8 with 60–90 sec. rest between paired sets
7a. Bent-over dumbbell shoulder fly	130	3 × 10–12	2 × 15–20	4 × 6–8
7b. Cable compound straight-arm pull-down	135	3 × 10–12 with 60–90 sec. rest between paired sets	2 × 15–20 with 60–90 sec. rest between paired sets	4 × 6–8 with 60–90 sec. rest between paired sets
CARDIO CONDITIONING		MCP**: unilateral leg complex— × 1 or 2 sets with 2 min. rest between sets (page 34)	Steady-state cardio on elliptical trainer or upright bike— 25–35 min. (page 29-30)	SMIT***: shuttle run—4 or 5 × 250 yd. with 2.5 min. rest between sets (page 25)

*(−1) means to stop the set one rep before failure; (−2) means to stop two reps before failure.

**MCP = metabolic conditioning protocol.

***SMIT = supramaximal interval training.

TABLE 10.18   **Two-Day Performance Program 1: Workout B—Lower Body and Core**

	Page	Days 1 and 4	Days 2 and 5	Days 3 and 6
SPEED				
1. 25-yard dash	141	5 or 6 sets with 60 sec. rest between sets	5 or 6 sets with 60 sec. rest between sets	5 or 6 sets with 60 sec. rest between sets
2a. Squat jump with arm drive	144	5 × 4 or 5	5 × 4 or 5	5 × 4 or 5
2b. Medicine-ball side-scoop diagonal throw (3–5 kg or 6.5–11 lbs.)	194	4 × 3 or 4 each side with 90 sec. rest between paired sets	4 × 3 or 4 each side with 90 sec. rest between paired sets	4 × 3 or 4 each side with 90 sec. rest between paired sets
STRENGTH				
3a. Trap-bar squat	164	5 × 1–5	5 × 1–5	5 × 1–5
3b. Ab snail	210	4 × 5–8 with 2 min. rest between paired sets	4 × 5–8 with 2 min. rest between paired sets	4 × 5–8 with 2 min. rest between paired sets
SIZE				
4a. One-leg one-arm dumbbell Romanian deadlift	149	2 × 14 or 15 each side	4 × 6–8 each side	3 × 10–12 each side
4b. Dumbbell plank row	197	2 × 14 or 15 each side with 60–90 sec. rest between paired sets	4 × 6–8 each side with 60–90 sec. rest between paired sets	3 × 10–12 each side with 60–90 sec. rest between paired sets
5a. Bench step-up	172	2 × 15–20 each side	4 × 6–8 each side	3 × 10–12 each side
5b. Leg lowering with band*	212	2 × 15–20 with 60–90 sec. rest between paired sets	4 × 6–8 with 60–90 sec. rest between paired sets	3 × 10–12 with 60–90 sec. rest between paired sets
6. 45-degree hip extension	182	2 × 15–20 with 60–90 sec. rest between sets	4 × 6–8 with 60–90 sec. rest between sets	3 × 10–12 with 60–90 sec. rest between sets
CARDIO CONDITIONING		Steady-state cardio: brisk walking outside or on treadmill—25–35 min. (page 29)	SMIT**: rower—4–6 sets of 45–60 sec. as fast as possible with 90 sec. to 2 min. rest between sets (page 28)	MCP***: bilateral farmer's-walk complex—2 or 3 sets with 2 min. between sets (page 57)

*There is an inverse relation between the amount of reps indicated and the resistance load of band you use or how far you extend your legs. Extend your legs the farthest you can control on the days you perform 6 to 8 reps or use the heaviest band, and use the lightest band or don't extend your legs out as far on the days you perform 15 to 20 reps.

**SMIT = supramaximal interval training.

***MCP = metabolic conditioning protocol.

TABLE 10.19 Two-Day Performance Program 2: Workout A—Pulling and Pushing

	Page	Days 1 and 4	Days 2 and 5	Days 3 and 6
SPEED				
1a. Medicine-ball rainbow slam (3 or 4 kg or 6.5–9 lbs.)	105	5 × 3 or 4 each side	5 × 3 or 4 each side	5 × 3 or 4 each side
1b. Medicine-ball sidescoop horizontal throw (3 or 4 kg)	193	4 × 3 or 4 each side with 90 sec. rest between paired sets	4 × 3 or 4 each side with 90 sec. rest between paired sets	4 × 3 or 4 each side with 90 sec. rest between paired sets
2. Lateral bound	148	4 × 3 or 4 each side with 90 sec. rest between sets	4 × 3 or 4 each side with 90 sec. rest between sets	4 × 3 or 4 each side with 90 sec. rest between sets
3. Power skip	142	4 × 8–10 each leg with 60 sec. rest between sets	4 × 8–10 each leg with 60 sec. rest between sets	4 × 8–10 each leg with 60 sec. rest between sets
STRENGTH				
4a. One-arm freestanding dumbbell row	112	4 × 3–5 each side	4 × 3–5 each side	4 × 3–5 each side
4b. One-arm dumbbell rotational push press	80	4 × 3 or 4 each side with 90 sec. rest between paired sets	4 × 3 or 4 each side with 90 sec. rest between paired sets	4 × 3 or 4 each side with 90 sec. rest between paired sets
SIZE				
5a. Seated row	125	3 × 10–12	2 × 15–20	4 × 6–8
5b. Push-up	92	3 × max (–1)* with 90 sec. rest between sets	2 × max with 90 sec. rest between sets	4 × max (–2)* with 90 sec. rest between sets
6a. Standing cable chest press	95	4 × 6–8	3 × 10–12	2 × 15–20
6b. Dumbbell shoulder A	131	4 × 10 with 60 sec. rest between sets	3 × 13 with 60 sec. rest between sets	2 × 15 with 60 sec. rest between sets
7a. Suspension biceps curl	138	4 × 6–8	3 × 10–12	2 × 15–20
7b. Suspension triceps skull crusher	101	4 × 6–8 with 60 sec. rest between sets	3 × 10–12 with 60 sec. rest between sets	2 × 15–20 with 60 sec. rest between sets
CARDIO CONDITIONING		SMIT**: gasser—1–3 with 3–4 min. rest between sets (page 26)	MCP***: Six-min. body-weight complex—2 or 3 sets with 2 min. rest between sets (page 32)	Steady-state cardio: brisk walking outside or on treadmill—25–35 min. (page 29)

*(–1) means to stop the set one rep before failure; (–2) means to stop two reps before failure.

**SMIT = supramaximal interval training.

***MCP = metabolic conditioning protocol.

TABLE 10.20   **Two-Day Performance Program 2: Workout B—Lower Body and Core**

	Page	Days 1 and 4	Days 2 and 5	Days 3 and 6
SPEED				
1. 30-yard shuttle	142	5 or 6 sets with 1 min. rest between sets	5 or 6 sets with 1 min. rest between sets	5 or 6 sets with 1 min. rest between sets
2a. Broad jump	146	5 × 3	5 × 3	5 × 3
2b. Medicine-ball downward-chop throw (3 or 4 kg or 6.5–9 lbs.)	196	4 × 5 or 6 each side with 2 min. rest between paired sets	4 × 5 or 6 each side with 2 min. rest between paired sets	4 × 5 or 6 each side with 2 min. rest between paired sets
STRENGTH				
3a. Barbell hybrid deadlift	158	5 × 2–4	5 × 2–4	5 × 2–4
3b. One-arm plank	201	4 × 10–20 secs. each side with 2 min. rest between paired sets	4 × 10–20 secs. each side with 2 min. rest between paired sets	4 × 10–20 secs. each side with 2 min. rest between paired sets
SIZE				
4a. Lateral lunge with cross-body reach	152	2 × 14 or 15 each side	4 × 6–8 each side	3 × 10–12 each side
4b. Stability-ball plate crunch	211	2 × 15–20 with 60–90 sec. rest between paired sets	4 × 6–8 with 60–90 sec. rest between paired sets	3 × 10–12 with 60–90 sec. rest between paired sets
5a. Elevated barbell reverse lunge	163	2 × 14 or 15 each side	4 × 6–8 each side	3 × 10–12 each side
5b. Stability-ball abdominal exercise indicated	204, 206, 205	Stability-ball knee tuck 2 × 15–20 with 60–90 sec. rest between paired sets	Stability-ball pike rollout 4 × 6–8 with 60–90 sec. rest between paired sets	Stability-ball pike 3 × 10–12 with 60–90 sec. rest between paired sets
6. Leg curl exercise variation indicated	184, 184, 178	Stability-ball leg curl 2 × 15–20 with 60 sec. rest between sets	One-leg stability-ball leg curl 4 × 6–8 with 60 sec. rest between sets	Hip thrust hamstring curl combo 3 × 10–12 with 60 sec. rest between sets
CARDIO CONDITIONING		Steady-state cardio: elliptical trainer or upright bike—25–35 min. (page 29-30)	SMIT*: treadmill—5–7 sets running at top speed for 15–30 sec. with 60 sec. rest between sets (page 28)	MCP**: boxing and kickboxing with heavy bag—4–6 2-min. rounds with 60 sec. rest between rounds (page 30)

*SMIT = supramaximal interval training.

**MCP = metabolic conditioning protocol.

TABLE 10.21 **Two-Day Performance Program 3: Workout A—Pulling and Pushing**

	Page	Days 1 and 4	Days 2 and 5	Days 3 and 6
SPEED				
1a. Medicine-ball step and overhead throw (3 or 4 kg or 6.5–9 lbs.)	104	5 × 6–8	5 × 6–8	5 × 6–8
1b. Medicine-ball step and push throw (3 or 4 kg)	77	5 × 4–6 with 90 sec. rest between paired sets	5 × 4–6 with 90 sec. rest between paired sets	5 × 4–6 with 90 sec. rest between paired sets
2a. Medicine-ball front-scoop horizontal throw (3–5 kg or 6.5–11 lbs.)	195	4 × 4 or 5 each side	4 × 4 or 5 each side	4 × 4 or 5 each side
2b. Power skip	142	4 × 8–10 each leg with 90 sec. rest between paired sets	4 × 8–10 each leg with 90 sec. rest between paired sets	4 × 8–10 each leg with 90 sec. rest between paired sets
STRENGTH				
3a. One-arm compound cable row	116	4 × 3–5 each side	4 × 3–5 each side	4 × 3–5 each side
3b. One-arm push-up or one-arm cable press	85, 84	4 × 1–5 or 4 × 3–6 each side with 90 sec. rest paired sets	4 × 1–5 or 4 × 3–6 each side with 90 sec. rest paired sets	4 × 1–5 or 4 × 3–6 each side with 90 sec. rest paired sets
SIZE				
4a. Dumbbell overhead press	90	3 × 10–12	2 × 15–20	4 × 6–8
4b. Wide-elbow suspension row	128	3 × 10–12	2 × 15–20	4 × 6–8
4c. Suspension biceps curl	138	3 × 10–12 with 60–90 sec. rest between tri-sets	2 × 15–20 with 60–90 sec. rest between tri-sets	4 × 6–8 with 60–90 sec. rest between tri-sets
5a. Cable compound straight-arm pull-down	135	3 × 10–12	2 × 15–20	4 × 6–8
5b. Cable triceps rope extension	101	3 × 10–12 with 60 sec. rest between paired sets	2 × 15–20 with 60 sec. rest between paired sets	4 × 6–8 with 60 sec. rest between paired sets
CARDIO CONDITIONING		MCP*: 20-20-10-10 leg complex—2 or 3 sets with 2 min. rest between sets (page 37)	Steady-state cardio: elliptical trainer or upright bike—25–35 min. (page 29-30)	SMIT**: shuttle run—2 or 3 × 300 yd. with 3 min. rest between sets (page 25)

*MCP = metabolic conditioning protocol.

**SMIT = supramaximal interval training.

TABLE 10.22 **Two-Day Performance Program 3: Workout B—Lower Body and Core**

	Page	Days 1 and 4	Days 2 and 5	Days 3 and 6
SPEED				
1. Broad jump	146	5 × 3 or 4 with 90 sec. rest between sets	5 × 3 or 4 with 90 sec. rest between sets	5 × 3 or 4 with 90 sec. rest between sets
2a. Anterior-leaning lunge scissor jump	147	4 × 2 or 3 each leg	4 × 2 or 3 each leg	4 × 2 or 3 each leg
2b. Medicine-ball side-scoop horizontal throw (3–5 kg or 6.5–11 lbs.)	193	4 × 4 or 5 each side with 90 sec. rest between paired sets	4 × 4 or 5 each side with 90 sec. rest between paired sets	4 × 4 or 5 each side with 90 sec. rest between paired sets
STRENGTH				
3a. Barbell Romanian deadlift	156	4 × 3–5	4 × 3–5	4 × 3–5
3b. Stability-ball stir-the-pot	207	3 × 4–8 each direction with 90 sec. rest between paired sets	3 × 4–8 each direction with 90 sec. rest between paired sets	3 × 4–8 each direction with 90 sec. rest between paired sets
SIZE				
4a. Angled barbell cross-shoulder reverse lunge	155	2 × 14 or 15 each side	4 × 6–8 each side	3 × 10–12 each side
4b. Angled barbell tight rainbow	202	2 × 15–20 each side with 90 sec. rest between paired sets	4 × 6–8 each side with 90 sec. rest between paired sets	3 × 10–12 each side with 90 sec. rest between paired sets
5a. Bulgarian split squat and Romanian deadlift combination	168	2 × 12–14 each side	4 × 5–7 each side	3 × 8–10 each side
5b. Reverse crunch*	211	2 × 15–20 with 90 sec. rest between paired sets	4 × 6–8 with 90 sec. rest between paired sets	3 × 10–12 with 90 sec. rest between paired sets
6. One-leg dumbbell bench hip thrust	177	2 × 15–20 each side with 60 sec. rest between sets	4 × 6–8 each side with 60 sec. rest between sets	3 × 10–12 each side with 60 sec. rest between sets
CARDIO CONDITIONING		Steady-state cardio: brisk walking outside or on treadmill—25–35 min. (page 29)	SMIT**: rower—4–6 sets of 45–60 sec. as fast as possible with 90 sec. to 2 min. rest between sets (page 28)	MCP***: unilateral farmer's-walk complex—2 or 3 sets with 2 min. rest between sets (page 59)

*There is an inverse relation between the amount of reps indicated and the weight you'll use as an anchor, as the heavier the anchor the easier the exercise becomes. Use the lightest dumbbell, kettlebell, or medicine ball as an anchor on the days you perform 6 to 8 reps, and use the heaviest anchor on the days you perform 15 to 20 reps.

**SMIT = supramaximal interval training.

***MCP = metabolic conditioning protocol.

The workout programs provided in this chapter show you how to build muscle while *focusing* on improving your hustle. The emphasis of the workout programs presented in the next chapter is just the opposite—to help you work on your hustle while focusing on muscle gains.

11

Muscle Programming

The functional-spectrum workout programs featured in this chapter focus on helping you improve muscular development without neglecting athletic ability or functional capacity. Therefore, the programs presented here include more exercise applications in the size component than do the programs featured in chapters 10 and 12.

In addition, whereas the performance-oriented workout programs presented in chapter 10 focus on specific exercises, the muscle-oriented programs featured here prioritize general exercises. As a result, compound and isolation exercises are placed earlier in these workout programs and total-body power exercises and cross-body exercises later in the programs. Naturally, you bring more physical energy and mental focus to the exercises that you perform earlier in a workout than to those that you perform later, when you're physically (and mentally) fatigued. This reality is the reason that the functional-spectrum workout programs manipulate the order of exercise applications to train each of the three S's—speed, strength, and size—depending on the main training focus of choice.

Muscle Workout Program Guidelines

As with the performance training program featured in chapter 10, each of the five functional-spectrum training programs presented here consists of three workouts: workout A, workout B, and workout C. Workout A focuses on pulling exercises, workout B focuses on lower-body and core exercises, and workout C focuses on pushing exercises.

You alternate workouts and perform them three, four, or five times per week depending on your preference and training schedule—but no more than three days in a row to maximize recovery and minimize the risk of overtraining. I recommend training at least three times per week for best results. Perform the workouts in each program six times before moving on to a new program. Table 11.1 guides you in setting up your training based on the number of times you train per week.

TABLE 11.1 **Weekly Training Frequency Guide**

Training frequency	Program length	Weekly setup examples
3 × per week	6 weeks	Monday (A), Wednesday (B), Friday (C)
4 × per week	4.5 weeks	Week 1: Monday (A), Tuesday (B), Thursday (C), Friday or Saturday (A) Week 2: B, C, A, B Week 3: C, A, B, C Week 4: A, B, C, A Week 5: B, C
5 × per week	3.5 weeks	Week 1: Monday (A), Tuesday (B), Wednesday (C), Friday (A), Saturday (B) Week 2: C, A, B, C, A Week 3: B, C, A, B, C Week 4: A, B, C

Focusing on Your Muscle Without Losing Your Hustle

It's often said that performing size-oriented (i.e., bodybuilding) workouts causes you to lose functional performance ability. In reality, bodybuilding-type workouts do not directly cause you to lose athleticism; however, if you *only* do bodybuilding, then you're likely to lose athleticism because you're not using it.

In other words, you don't lose athletic ability if you're regularly doing athletic stuff! This is precisely why the functional-spectrum training workout programs provided in this chapter incorporate speed and power exercise applications, as well as some cross-body exercises. They provide you with that more athletic (i.e., specific) exercise component to ensure that you keep your hustle while focusing most of your effort on building muscle.

Muscle Workout Programs

The training focus of the programs provided in this chapter is the opposite of the programs provided in chapter 10. Therefore, although all of the functional-spectrum workout programs allow you to train both your hustle (performance) and your muscle (strength and size), the programs presented here focus on gaining muscle.

Here are a few key points to remember when performing the exercises:

Speed Exercises

- Perform each rep as explosively as possible.
- If the exercise involves jumping, land as quietly as possible.
- If the workout calls for throwing a medicine ball (outside or against a solid wall) and your training environment prevents you from doing so; simply choose an alternative, non-medicine ball exercise option from the Total-Body Power Exercises section of chapter 4 or 5. Perform the alternative exercise for roughly the same amount of sets and reps that were recommended for the original exercise.

Strength Exercises

- While maintaining optimal technique, perform the concentric lifting portion of each rep as forcefully as you can; during the eccentric (lowering) portion, maintain good control.
- Use a weight load that allows you to perform the indicated number of reps in the fashion described in the preceding point. In each workout, you ensure improvement in strength either by adding weight and performing the same number of reps as in the preceding workout or by performing more reps with the same weight.

Size Exercises

- Focus on the working muscles in each exercise and maintain strict form without "cheating" by using additional movements or momentum.
- Perform the concentric lifting portion of each exercise at a normal tempo and maintain control during the eccentric (lowering) portion.
- The set and rep numbers used for the exercises in this section are undulated with three schemes. Regardless of the scheme you're on, use a weight load that leaves you unable to perform any more reps than indicated while maintaining proper control and technique.

Cardio conditioning

- If the workout calls for a particular supramaximal interval training (SMIT), steady-state cardio, or metabolic conditioning protocol (MCP) that your training environment prevents you from performing, simply choose a comparable alternative from chapter 3. Perform the alternative exercise for roughly the same amount of reps, rounds, or time that were recommended for the original exercise.
- Only workouts A and C of each program involve a Cardio conditioning component.

Muscle Workout Programs (Three to Five Days Per Week)

In the following programs, perform *a* and *b* exercises as paired-sets. Perform all indicated sets and reps of a given paired set before moving on to the next set. If necessary, rest a bit longer than indicated between sets in order to complete the designated number of reps with good control. This program emphasizes movement quality over quantity! To help you personalize these workouts to *best* fit you, refer to chapter 12.

TABLE 11.2 **Muscle Program 1: Workout A—Pulling**

	Page	Days 1 and 4	Days 2 and 5	Days 3 and 6
STRENGTH				
1. Barbell bent-over row	123	5 × 3–5 with 2 min. rest between sets	5 × 3–5 with 2 min. rest between sets	5 × 3–5 with 2 min. rest between sets
SIZE				
2. Leaning lat pull-down	122	4 × 6–8 with 90 sec. rest between sets	3 × 10–12 with 90 sec. rest between sets	2 × 15–20 with 90 sec. rest between sets
3. Wide-grip seated row	126	4 × 6–8 with 90 sec. rest between sets	3 × 10–12 with 90 sec. rest between sets	2 × 15–20 with 90 sec. rest between sets
4a. Suspension biceps curl	138	4 × 6–8	3 × 10–12	2 × 15–20
4b. Bent-over dumbbell shoulder fly	130	4 × 6–8 with 60 sec. rest between paired sets	3 × 10–12 with 60 sec. rest between paired sets	2 × 15–20 with 60 sec. rest between paired sets
5. One-arm cable row	114	4 × 6–8 each side with 60 sec. rest between sets	3 × 10–12 each side with 60 sec. rest between sets	2 × 15–20 each side with 60 sec. rest between sets
SPEED				
6. Medicine-ball step and overhead throw (3–4 kg or 6.5–9 lbs.)	104	4 × 8–10 with 90 sec. rest between sets	4 × 8–10 with 90 sec. rest between sets	4 × 8–10 with 90 sec. rest between sets
CARDIO CONDITIONING		SMIT*: shuttle run—200 yd. × 5 or 6 with 2 min. rest between sets (page 25)	MCP**: bilateral farmer's-walk complex—2 or 3 sets with 2 min. rest between sets (page 57)	Steady-state cardio: elliptical trainer or upright bike—25–35 min. (page 29-30)

*SMIT = supramaximal interval training.

**MCP = metabolic conditioning protocol.

TABLE 11.3 **Muscle Program 1: Workout B—Lower Body and Core**

	Page	Days 1 and 4	Days 2 and 5	Days 3 and 6
STRENGTH				
1a. Trap-bar squat	164	5 × 2–5	5 × 2–5	5 × 2–5
1b. Ab snail	210	4 × 5–8 with 2 min. rest between paired sets	4 × 5–8 with 2 min. rest between paired sets	4 × 5–8 with 2 min. rest between paired sets
SIZE				
2a. Barbell calf raise	188	3 × 10–12	2 × 15–20	4 × 6–8
2b. Dumbbell plank row	197	3 × 10–12 each side with 90 sec. rest between paired sets	2 × 15–20 each side with 90 sec. rest between paired sets	4 × 6–8 each side with 90 sec. rest between paired sets
3a. Machine leg press	165	3 × 10–12	2 × 15–20	4 × 6–8
3b. Leg lowering with band*	212	3 × 10–12 with 90 sec. rest between paired sets	2 × 15–20 with 90 sec. rest between paired sets	4 × 6–8 with 90 sec. rest between paired sets
4. 45-degree hip extension	182	3 × 10–12	2 × 15–20	4 × 6–8
5. One-leg one-arm dumbbell Romanian deadlift	149	3 × 10–12 each side with 90 sec. rest between sets	2 × 15–20 each side with 90 sec. rest between sets	4 × 6–8 each side with 90 sec. rest between sets
SPEED				
6. Squat jump with arm drive	144	4 × 6–8 with 90 sec. rest between sets	4 × 6–8 with 90 sec. rest between sets	4 × 6–8 with 90 sec. rest between sets

*There is an inverse relation between the amount of reps indicated and the resistance load of band you use or how far you extend your legs. Extend your legs the farthest you can control on the days you perform 6 to 8 reps or use the heaviest band, and use the lightest band or don't extend your legs out as far on the days you perform 15 to 20 reps.

TABLE 11.4 Muscle Program 1: Workout C—Pushing

	Page	Days 1 and 4	Days 2 and 5	Days 3 and 6
STRENGTH				
1. Dumbbell bench press	88	5 × 2–5 with 2 min. rest between sets	5 × 2–5 with 2 min. rest between sets	5 × 2–5 with 2 min. rest between sets
SIZE				
2. Incline dumbbell bench press	89	2 × 15–20 with 90 sec. rest between sets	4 × 6–8 with 90 sec. rest between sets	3 × 10–12 with 90 sec. rest between sets
3. Dumbbell overhead press	90	2 × 15–20 with 90 sec. rest between sets	4 × 6–8 with 90 sec. rest between sets	3 × 10–12 with 90 sec. rest between sets
4a. Cable triceps rope extension	101	2 × 15–20	4 × 6–8	3 × 10–12
4b. Dumbbell side shoulder raise	99	2 × 15–20 with 60 sec. rest between paired sets	4 × 6–8 with 60 sec. rest between paired sets	3 × 10–12 with 60 sec. rest between paired sets
5. One-arm cable press	84	2 × 15–20 each side with 90 sec. rest between sets	4 × 6–8 each side with 90 sec. rest between sets	3 × 10–12 each side with 90 sec. rest between sets
SPEED				
6. Medicine-ball vertical squat push throw (3–4 kg or 6.5–9 lbs.)	73	4 × 5 or 6 with 90 sec. rest between sets	4 × 5 or 6 with 90 sec. rest between sets	4 × 5 or 6 with 90 sec. rest between sets
CARDIO CONDITIONING		Steady-state cardio: elliptical trainer or upright bike—25–35 min. (page 29-30)	SMIT*: rower—4–6 sets of 45–60 sec. as fast as possible with 90 sec. to 2 min. rest between sets (page 28)	MCP**: Six-min. body-weight complex—2 or 3 sets with 2 min. rest between sets (page 32)

*SMIT = supramaximal interval training.

**MCP = metabolic conditioning protocol.

TABLE 11.5   Muscle Program 2: Workout A—Pulling

	Page	Days 1 and 4	Days 2 and 5	Days 3 and 6
STRENGTH				
1. Pull-up or lat pull-down	120, 121	5 × 1–with 2 min. rest	5 × 1–5 with 2 min. rest	5 × 1–5 with 2 min. rest
SIZE				
2. Seated row	125	4 × 6–8 with 90 sec. rest between sets	3 × 10–12 with 90 sec. rest between sets	2 × 15–20 with 90 sec. rest between sets
3. Wide-grip seated row	126	4 × 6–8 with 90 sec. rest between sets	3 × 10–12 with 90 sec. rest between sets	2 × 15–20 with 90 sec. rest between sets
4a. Cable biceps curl	137	4 × 6–8	3 × 10–12	2 × 15–20
4b. Rope face pull	134	4 × 6–8 with 60 sec. rest between paired sets	3 × 10–12 with 60 sec. between paired sets	2 × 15–20 with 60 sec. between paired sets
5. One-arm one-leg dumbbell bench row	113	4 × 6–8 each side with 90 sec. rest between sets	3 × 10–12 each side with 90 sec. rest between sets	2 × 15–20 each side with 90 sec. rest between sets
SPEED				
6. Medicine-ball rainbow slam (3–4 kg or 6.5–9 lbs.)	105	4 × 5 or 6 each side with 90 sec. rest between sets	4 × 5 or 6 each side with 90 sec. rest between sets	4 × 5 or 6 each side with 90 sec. rest between sets
CARDIO CONDITIONING		SMIT*: gasser—1–3 with 3–4 min. rest between sets (page 26)	MCP**: boxing and kickboxing with heavy bag—4–6 2-min. rounds with 60 sec. rest between rounds (page 30)	Steady-state cardio: brisk walking outside or on treadmill—25–35 min. (page 29)

*SMIT = supramaximal interval training.

**MCP = metabolic conditioning protocol.

TABLE 11.6 **Muscle Program 2: Workout B—Lower Body and Core**

	Page	Days 1 and 4	Days 2 and 5	Days 3 and 6
STRENGTH				
1a. Barbell hybrid dead-lift	158	5 × 2–5	5 × 2–5	5 × 2–5
1b. One-arm plank	201	4 × 10–20 sec. each side with 90 sec. rest between paired sets	4 × 10–20 sec. each side with 90 sec. rest between paired sets	4 × 10–20 sec. each side with 90 sec. rest between paired sets
SIZE				
2a. Barbell squat and calf raise	160	3 × 10–12	2 × 15–20	4 × 6–8
2b. Stability-ball plate crunch	211	3 × 10–12 with 90 sec. rest between paired sets	2 × 15–20 with 90 sec. rest between paired sets	4 × 6–8 with 90 sec. rest between paired sets
3a. Elevated barbell reverse lunge	163	3 × 10–12 each side	2 × 14 or 15 each side	4 × 6–8 each side
3b. Stability-ball abdominal exercise indicated	205, 204, 206	Stability-ball pike 3 × 10–12 with 90 sec. rest between paired sets	Stability-ball knee tuck 2 × 15–20 with 90 sec. rest between paired sets	Stability-ball pike roll-out 4 × 6–8 with 90 sec. rest between paired sets
4. Leg-curl exercise variation indicated	178, 184, 184	Hip thrust hamstring curl combo 3 × 10–12 with 60 sec. rest between sets	Stability-ball leg curl 2 × 15–20 with 60 sec. rest between sets	One-leg stability-ball leg curl 4 × 6–8 with 60 sec. rest between sets
5. Lateral lunge with cross-body reach	152	3 × 8–10 each side with 60 sec. rest between sets	2 × 12–14 each side with 60 sec. rest between sets	3 × 6 or 7 each side with 60 sec. rest between sets
SPEED				
6. Lateral bound	148	4 × 4–6 each side with 90 sec. rest between sets	4 × 4–6 each side with 90 sec. rest between sets	4 × 4–6 each side with 90 sec. rest between sets

TABLE 11.7 **Muscle Program 2: Workout C—Pushing**

	Page	Days 1 and 4	Days 2 and 5	Days 3 and 6
STRENGTH				
1. Barbell overhead push press	79	4 × 2–5 with 90 sec. rest between sets	4 × 2–5 with 90 sec. rest between sets	4 × 2–5 with 90 sec. rest between sets
SIZE				
2. Standing cable chest press	95	2 × 15–20 with 90 sec. rest between sets	4 × 6–8 with 90 sec. rest between sets	3 × 10–12 with 90 sec. rest between sets
3a. Dumbbell wide-arm upright row	100	2 × 15–20	4 × 6–8	3 × 10–12
3b. Dumbbell triceps skull crusher	100	2 × 15–20 with 60 sec. rest between paired sets	4 × 6–8 with 60 sec. rest between paired sets	3 × 10–12 with 60 sec. rest between paired sets
4. Box crossover push-up	86	2 × max with 90 sec. rest between sets	4 × max (–2)* with 90 sec. rest between sets	3 × max (–1)* with 90 sec. rest between sets
5. Angled barbell press	82	2 × 15–20 each side with 90 sec. rest between sets	4 × 6–8 each side with 90 sec. rest between sets	3 × 10–12 each side with 90 sec. rest between sets
SPEED				
6. Medicine-ball side-scoop horizontal throw (3–5 kg or 6.5–11 lbs.)	193	4 × 5 or 6 each side with 90 sec. rest between sets	4 × 5 or 6 each side with 90 sec. rest between sets	4 × 5 or 6 each side with 90 sec. rest between sets
CARDIO CONDITIONING		Steady-state cardio: brisk walking outside or on treadmill—25–35 min. (page 29)	SMIT**: treadmill—5–7 sets running at top speed for 15–30 sec. with 60 sec. rest between sets (page 28)	MCP***: unilateral leg complex—1 or 2 sets with 2 min. rest between sets (page 34)

*(–1) means to stop the set one rep before failure; (–2) means to stop two reps before failure.

**SMIT = supramaximal interval training.

***MCP = metabolic conditioning protocol.

TABLE 11.8   **Muscle Program 3: Workout A—Pulling**

	Page	Days 1 and 4	Days 2 and 5	Days 3 and 6
STRENGTH				
1. Barbell high pull	106	5 × 3–5 with 2 min. rest between sets	5 × 3–5 with 2 min. rest between sets	5 × 3–5 with 2 min. rest between sets
SIZE				
2. Fighter's cable lat pull-down	122	4 × 6–8 each side with 60 sec. rest between sets	3 × 10–12 each side with 60 sec. rest between sets	2 × 14 or 15 each side with 60 sec. rest between sets
3. Cable compound straight-arm pull-down	135	4 × 6–8 with 60 sec. rest between sets	3 × 10–12 with 60 sec. rest between sets	2 × 15–20 with 60 sec. rest between sets
4a. Wide-elbow suspension row	128	4 × 6–8	3 × 10–12	2 × 15–20
4b. Suspension biceps curl	138	4 × 6–8 with 60 sec. rest between paired sets	3 × 10–12 with 60 sec. rest between paired sets	2 × 15–20 with 60 sec. rest between paired sets
5. One-arm compound cable row	116	4 × 6–8 each side with 60 sec. rest between sets	3 × 10–12 each side with 60 sec. rest between sets	2 × 15–20 each side with 60 sec. rest between sets
SPEED				
6. Medicine-ball step and overhead throw (3–4 kg or 6.5–9 lbs.)	104	4 × 8–10 with 90 sec. rest between sets	4 × 8–10 with 90 sec. rest between sets	4 × 8–10 with 90 sec. rest between sets
CARDIO CONDITIONING		SMIT*: rower—4–6 sets of 45–60 secs. as fast as possible with 90 sec. to 2 min. rest between sets (page 28)	MCP**: Six-min. body-weight complex—2 or 3 sets with 2 min. rest between sets (page 32)	Steady-state cardio: elliptical trainer or upright bike—25–35 min. (page 29-30)

*SMIT = supramaximal interval training.

**MCP = metabolic conditioning protocol.

TABLE 11.9　**Muscle Program 3: Workout B—Lower Body and Core**

	Page	Days 1 and 4	Days 2 and 5	Days 3 and 6
STRENGTH				
1a. Machine leg press	165	5 × 3–5	5 × 3–5	5 × 3–5
1b. Stability-ball stir-the-pot	207	4 × 4–6 each direction with 90 sec. rest between paired sets	4 × 4–6 each direction with 90 sec. rest between paired sets	4 × 4–6 each direction with 90 sec. rest between paired sets
SIZE				
2a. Barbell front squat	161	3 × 10–12	2 × 15–20	4 × 6–8
2b. Reverse crunch*	211	3 × 10–12 with 90 sec. rest between paired sets	2 × 15–20 with 90 sec. rest between paired sets	4 × 6–8 with 90 sec. rest between paired sets
3a. Bulgarian split squat and Romanian deadlift combination	168	3 × 7–9 each side	2 × 10–12 each side	4 × 5 or 6 each side
3b. Angled barbell tight rainbow	202	3 × 10–12 each side with 90 sec. rest between paired sets	2 × 14 or 15 each side with 90 sec. rest between paired sets	4 × 6–8 each side with 90 sec. rest between paired sets
4. One-leg dumbbell bench hip thrust	177	3 × 10–12 each side with 60 sec. rest between sets	2 × 15–20 each side with 60 sec. rest between sets	4 × 6–8 each side with 60 sec. rest between sets
5. Angled barbell cross-shoulder reverse lunge	155	3 × 7–9 each side with 90 sec. rest between sets	2 × 10–12 each side with 90 sec. rest between sets	4 × 5 or 6 each side with 90 sec. rest between sets
SPEED				
6. Anterior-leaning lunge scissor jump	147	4 × 3–5 each side with 90 sec. rest between sets	4 × 3–5 each side with 90 sec. rest between sets	4 × 3–5 each side with 90 sec. rest between sets

*There is an inverse relation between the amount of reps indicated and the weight you'll use as an anchor, as the heavier the anchor the easier the exercise becomes. Use the lightest dumbbell, kettlebell, or medicine ball as an anchor on the days you perform 6 to 8 reps, and use the heaviest anchor on the days you perform 15 to 20 reps.

TABLE 11.10 **Muscle Program 3: Workout C—Pushing**

	Page	Days 1 and 4	Days 2 and 5	Days 3 and 6
STRENGTH				
1. Incline barbell bench press	276	4 × 2–5 with 2 min. rest between sets	4 × 2–5 with 2 min. rest between sets	4 × 2–5 with 2 min. rest between sets
SIZE				
2. Dumbbell overhead press	90	2 × 15–20 with 90 sec. rest between sets	4 × 6–8 with 90 sec. rest between sets	3 × 10–12 with 90 sec. rest between sets
3. Close-grip push-up	95	2 × max with 90 sec. rest between sets	4 × max (–2)* with 90 sec. rest between sets	3 × max (–1)* with 90 sec. rest between sets
4a. Cable triceps rope extension	101	2 × 15–20	4 × 6–8	3 × 10–12
4b. Dumbbell front shoulder raise	99	2 × 15–20 with 60 sec. rest between paired sets	4 × 6–8 with 60 sec. rest between paired sets	3 × 10–12 with 60 sec. rest between paired sets
5. One-arm cable press	84	2 × 15–20 each side with 60 sec. rest between sets	4 × 6–8 each side with 60 sec. rest between sets	3 × 10–12 each side with 60 sec. rest between sets
SPEED				
6. Medicine-ball diagonal squat push throw (3–4 kg or 6.5–9 lbs.)	74	4 × 4–6 with 90 sec. rest between sets	4 × 4–6 with 90 sec. rest between sets	4 × 4–6 with 90 sec. rest between sets
CARDIO CONDITIONING		Steady-state cardio: elliptical trainer or upright bike—25–35 min. (page 29-30)	SMIT**: shuttle run—250 yd. × 4 or 5 with 2.5 min. rest between sets (page 25)	MCP***: unilateral farmer's walk complex—2 or 3 sets with 2 min. rest between sets (page 59)

*(–1) means to stop the set one rep before failure; (–2) means to stop two reps before failure.

**SMIT = supramaximal interval training.

***MCP = metabolic conditioning protocol.

TABLE 11.11 **Muscle Program 4: Workout A—Pulling**

	Page	Days 1 and 4	Days 2 and 5	Days 3 and 6
STRENGTH				
1. One-arm freestanding dumbbell row	112	4 × 2–4 each side with 90 sec. rest between sets	4 × 2–4 each side with 90 sec. rest between sets	4 × 2–4 each side with 90 sec. rest between sets
SIZE				
2. Wide-grip barbell bent-over row	123	4 × 6–8 with 60–90 sec. rest between sets	3 × 10–12 with 60–90 sec. rest between sets	2 × 15–20 with 60–90 sec. rest between sets
3. Lat pull-down	121	4 × 6–8 with 60–90 sec. rest between sets	3 × 10–12 with 60–90 sec. rest between sets	2 × 15–20 with 60–90 sec. rest between sets
4a. Dumbbell biceps curl	136	4 × 6–8	3 × 10–12	2 × 15–20
4b. Bent-over dumbbell shoulder fly	130	4 × 6–8 with 60 sec. rest between paired sets	3 × 10–12 with 60 sec. rest between paired sets	2 × 15–20 with 60 sec. rest between paired sets
5. One-arm cable row with hip rotation	115	4 × 6–8 each side with 60 sec. rest between sets	3 × 10–12 each side with 60 sec. rest between sets	2 × 15–20 each side with 60 sec. rest between sets
SPEED				
6. Rope slam	111	4 × 12–15 with 90 sec. rest between sets	4 × 12–15 with 90 sec. rest between sets	4 × 12–15 with 90 sec. rest between sets
CARDIO CONDITIONING		SMIT*: treadmill—5–7 sets running at top speed for 15–30 sec. with 60 sec. rest between sets (page 28)	MCP**: Four-min. rope complex—2 or 3 sets with 2–3 min. rest between sets (page 47)	Steady-state cardio: brisk walking outside or on treadmill—25–35 min. (page 29)

*SMIT = supramaximal interval training.

**MCP = metabolic conditioning protocol.

TABLE 11.12 **Muscle Program 4: Workout B—Lower Body and Core**

	Page	Days 1 and 4	Days 2 and 5	Days 3 and 6
STRENGTH				
1a. Barbell sumo dead-lift	157	5 × 2–5	5 × 2–5	5 × 2–5
2a. Stability-ball pike rollout	206	4 × 8–12 with 90 sec. rest between paired sets	4 × 8–12 with 90 sec. rest between paired sets	4 × 8–12 with 90 sec. rest between paired sets
SIZE				
3a. Machine leg extension	187	3 × 10–12	2 × 15–20	4 × 6–8
3b. Stability-ball plate crunch	211	3 × 10–12 with 90 sec. rest between paired sets	2 × 15–20 with 90 sec. rest between paired sets	4 × 6–8 with 90 sec. rest between paired sets
4a. Dumbbell fighter's lunge	170	3 × 10–12 each side	2 × 14 or 15 each side	4 × 6–8 each side
4b. One-arm dumbbell farmer's walk	197	3 × 45 sec. each side with 90 sec. rest between paired sets	2 × 60 sec. each side with 90 sec. rest between paired sets	4 × 30 sec. each side with 90 sec. rest between paired sets
5. Machine seated hamstring curl	186	3 × 10–12 with 60 sec. rest between sets	2 × 15–20 with 60 sec. rest between sets	4 × 6–8 with 60 sec. rest between sets
6. One-leg 45-degree cable Romanian deadlift	150	3 × 10–12 each side with 60 sec. rest between sets	2 × 15–20 each side with 60 sec. rest between sets	4 × 6–8 each side with 60 sec. rest between sets
SPEED				
7. Deadlift jump with arm drive	145	4 × 4–6 with 90 sec. rest between sets	4 × 4–6 with 90 sec. rest between sets	4 × 4–6 with 90 sec. rest between sets

TABLE 11.13 Muscle Program 4: Workout C—Pushing

	Page	Days 1 and 4	Days 2 and 5	Days 3 and 6
STRENGTH				
1. Barbell bench press	87	5 × 1–5 with 2 min. rest between sets	5 × 1–5 with 2 min. rest between sets	5 × 1–5 with 2 min. rest between sets
SIZE				
2. Incline dumbbell bench press	89	2 × 15–20 with 60–90 sec. rest between sets	4 × 6–8 with 60–90 sec. rest between sets	3 × 10–12 with 60–90 sec. rest between sets
3. Cable pec fly	97	2 × 15–20 with 60–90 sec. rest between sets	4 × 6–8 with 60–90 sec. rest between sets	3 × 10–12 with 60–90 sec. rest between sets
4a. Cable triceps rope extension	101	2 × 15–20	4 × 6–8	3 × 10–12
4b. Dumbbell side shoulder raise	99	2 × 15–20 with 90 sec. rest between paired sets	4 × 6–8 with 90 sec. rest between paired sets	3 × 10–12 with 90 sec. rest between paired sets
5. One-arm dumbbell rotational push press	80	2 × 11 or 12 each side with 90 sec. rest between sets	4 × 5 or 6 each side with 90 sec. rest between sets	3 × 8 or 9 each side with 90 sec. rest between sets
SPEED				
6. Medicine-ball horizontal punch throw (3–4 kg or 6.5–9 lbs.)	191	4 × 4 or 5 each side with 90 sec. rest between sets	4 × 4 or 5 each side with 90 sec. rest between sets	4 × 4 or 5 each side with 90 sec. rest between sets
CARDIO CONDITIONING		Steady-state cardio: brisk walking outside or on treadmill—25–35 min. (page 29)	SMIT*: gasser—1–3 with 3–4 min. rest between sets (page 26)	MCP**: 20-20-10-10 leg complex—2 or 3 sets with 2 min. rest between sets (page 37)

*SMIT = supramaximal interval training.

**MCP = metabolic conditioning protocol.

TABLE 11.14 **Muscle Program 5: Workout A—Pulling**

	Page	Days 1 and 4	Days 2 and 5	Days 3 and 6
STRENGTH				
1. Chin-up or under-hand-grip lat pull-down	119, 121	5 × 1–5 with 2 min. rest between sets	5 × 1–5 with 2 min. rest between sets	5 × 1–5 with 2 min. rest between sets
SIZE				
2. Smith-bar under-hand-grip row or suspension row	128, 127	4 × 6–8 with 60–90 sec. rest between sets	3 × 10–12 with 60–90 sec. rest between sets	2 × 15–20 with 60–90 sec. rest between sets
3. Cable compound straight-arm pull-down	135	4 × 6–8 with 60 sec. rest between sets	3 × 10–12 with 60 sec. rest between sets	2 × 15–20 with 60 sec. rest between sets
4a. Cable biceps curl	137	4 × 6–8	3 × 10–12	2 × 15–20
4b. Bent-over dumbbell shoulder fly	130	4 × 6–8 with 60 sec. rest between paired sets	3 × 10–12 with 60 sec. rest between paired sets	2 × 15–20 with 60 sec. rest between paired sets
5. One-arm anti-rotation suspension row	117	4 × 6–8 each side with 60 sec. rest between sets	3 × 10–12 each side with 60 sec. rest between sets	2 × 15–20 each side with 60 sec. rest between sets
SPEED				
6. Medicine-ball rainbow slam (3–4 kg or 6.5–9 lbs.)	105	4 × 5 or 6 each side with 90 sec. rest between sets	4 × 5 or 6 each side with 90 sec. rest between sets	4 × 5 or 6 each side with 90 sec. rest between sets
CARDIO CONDITIONING		SMIT*: shuttle run—300 yd. × 2 or 3 with 3 min. rest between sets (page 25)	MCP**: weight-plate push—4–6 sets × 40–50 yd. per set with 90 sec. rest between sets (page 50)	Steady-state cardio: elliptical trainer or upright bike—25–35 min. (page 29-30)

*SMIT = supramaximal interval training.

**MCP = metabolic conditioning protocol.

TABLE 11.15 Muscle Program 5: Workout B—Lower Body and Core

	Page	Days 1 and 4	Days 2 and 5	Days 3 and 6
STRENGTH				
1a. Barbell hybrid dead-lift	158	5 × 2–5	5 × 2–5	5 × 2–5
1b. Leg lowering with band	212	4 × 10–15 with 90 sec. rest between paired sets	4 × 10–15 with 90 sec. rest between paired sets	4 × 10–15 with 90 sec. rest between paired sets
SIZE				
2a. Barbell squat and calf raise	160	3 × 10–12	2 × 15–20	4 × 6–8
2b. Rollout exercise variation indicated	208, 204, 208	Arm walkout 3 × 10–12 with 60 to 90 sec. rest between paired sets	Stability-ball rollout 2 × 15–20 with 60 to 90 sec. rest between paired sets	Medicine-ball walkout 4 × 6–8 with 60 to 90 sec. rest between paired sets
3a. Dumbbell anterior lunge	172	3 × 10–12 each side	2 × 14 or 15 each side	4 × 6–8 each side
3b. Low-to-high cable chop	198	3 × 10–12 each side with 90 sec. rest between paired sets	2 × 14 or 15 each side with 90 sec. rest between paired sets	4 × 6–8 each side with 90 sec. rest between paired sets
4. Leg-curl exercise variation indicated	178, 184, 184	Hip thrust hamstring curl combo 3 × 10–12 with 60 sec. rest between sets	Stability-ball leg curl 2 × 15–20 with 60 sec. rest between sets	One-leg stability-ball leg curl 4 × 6–8 with 60 sec. rest between sets
5. One-leg offset traveling lunge	154	3 × 8–10 each side with 90 sec. rest between sets	2 × 12–14 each side with 90 sec. rest between sets	4 × 5–7 each side with 90 sec. rest between sets
SPEED				
6. Squat jump with arm drive	144	4 × 4–6 with 90 sec. rest between sets	4 × 4–6 with 90 sec. rest between sets	4 × 4–6 with 90 sec. rest between sets

TABLE 11.16 Muscle Program 5: Workout C—Pushing

	Page	Days 1 and 4	Days 2 and 5	Days 3 and 6
STRENGTH				
1. One-arm dumbbell rotational push press	80	4 × 2–4 each side with 90 sec. rest between sets	4 × 2–4 each side with 90 sec. rest between sets	4 × 2–4 each side with 90 sec. rest between sets
SIZE				
2. Barbell bench press	87	2 × 15–20 with 60–90 sec. rest between sets	4 × 6–8 with 60–90 sec. rest between sets	3 × 10–12 with 60–90 sec. rest between sets
3. Cable pec fly	97	2 × 15–20 with 60–90 sec. rest between sets	4 × 6–8 with 60–90 sec. rest between sets	3 × 10–12 with 60–90 sec. rest between sets
4. Box crossover push-up	86	2 × max with 90 sec. rest between sets	4 × max (–2)* with 90 sec. rest between sets	3 × max (–1)* with 90 sec. rest between sets
5. Suspension triceps skull crusher	101	2 × 15–20 with 60–90 sec. rest between sets	4 × 6–8 with 60–90 sec. rest between sets	3 × 10–12 with 60–90 sec. rest between sets
6. Angled barbell rotational push press	83	2 × 14 or 15 each side with 60–90 sec. rest between sets	4 × 6–8 each side with 60–90 sec. rest between sets	3 × 10–12 each side with 60–90 sec. rest between sets
SPEED				
7. Power skip	142	4 × 8–10 each leg with 60–90 sec. rest between sets	4 × 8–10 each leg with 60–90 sec. rest between sets	4 × 8–10 each leg with 60–90 sec. rest between sets
CARDIO CONDITIONING		Steady-state cardio: elliptical trainer or upright bike—25–35 min. (page 29-30)	SMIT**: rower—4–6 sets of 45–60 sec. as fast as possible with 90 sec. to 2 min. rest between sets (page 28)	MCP***: boxing and kickboxing with heavy bag—3–5 3 min. rounds with 90 sec. rest between rounds (page 30)

*(–1) means to stop the set one rep before failure; (–2) means to stop two reps before failure.

**SMIT = supramaximal interval training.

***MCP = metabolic conditioning protocol.

Muscle Workout Programs (Two Days Per Week)

Although I recommend training at least three times per week, you can still get positive results if your schedule allows only two training days per week. Designed to meet that need, the following programs are alternative versions of the programs provided in the preceding sections of the chapter.

Each of the following three programs consists of either two or three workouts: workout A and workout B or workout A, B, and C. Workout A focuses on pulling and pushing exercises, and workout B focuses on lower-body and core exercises. Perform the workouts in each program six times before moving on to a new program. In other words, if you're training twice per week, use the same program for six weeks before switching to the next program and performing that one for another six weeks, and so on.

In each of the following programs, workout B (lower body and core) is almost identical to the corresponding workout in the preceding sections, with the exception of an additional exercise application in the speed category. On the other hand, the version of workout A used in these programs is a combination of the corresponding workout A and workout C in the preceding sections. Therefore, although they feature exercises also found in the preceding sections, each workout A presented here involves performing several more exercises.

TABLE 11.17 Two-Day Muscle Program 1: Workout A—Pulling and Pushing

	Page	Days 1 and 4	Days 2 and 5	Days 3 and 6
STRENGTH				
1a. Barbell bent-over row	123	5 × 3–5	5 × 3–5	5 × 3–5
1b. Dumbbell bench press	88	5 × 2–5 with 90 sec. rest between paired sets	5 × 2–5 with 90 sec. rest between paired sets	5 × 2–5 with 90 sec. rest between paired sets
SIZE				
2a. Leaning lat pull-down	122	4 × 6–8	3 × 10–12	2 × 15–20
2b. Dumbbell side shoulder raise	99	4 × 6–8 with 60 sec. rest between paired sets	3 × 10–12 with 60 sec. rest between paired sets	2 × 15–20 with 60 sec. rest between paired sets
3a. Wide-grip seated row	126	4 × 6–8	3 × 10–12	2 × 15–20
3b. Close-grip push-up	95	4 × max (–2)* with 60 sec. rest between paired sets	3 × max (–1)* with 60 sec. rest between paired sets	2 × max with 60 sec. rest between paired sets
4a. Cable biceps curl	137	4 × 6–8	3 × 10–12	2 × 15–20
4b. Cable triceps rope extension	101	4 × 6–8 with 60 sec. rest between paired sets	3 × 10–12 with 60 sec. rest between paired sets	2 × 15–20 with 60 sec. rest between paired sets
5. One-arm cable press	84	4 × 6–8 each side with 60 sec. rest between sets	3 × 10–12 each side with 60 sec. rest between sets	2 × 15–20 each side with 60 sec. rest between sets
SPEED				
6a. Medicine-ball step and overhead throw (3–4 kg or 6.5–9 lbs.)	104	4 × 8–10	4 × 8–10	4 × 8–10
6b. Medicine-ball vertical squat push throw (3–4 kg)	73	4 × 5 or 6 with 90 sec. rest between paired sets	4 × 5 or 6 with 90 sec. rest between paired sets	4 × 5 or 6 with 90 sec. rest between paired sets
CARDIO CONDITIONING		SMIT**: shuttle run—250 yd. × 4 or 5 with 2.5 min. rest between sets (page 25)	MCP***: unilateral leg complex—1 or 2 sets with 2 min. rest between sets (page 34)	Steady-state cardio: elliptical trainer or upright bike—25–35 min. (page 29-30)

*(–1) means to stop the set one rep before failure; (–2) means to stop two reps before failure.

**SMIT = supramaximal interval training.

***MCP = metabolic conditioning protocol.

TABLE 11.18 Two-Day Muscle Program 1: Workout B—Lower Body and Core

	Page	Days 1 and 4	Days 2 and 5	Days 3 and 6
STRENGTH				
1a. Trap-bar squat	164	5 × 2–5	5 × 2–5	5 × 2–5
1b. Ab snail	210	4 × 4–8 with 90 sec. rest between paired sets	4 × 4–8 with 90 sec. rest between paired sets	4 × 4–8 with 90 sec. rest between paired sets
SIZE				
2a. Barbell calf raise	188	3 × 10–12	2 × 15–20	4 × 6–8
2b. Dumbbell plank row	197	3 × 10–12 each side with 60 sec. rest between paired sets	2 × 14 or 15 each side with 60 sec. rest between paired sets	4 × 6–8 each side with 60 sec. rest between paired sets
3a. Machine leg press	165	3 × 10–12	2 × 15–20	4 × 6–8
3b. Leg lowering with band*	212	3 × 10–12 with 60 sec. rest between paired sets	2 × 15–20 with 60 sec. rest between paired sets	4 × 6–8 with 60 sec. rest between paired sets
4. 45-degree hip extension	182	3 × 10–12 with 60 sec. rest between sets	2 × 15–20 with 60 sec. rest between sets	4 × 6–8 with 60 sec. rest between sets
5. One-leg one-arm dumbbell Romanian deadlift	149	3 × 10–12 each side with 60 sec. rest between sets	2 × 15–20 each side with 60 sec. rest between sets	4 × 6–8 each side with 60 sec. rest between sets
SPEED				
6. Squat jump with arm drive	144	4 × 5 or 6 with 90 sec. rest between sets	4 × 5 or 6 with 90 sec. rest between sets	4 × 5 or 6 with 90 sec. rest between sets
CARDIO CONDITIONING		MCP**: bilateral farmer's-walk complex—2 or 3 sets with 2 min. rest between sets (page 57)	Steady-state cardio: brisk walking outside or on treadmill—25–35 min. (page 29)	SMIT***: rower— 4–6 sets of 45–60 sec. as fast as possible with 90 sec. to 2 min. rest between sets (page 28)

*There is an inverse relation between the amount of reps indicated and the resistance load of band you use or how far you extend your legs. Extend your legs the farthest you can control on the days you perform 6 to 8 reps or use the heaviest band, and use the lightest band or don't extend your legs out as far on the days you perform 15 to 20 reps.

**MCP = metabolic conditioning protocol.

***SMIT = supramaximal interval training.

TABLE 11.19 Two-Day Muscle Program 2: Workout A—Pulling and Pushing

	Page	Days 1 and 4	Days 2 and 5	Days 3 and 6
STRENGTH				
1a. Pull-up or lat pull-down	120, 121	5 × 1–5	5 × 1–5	5 × 1–5
1b. Barbell overhead push press	79	4 × 2–5 with 90 sec. rest between paired sets	4 × 2–5 with 90 sec. rest between paired sets	4 × 2–5 with 90 sec. rest between paired sets
SIZE				
2a. Wide-grip barbell bent-over row	123	4 × 6–8	3 × 10–12	2 × 15–20
2b. Feet-elevated push-up	94	4 × max (–2)* with 60 sec. rest between paired sets	3 × max (–1)* with 60 sec. rest between paired sets	2 × max with 60 sec. rest between paired sets
3a. Wide-elbow Smith-bar row	129	4 × 6–8	3 × 10–12	2 × 15–20
3b. Angled barbell press	82	2 × 15–20 each side with 60 sec. rest between paired sets	4 × 6–8 each side with 60 sec. rest between paired sets	3 × 10–12 each side with 60 sec. rest between paired sets
4a. Cable biceps curl	137	4 × 6–8	3 × 10–12	2 × 15–20
4b. Cable triceps rope extension	101	4 × 6–8	3 × 10–12	2 × 15–20
4c. Rope face pull	134	4 × 6–8 with 60 sec. rest between tri-sets	3 × 10–12 with 60 sec. rest between tri-sets	2 × 15–20 with 60 sec. rest between tri-sets
5. One-arm one-leg dumbbell bench row	113	4 × 6–8 each side with 60 sec. rest between sets	3 × 10–12 each side with 60 sec. rest between sets	2 × 15–20 each side with 60 sec. rest between sets
SPEED				
6a. Medicine-ball rain-bow slam	105	4 × 5 or 6 each side	4 × 5 or 6 each side	4 × 5 or 6 each side
6b. Medicine-ball side-scoop horizontal throw (3–5 kg or 6.5–11 lbs.)	193	4 × 5 or 6 each side with 90 sec. rest between paired sets	4 × 5 or 6 each side with 90 sec. rest between paired sets	4 × 5 or 6 each side with 90 sec. rest between paired sets
CARDIO CONDITIONING		SMIT**: gasser—1–3 with 3–4 min. rest between sets (page 26)	MCP***: Six min. body-weight complex—2 or 3 sets with 2 min. rest between sets (page 32)	Steady-state cardio: brisk walking outside or on treadmill—25–35 min. (page 29)

*(–1) means to stop the set one rep before failure; (–2) means to stop two reps before failure.

**SMIT = supramaximal interval training.

***MCP = metabolic conditioning protocol.

TABLE 11.20 Two-Day Muscle Program 2: Workout B—Lower Body and Core

	Page	Days 1 and 4	Days 2 and 5	Days 3 and 6
STRENGTH				
1a. Barbell hybrid dead-lift	158	5 × 2–5	5 × 2–5	5 × 2–5
1b. One-arm plank	201	4 × 10–20 sec. each side with 90 sec. rest between paired sets	4 × 10–20 sec. each side with 90 sec. rest between paired sets	4 × 10–20 sec. each side with 90 sec. rest between paired sets
SIZE				
2a. Barbell squat and calf raise	160	3 × 10–12	2 × 15–20	4 × 6–8
2b. Stability-ball plate crunch	211	3 × 10–12 with 90 sec. rest between paired sets	2 × 15–20 with 90 sec. rest between paired sets	4 × 6–8 with 90 sec. rest between paired sets
3a. Elevated barbell reverse lunge	163	3 × 10–12 each side	2 × 14 or 15 each side	4 × 6–8 each side
3b. Stability-ball abdominal exercise indicated	205, 204, 206	Stability-ball pike 3 × 10–12 with 90 sec. rest between paired sets	Stability-ball knee-tuck 2 × 15–20 with 90 sec. rest between paired sets	Stability-ball pike roll-out 4 × 6–8 with 90 sec. rest between paired sets
4. Machine seated hamstring curl	186	3 × 10–12 with 60 sec. rest between sets	2 × 15–20 with 60 sec. rest between sets	4 × 6–8 with 60 sec. rest between sets
5. Lateral lunge with cross-body reach	152	3 × 8–10 each side with 60 sec. rest between sets	2 × 12–14 each side with 60 sec. rest between sets	4 × 6 or 7 each side with 60 sec. rest between sets
SPEED				
6. Lateral bound	148	4 × 4–6 each side with 90 sec. rest between sets	4 × 4–6 each side with 90 sec. rest between sets	4 × 4–6 each side with 90 sec. rest between sets
CARDIO CONDITIONING		MCP*: boxing and kickboxing with heavy bag—4–6 2 min. rounds with 60 sec. rest between rounds (page 30)	Steady-state cardio: elliptical trainer or upright bike—25–35 min. (page 29-30)	SMIT**: treadmill—5–7 sets running at top speed for 15–30 sec. with 60 sec. rest between sets (page 28)

*MCP = metabolic conditioning protocol.

**SMIT = supramaximal interval training.

TABLE 11.21 Two-Day Muscle Program 3: Workout A—Pulling

	Page	Days 1 and 4	Days 2 and 5	Days 3 and 6
STRENGTH				
1a. Barbell high pull	106	5 × 3–5	5 × 3–5	5 × 3–5
1b. Incline barbell bench press	88	4 × 2–5 Rest 90 sec. between paired sets	4 × 2–5 Rest 90 sec. between paired sets	4 × 2–5 Rest 90 sec. between paired sets
SIZE				
2a. Fighter's cable lat pull-down	122	4 × 6–8 each side	3 × 10–12 each side	2 × 15–20 each side
2b. Dumbbell rotational shoulder press	81	4 × 6–8 each side with 60 sec. rest between paired-sets	3 × 10–12 each side with 60 sec. rest between paired-sets	2 × 15–20 each side with 60 sec. rest between paired-sets
3a. Cable compound straight-arm pull-down	135	4 × 6–8	3 × 10–12	2 × 15–20
3b. Dumbbell front shoulder raise	99	4 × 6–8 with 60 sec. rest between paired-sets	3 × 10–12 with 60 sec. rest between paired-sets	2 × 15–20 with 60 sec. rest between paired-sets
4a. Suspension triceps skull crusher	101	4 × 6–8	3 × 10–12	2 × 15–20
4b. Wide-elbow suspension row	128	4 × 6–8	3 × 10–12	2 × 15–20
4c. Suspension biceps curl	138	4 × 6–8 with 60 sec. between tri-sets	3 × 10–12 with 60 sec. between tri-sets	2 × 15–20 with 60 sec. between tri-sets
5. Angled barbell press	82	4 × 6–8 each side with 60 sec. between sets	3 × 10–12 each side with 60 sec. between sets	2 × 15–20 each side with 60 sec. between sets
SPEED				
6a. Medicine-ball step and overhead throw (3–4 kg or 6.5–9 lbs.)	104	4 × 5–6	4 × 5–6	4 × 5–6
6b. Medicine ball diagonal squat push throw (3–5 kg or 6.5–11 lbs.)	74	4 × 5–6 with 90 sec. rest between paired-sets	4 × 5–6 with 90 sec. rest between paired-sets	4 × 5–6 with 90 sec. rest between paired-sets
CARDIO CONDITIONING		SMIT*: gasser—1–3 with 3–4 min. rest between sets (page 26)	MCP**: Six-min. body-weight complex—2 or 3 sets with 2 min. rest between sets (page 32)	Steady-state cardio: brisk walking outside or on treadmill—25–35 min. (page 29)

*SMIT = supramaximal interval training.

**MCP = metabolic conditioning protocol.

TABLE 11.22 Two-Day Muscle Program 3: Workout B—Lower Body and Core

	Page	Days 1 and 4	Days 2 and 5	Days 3 and 6
STRENGTH				
1a. Barbell sumo deadlift	157	5 × 3–5	5 × 3–5	5 × 3–5
1b. Stability-ball stir-the-pot	207	4 × 10–20 sec. each side with 90 sec. rest between paired-sets	4 × 10–20 sec. each side with 90 sec. rest between paired-sets	4 × 10–20 sec. each side with 90 sec. rest between paired-sets
SIZE				
2a. Barbell front squat	161	3 × 10–12	2 × 15–20	4 × 6–8
2b. Rollout exercise variation indicated	208, 204, 208	Arm Walkout: 3 × 10–12 with 60–90 sec. rest between paired sets	Stability-ball rollout: 2 × 15–20 with 60–90 sec. rest between paired sets	Medicine-Ball Walkout: 4 × 6–8 with 60–90 sec. rest between paired sets
3a. Bulgarian split squat and Romanian deadlift combination	168	3 × 10–12 each side	2 × 14–15 each side	4 × 6–8 each side
3b. Reverse crunch*	211	3 × 10–12 Rest 90 sec between paired-sets	2 × 15–20 Rest 90 sec between paired-sets	4 × 6–8 Rest 90 sec between paired-sets
4. One-leg dumbbell bench hip thrust	177	3 × 10–12 each side with 60 sec. between sets	2 × 15–20 each side with 60 sec. between sets	4 × 6–8 each side with 60 sec. between sets
5. Angled barbell cross- shoulder reverse lunge	155	3 × 8–10 each side with 60 sec. between sets	2 × 12–14 each side with 60 sec. between sets	4 × 6–7 each side with 60 sec. between sets
SPEED				
6. Anterior-leaning lunge scissor jump	147	4 × 3–5 each side with 90 sec. rest between sets	4 × 3–5 each side with 90 sec. rest between sets	4 × 3–5 each side with 90 sec. rest between sets
CARDIO CONDITIONING		MCP**: boxing and kickboxing with heavy bag—4–6 2 min. rounds with 60 sec. rest between rounds (page 30)	Steady-state cardio on elliptical trainer (page 29) or upright bike (page 30) for 25–35 min.	SMIT***: treadmill (page 28)—× 5–7 sets running at top speed for 15–30 sec. with 60 sec. rest between sets

*There is an inverse relation between the amount of reps indicated and the weight you'll use as an anchor, as the heavier the anchor the easier the exercise becomes. Use the lightest dumbbell, kettlebell, or medicine ball as an anchor on the days you perform 6 to 8 reps, and use the heaviest anchor on the days you perform 15 to 20 reps.

**MCP = metabolic conditioning protocol.

***SMIT = supramaximal interval training.

The muscle training programs provided in this chapter and the performance training programs provided in the previous chapter emphasize different ends of the training spectrum, but they share the fact that they each focus on one end of the spectrum. If you're looking to use the functional-spectrum training system *without* focusing your efforts on training one aspect over the other, then the performance-and-muscle programs provided in the next chapter are just what the doctor ordered!

12

Performance and Muscle Programming

So far you've been provided with two kinds of functional-spectrum programming: first, in chapter 10, training focused mostly on improving your hustle while still training your muscle; and second, in chapter 11, training focused mostly on making gains in your muscle while still training your hustle. In contrast, the programs provided in this chapter do *not* focus on improving muscle over performance, or vice versa. Instead, they occupy a middle ground between the other two approaches.

As a result, the programs presented in this chapter include more exercises in the size category than do the performance-focused programs but fewer than do the muscle-focused programs. On the flip side, the programs presented here—specifically, in the day-A pulling and day-B pushing workouts—include more exercises in the speed and power category than do the muscle-oriented programs but fewer than do the performance-oriented programs.

Although the muscle- and performance-focused programs provided in chapters 10 and 11 emphasize different ends of the training spectrum, they are characterized more by similarity than by difference. The reason for this commonality is two-fold:

1. Exercise applications aren't mutually exclusive in their functional transfer, which is why, as established in chapter 1, the functional-spectrum training system integrates general and specific exercise applications in all programs.

2. The functional-spectrum workout programs provided in this book are designed to be complementary in order to help you quickly and easily see how exercise applications for each of the three S's—speed, strength, and size—are manipulated in each chapter. This approach prepares you to design your own functional-spectrum training workouts.

Let's look a bit more closely at what it means that the functional-spectrum training programs provided in the three programming chapters (i.e., chapters 10, 11, and 12) are complementary. Each program presented in a given programming chapter uses many of the same exercises as—and thus complements—the corresponding program in the other programming chapters. However, the order and number of exercises used in each of the three S's differ based on whether the program emphasizes muscle gains, performance gains, or both—which is the case for the workouts provided in this chapter. For example, the A workouts presented in program 1 of each programming chapter incorporate many of the same exercises, but the number and order vary depending on which training element is emphasized.

Performance and Muscle Workout Program Guidelines

As with the programs provided in chapters 10 and 11, each of the five functional-spectrum performance-and muscle-training programs presented here consists of three workouts: workout A, workout B, and workout C. Workout A focuses on pulling exercises, workout B focuses on lower-body and core exercises, and workout C focuses on pushing exercises.

You alternate workouts and perform them three, four, or five times per week depending on your preference and training schedule—but no more than three days in a row, to maximize recovery and minimize the risk of overtraining. I recommend training at least three times per week for best results. Perform the workouts in each program six times before moving on to a new program. Table 12.1 guides you in setting up your training based on the number of times you train per week.

TABLE 12.1 **Weekly Training Frequency Guide**

Training frequency	Program length	Weekly setup examples
3 × per week	6 weeks	Monday (A), Wednesday (B), Friday (C)
4 × per week	4.5 weeks	Week 1: Monday (A), Tuesday (B), Thursday (C), Friday or Saturday (A) Week 2: B, C, A, B Week 3: C, A, B, C Week 4: A, B, C, A Week 5: B, C
5 × per week	3.5 weeks	Week 1: Monday (A), Tuesday (B), Wednesday (C), Friday (A), Saturday (B) Week 2: C, A, B, C, A Week 3: B, C, A, B, C Week 4: A, B, C

Performance and Muscle Workout Programs

Whereas the workout programs featured in chapter 10 emphasize muscle gains and the programs presented in chapter 11 emphasize performance gains, the programs presented here are more neutral. Of course, all functional-spectrum training programs allow you to train both your hustle (performance) and your muscle (strength and size), but the programs presented in this chapter allow you to do so without emphasizing one component over the other.

Because the following workout programs are relatively balanced, you won't see results as fast or as much at either end of the functional spectrum—performance or muscle—as you would if you followed one of the programs emphasizing one aspect over the other.

Here are a few key points to remember when performing the exercises:

Speed Exercises

- Perform each rep as explosively as possible.
- In addition, if the exercise involves jumping, land as quietly as possible.
- If the workout calls for throwing a medicine ball (outside or against a solid wall) and your training environment prevents you from doing so; simply choose an alternative, non-medicine ball exercise option from the Total-Body Power Exercises section of chapter 4 or 5. Perform the alternative exercise for roughly the same amount of sets and reps that were recommended for the original exercise.

Strength Exercises

- While maintaining optimal technique, perform the concentric lifting portion of each rep as forcefully as you can; during the eccentric (lowering) portion, maintain good control.
- Use a weight load that allows you to perform the indicated number of reps in the fashion described in the preceding point. In each workout, you ensure improvement in strength either by adding weight and performing the same number of reps as in the preceding workout or by performing more reps with the same weight.

Size Exercises

- Focus on the working muscles in each exercise and maintain strict form without "cheating" by using additional movements or momentum.
- Perform the concentric lifting portion of each rep at a normal tempo and maintain control during the eccentric (lowering) portion.
- The set and rep numbers used for exercises in this section are undulated with three schemes. Regardless of the scheme you're on, use a weight load that leaves you unable to perform any more reps than indicated while maintaining proper control and technique.

Cardio Conditioning

- If the workout calls for a particular supramaximal interval training (SMIT), steady-state cardio, or metabolic conditioning protocol (MCP) that your training environment prevents you from performing, simply choose a comparable alternative from chapter 3. Perform the alternative exercise for roughly the same amount of reps, rounds, or time that were recommended for the original exercise.
- Only workouts A and C of each program involve a cardio conditioning component.

Performance and Muscle Workout Programs (Three to Five Days Per Week)

In the following programs, perform *a* and *b* exercises as paired sets. Perform all indicated sets and reps of a given paired set before moving on to the next set. If necessary, rest a bit longer than indicated between sets in order to complete the designated number of reps with good control. This program emphasizes movement quality over quantity! To help you personalize these workouts to *best* fit you, refer to this chapter.

TABLE 12.2 **Performance and Muscle Program 1: Workout A—Pulling**

	Page	Days 1 and 4	Days 2 and 5	Days 3 and 6
SPEED				
1a. Medicine-ball step and overhead throw (3–4 kg or 6.5–9 lbs.)	104	5 × 6–8	5 × 6–8	5 × 6–8
1b. Medicine-ball front-scoop horizontal throw (3–5 kg or 6.5–11 lbs.)	195	4 × 5 or 6 each side with 90 sec. rest between paired sets	4 × 5 or 6 each side with 90 sec. rest between paired sets	4 × 5 or 6 each side with 90 sec. rest between paired sets
STRENGTH				
2. One-arm cable row	114	5 × 4–6 each side with 90 sec. rest between sets	5 × 4–6 each side with 90 sec. rest between sets	5 × 4–6 each side with 90 sec. rest between sets
SIZE				
3. Leaning lat pull-down	122	3 × 10–12 with 60–90 sec. rest between sets	2 × 15–20 with 60–90 sec. rest between sets	4 × 6–8 with 60–90 sec. rest between sets
4. Wide-grip seated row	126	3 × 10–12 with 60–90 sec. rest between sets	2 × 15–20 with 60–90 sec. rest between sets	4 × 6–8 with 60–90 sec. rest between sets
5a. Dumbbell biceps curl	136	3 × 10–12	2 × 15–20	4 × 6–8
5b. Bent-over dumbbell shoulder fly	130	3 × 10–12 with 60 sec. rest between paired sets	2 × 15–20 with 60 sec. rest between paired sets	4 × 6–8 with 60 sec. rest between paired sets
CARDIO CONDITIONING		MCP*: bilateral farmer's-walk complex—2 or 3 sets with 2 min. rest between sets (page 57)	Steady-state cardio: elliptical trainer or upright bike—25–35 min. (page 29-30)	SMIT**: shuttle run—200 yd. × 5 or 6 with 2 min. rest between sets (page 25)

*MCP = metabolic conditioning protocol.

**SMIT = supramaximal interval training.

TABLE 12.3 **Performance and Muscle Program 1: Workout B—Lower Body and Core**

	Page	Days 1 and 4	Days 2 and 5	Days 3 and 6
SPEED				
1. 25-yard dash	141	5–8 sets with 60 sec. rest between sets	5–8 sets with 60 sec. rest between sets	5–8 sets with 60 sec. rest between sets
STRENGTH				
2a. Trap-bar squat	164	5 × 1–5	5 × 1–5	5 × 1–5
2b. Ab snail	210	4 × 6–10 with 2 min. rest between paired sets	4 × 6–10 with 2 min. rest between paired sets	4 × 6–10 with 2 min. rest between paired sets
SIZE				
3a. One-leg one-arm dumbbell Romanian deadlift	149	2 × 15–20 each side	4 × 6–8 each side	3 × 10–12 each side
3b. Dumbbell plank row	197	2 × 14 or 15 each side with 60–90 sec. rest between paired sets	4 × 6–8 each side with 60–90 sec. rest between paired sets	3 × 10–12 each side with 60–90 sec. rest between paired sets
4a. Bench step-up	172	2 × 14 or 15 each side	4 × 6–8 each side	3 × 10–12 each side
4b. Leg lowering with band*	212	2 × 15–20 with 60–90 sec. rest between paired sets	4 × 6–8 with 60–90 sec. rest between paired sets	3 × 10–12 with 60–90 sec. rest between paired sets
5. 45-degree hip extension	182	2 × 15–20 with 60–90 sec. rest between sets	4 × 6–8 with 60–90 sec. rest between sets	3 × 10–12 with 60–90 sec. rest between sets
6. Barbell calf raise	188	2 × 15–20 with 60–90 sec. rest between sets	4 × 6–8 with 60–90 sec. rest between sets	3 × 10–12 with 60–90 sec. rest between sets

*There is an inverse relation between the amount of reps indicated and the resistance load of band you use or how far you extend your legs. Extend your legs the farthest you can control on the days you perform 6 to 8 reps or use the heaviest band, and use the lightest band or don't extend your legs out as far on the days you perform 15 to 20 reps.

TABLE 12.4 **Performance and Muscle Program 1: Workout C—Pushing**

	Page	Days 1 and 4	Days 2 and 5	Days 3 and 6
SPEED				
1a. Medicine-ball vertical squat push throw (3–4 kg or 6.5–9 lbs.)	73	5 × 4–6	5 × 4–6	5 × 4–6
1b. Medicine-ball downward-chop throw (3–4 kg)	196	4 × 4–6 each side with 90 sec. rest between paired sets	4 × 4–6 each side with 90 sec. rest between paired sets	4 × 4–6 each side with 90 sec. rest between paired sets
STRENGTH				
2. Angled barbell rotational push press	83	5 × 3–5 each side with 90 sec. rest between sets	5 × 3–5 each side with 90 sec. rest between sets	5 × 3–5 each side with 90 sec. rest between sets
SIZE				
3. One-arm cable press	84	4 × 6–8 each side with 60–90 sec. rest between sets	3 × 10–12 each side with 60–90 sec. rest between sets	2 × 15–20 each side with 60–90 sec. rest between sets
4. Box crossover push-up	86	4 × max (–2)* with 60–90 sec. rest between sets	3 × max (–1)* with 60–90 sec. rest between sets	2 × max with 60–90 sec. rest between sets
5a. Cable triceps rope extension	101	4 × 6–8 sets	3 × 10–12 sets	2 × 15–20 sets
5b. Dumbbell front shoulder raise	99	4 × 6–8 with 60 sec. rest between paired sets	3 × 10–12 with 60 sec. rest between paired sets	2 × 15–20 with 60 sec. rest between paired sets
CARDIO CONDITIONING		SMIT**: rower—4–6 sets of 45–60 sec. as fast as possible with 90 sec. to 2 min. rest between sets (page 28)	MCP***: Six-min. body-weight complex— 2 or 3 sets with 2 min. rest between sets (page 32)	Steady-state cardio: elliptical trainer or upright bike— 25–35 min. (page 29-30)

*(–1) means to stop the set one rep before failure; (–2) means to stop two reps before failure.

**SMIT = supramaximal interval training.

***MCP = metabolic conditioning protocol.

TABLE 12.5 **Performance and Muscle Program 2: Workout A—Pulling**

	Page	Days 1 and 4	Days 2 and 5	Days 3 and 6
SPEED				
1a. Medicine-ball rainbow slam (3–4 kg or 6.5–9 lbs.)	105	5 × 3 or 4 each side	5 × 3 or 4 each side	5 × 3 or 4 each side
1b. Medicine-ball side-scoop diagonal throw (3–4 kg)	193	4 × 4 or 5 each side with 90 sec. rest between paired sets	4 × 4 or 5 each side with 90 sec. rest between paired sets	4 × 4 or 5 each side with 90 sec. rest between paired sets
STRENGTH				
2. One-arm freestanding dumbbell row	112	5 × 2–4 each side with 90 sec. rest between sets	5 × 2–4 each side with 90 sec. rest between sets	5 × 2–4 each side with 90 sec. rest between sets
SIZE				
3. Wide-grip barbell bent-over row	123	3 × 10–12 with 60–90 sec. rest between sets	2 × 15–20 with 60–90 sec. rest between sets	4 × 6–8 with 60–90 sec. rest between sets
4. Wide-elbow Smith-bar row	129	3 × 10–12 with 60–90 sec. rest between sets	2 × 15–20 with 60–90 sec. rest between sets	4 × 6–8 with 60–90 sec. rest between sets
5a. Cable biceps curl	137	3 × 10–12 sets	2 × 15–20 sets	4 × 6–8 sets
5b. Rope face pull	134	3 × 10–12 with 60 sec. rest between paired sets	2 × 15–20 with 60 sec. rest between paired sets	4 × 6–8 with 60 sec. rest between paired sets
CARDIO CONDITIONING		MCP*: boxing and kickboxing with heavy bag— 4–6 2-min. rounds with 60 sec. rest between rounds (page 30)	Steady-state cardio: brisk walking outside or on treadmill—25–35 min. (page 28)	SMIT**: gasser— 1–3 with 3–4 min. rest between sets (page 26)

*MCP = metabolic conditioning protocol.

**SMIT = supramaximal interval training.

323

TABLE 12.6   **Performance and Muscle Program 2: Workout B—Lower Body and Core**

	Page	Days 1 and 4	Days 2 and 5	Days 3 and 6
SPEED				
1. 30-yard shuttle	142	× 4–8 sets with 60 sec. rest between sets	× 4–8 sets with 60 sec. rest between sets	× 4–8 sets with 60 sec. rest between sets
STRENGTH				
2a. Barbell hybrid dead-lift	158	5 × 2–5	5 × 2–5	5 × 2–5
2b. One-arm plank	201	4 × 15–20 sec. each side with 2 min. rest between paired sets	4 × 15–20 sec. each side with 2 min. rest between paired sets	4 × 15–20 sec. each side with 2 min. rest between paired sets
SIZE				
3a. Lateral lunge with cross-body reach	152	2 × 14 or 15 each side	4 × 6–8 each side	3 × 10–12 each side
3b. Stability-ball abdominal exercise indicated	204, 206, 205	Stability-ball knee tuck 2 × 15–20 with 60–90 sec. rest between paired sets	Stability-ball pike rollout 4 × 6–8 with 60–90 sec. rest between paired sets	Stability-ball pike 3 × 10–12 with 60–90 sec. rest between paired sets
4a. Elevated barbell reverse lunge	163	2 × 14 or 15 each side	4 × 6–8 each side	3 × 10–12 each side
4b. Stability-ball plate crunch	211	2 × 15–20 with 60–90 sec. rest between paired sets	4 × 6–8 with 60–90 sec. rest between paired sets	3 × 10–12 with 60–90 sec. rest between paired sets
5. Machine seated hamstring curl	186	2 × 15–20 with 60 sec. rest between sets	4 × 6–8 with 60 sec. rest between sets	3 × 10–12 with 60 sec. rest between sets
6. Barbell calf raise	188	2 × 15–20 with 60 sec. rest between sets	4 × 6–8 with 60 sec. rest between sets	3 × 10–12 with 60 sec. rest between sets

TABLE 12.7 **Performance and Muscle Program 2: Workout C—Pushing**

	Page	Days 1 and 4	Days 2 and 5	Days 3 and 6
SPEED				
1. Angled barbell press and catch	78	4 × 5 or 6 each side with 90 sec. rest between sets	4 × 5 or 6 each side with 90 sec. rest between sets	4 × 5 or 6 each side with 90 sec. rest between sets
2. Lateral power shuffle	143	4 × 6–8 each direction with 90 sec. rest between sets	4 × 6–8 each direction with 90 sec. rest between sets	4 × 6–8 each direction with 90 sec. rest between sets
STRENGTH				
3. One-arm dumbbell rotational push press	80	4 × 2–4 each side with 90 sec. rest between sets	4 × 2–4 each side with 90 sec. rest between sets	4 × 2–4 each side with 90 sec. rest between sets
SIZE				
4. One-arm cable press	84	4 × 6–8 each side with 90 sec. rest between sets	3 × 10–12 each side with 90 sec. rest between sets	2 × 15–20 each side with 90 sec. rest between sets
5. Close-grip push-up	95	4 × max (–2)* with 90 sec. rest between sets	3 × max (–1)* with 90 sec. rest between sets	2 × max with 90 sec. rest between sets
6. Dumbbell pec fly	98	4 × 6–8 with 90 sec. rest between sets	3 × 10–12 with 90 sec. rest between sets	2 × 15–20 with 90 sec. rest between sets
7. Dumbbell triceps skull crusher	100	4 × 6–8 sets	3 × 10–12 sets	2 × 15–20 sets
CARDIO CONDITIONING		SMIT**: treadmill— 5–7 sets running at top speed for 15–30 sec. with 60 sec. rest between sets (page 28)	MCP***: unilateral leg complex—1 or 2 sets with 2 min. rest between sets (page 34)	Steady-state cardio: brisk walking outside or on treadmill—25–35 min. (page 29)

*(–1) means to stop the set one rep before failure; (–2) means to stop two reps before failure.

**SMIT = supramaximal interval training.

***MCP = metabolic conditioning protocol.

TABLE 12.8 **Performance and Muscle Program 3: Workout A—Pulling**

	Page	Days 1 and 4	Days 2 and 5	Days 3 and 6
SPEED				
1a. Medicine-ball step and overhead throw (3–4 kg or 6.5–9 lbs.)	104	5 × 6–8	5 × 6–8	5 × 6–8
1b. Medicine-ball side-scoop horizontal throw (3–5 kg or 6.5–11 lbs.)	193	4 × 5 or 6 each side with 90 sec. rest between paired sets	4 × 5 or 6 each side with 90 sec. rest between paired sets	4 × 5 or 6 each side with 90 sec. rest between paired sets
STRENGTH				
2. One-arm compound cable row	116	4 or 5 × 3–5 each side with 90 sec. rest between sets	4 or 5 × 3–5 each side with 90 sec. rest between sets	4 or 5 × 3–5 each side with 90 sec. rest between sets
SIZE				
3. Fighter's cable lat pull-down	122	3 × 10–12 each side with 60–90 sec. rest between sets	2 × 14 or 15 each side with 60–90 sec. rest between sets	4 × 6–8 each side with 60–90 sec. rest between sets
4. Cable compound straight-arm pull-down	135	3 × 10–12 with 60–90 sec. rest between sets	2 × 15–20 with 60–90 sec. rest between sets	4 × 6–8 with 60–90 sec. rest between sets
5a. Wide-elbow suspension row	128	3 × 10–12	2 × 15–20	4 × 6–8
5b. Suspension biceps curl	138	3 × 10–12 with 60–90 sec. rest between paired sets	2 × 15–20 with 60–90 sec. rest between paired sets	4 × 6–8 with 60–90 sec. rest between paired sets
CARDIO CONDITIONING		MCP*: Six-min. body-weight complex—2 or 3 sets with 2 min. rest between sets (page 32)	Steady-state cardio: elliptical trainer or upright bike—25–35 min. (page 29-30)	SMIT**: rower—4–6 sets of 45–60 sec. as fast as possible with 90 sec. to 2 min. rest between sets (page 28)

*MCP = metabolic conditioning protocol.

**SMIT = supramaximal interval training.

TABLE 12.9 **Performance and Muscle Program 3: Workout B—Lower Body and Core**

	Page	Days 1 and 4	Days 2 and 5	Days 3 and 6
SPEED				
1. Broad jump	146	4 or 5 × 3 or 4 with 90 sec. rest between sets	4 or 5 × 3 or 4 with 90 sec. rest between sets	4 or 5 × 3 or 4 with 90 sec. rest between sets
STRENGTH				
2a. Barbell Romanian deadlift	156	5 × 3–5	5 × 3–5	5 × 3–5
2b. Stability-ball stir-the-pot	207	4 × 4–8 in each direction with 2 min. rest between paired sets	4 × 4–8 in each direction with 2 min. rest between paired sets	4 × 4–8 in each direction with 2 min. rest between paired sets
SIZE				
3a. Angled barbell cross-shoulder reverse lunge	155	2 × 14 or 15 each side	4 × 6–8 each side	3 × 10–12 each side
3b. Angled barbell tight rainbow	202	2 × 15–20 each side with 60–90 sec. rest between paired sets	4 × 6–8 each side with 60–90 sec. rest between paired sets	3 × 10–12 each side with 60–90 sec. rest between paired sets
4a. Bulgarian split squat and Romanian deadlift combination	168	2 × 12–14 each side	4 × 5–7 each side	3 × 8–10 each side
4b. Reverse crunch*	211	2 × 14 or 15 with 60–90 sec. rest between paired sets	4 × 6–8 with 60–90 sec. rest between paired sets	3 × 10–12 with 60–90 sec. rest between paired sets
5. One-leg dumbbell bench hip thrust	177	2 × 15–20 each side with 60 sec. rest between sets	4 × 6–8 each side with 60 sec. rest between sets	3 × 10–12 each side with 60 sec. rest between sets
6. Machine leg press	165	2 × 15–20	4 × 6–8	3 × 10–12

*There is an inverse relation between the amount of reps indicated and the weight you'll use as an anchor, as the heavier the anchor the easier the exercise becomes. Use the lightest dumbbell, kettlebell, or medicine ball as an anchor on the days you perform 6 to 8 reps, and use the heaviest anchor on the days you perform 15 to 20 reps.

TABLE 12.10 **Performance and Muscle Program 3: Workout C—Pushing**

	Page	Days 1 and 4	Days 2 and 5	Days 3 and 6
SPEED				
1a. Medicine-ball step and push throw (3–4 kg or 6.5–9 lbs.)	77	5 × 4–6	5 × 4–6	5 × 4–6
1b. 180-degree squat jump with cross-arm drive	144	4 × 2 or 3 each direction with 90 sec. rest between paired sets	4 × 2 or 3 each direction with 90 sec. rest between paired sets	4 × 2 or 3 each direction with 90 sec. rest between paired sets
STRENGTH				
2. One-arm push-up or one-arm cable press	85, 84	4 or 5 × 1–5 or 4 or 5 × 4–6 each side with 90 sec. rest between sets	4 or 5 × 1–5 or 4 or 5 × 4–6 each side with 90 sec. rest between sets	4 or 5 × 1–5 or 4 or 5 × 4–6 each side with 90 sec. rest between sets
SIZE				
3. Angled barbell press	82	4 × 6–8 with 60–90 sec. rest between sets	3 × 10–12 with 60–90 sec. rest between sets	2 × 15–20 with 60–90 sec. rest between sets
4. Incline barbell bench press	88	4 × 6–8 with 60–90 sec. rest between sets	3 × 10–12 with 60–90 sec. rest between sets	2 × 15–20 with 60–90 sec. rest between sets
5a. Dumbbell front-hold overhead press	90	4 × 6–8 sets	3 × 10–12 sets	2 × 15–20 sets
5b. Cable triceps rope extension	101	4 × 6–8 with 60 sec. rest between paired sets	3 × 10–12 with 60 sec. rest between paired sets	2 × 15–20 with 60 sec. rest between paired sets
CARDIO CONDITIONING		SMIT*: shuttle run—250 yd. × 4 or 5 with 2.5 min. rest between sets (page 25)	MCP**: unilateral farmer's-walk complex—× 2 or 3 sets with 2 min. rest between sets (page 59)	Steady-state cardio: elliptical trainer or upright bike—25–35 min. (page 29-30)

*SMIT = supramaximal interval training.

**MCP = metabolic conditioning protocol.

TABLE 12.11 Performance and Muscle Program 4: Workout A—Pulling

	Page	Days 1 and 4	Days 2 and 5	Days 3 and 6
SPEED				
1. Rope slam	111	4 × 12–15	4 × 12–15	4 × 12–15
2. Medicine-ball side-scoop horizontal throw (3–5 kg or 6.5–11 lbs.)	193	4 × 5 or 6 each side with 90 sec. rest between paired sets	4 × 5 or 6 each side with 90 sec. rest between paired sets	4 × 5 or 6 each side with 90 sec. rest between paired sets
STRENGTH				
3. One-arm freestanding dumbbell row	112	4 or 5 × 3–5 each side with 90 sec. rest between sets	4 or 5 × 3–5 each side with 90 sec. rest between sets	4 or 5 × 3–5 each side with 90 sec. rest between sets
SIZE				
4. Wide-grip barbell bent-over row	123	3 × 10–12 with 60–90 sec. rest between sets	2 × 15–20 with 60–90 sec. rest between sets	4 × 6–8 with 60–90 sec. rest between sets
5. Lat pull-down	121	3 × 10–12 with 60–90 sec. rest between sets	2 × 15–20 with 60–90 sec. rest between sets	4 × 6–8 with 60–90 sec. rest between sets
6a. Dumbbell biceps curl	136	3 × 10–12	2 × 15–20	4 × 6–8
6b. Dumbbell shoulder A	131	3 × 10–12 with 60 sec. rest between paired sets	2 × 15–20 with 60 sec. rest between paired sets	4 × 6–8 with 60 sec. rest between paired sets
CARDIO CONDITIONING		MCP*: Four-min. rope complex—2 or 3 sets with 2–3 min. rest between sets (page 47)	Steady-state cardio: brisk walking outside or on treadmill—25–35 min. (page 29)	SMIT**: treadmill—5–7 sets running at top speed for 15–30 sec. with 60 sec. rest between sets (page 28)

*MCP = metabolic conditioning protocol.

**SMIT = supramaximal interval training.

TABLE 12.12 **Performance and Muscle Program 4: Workout B—Lower Body and Core**

	Page	Days 1 and 4	Days 2 and 5	Workouts 3 and 6
SPEED				
1. 25-yard dash	141	5–8 with 60 sec. rest between sets	5–8 with 60 sec. rest between sets	5–8 with 60 sec. rest between sets
STRENGTH				
2a. Barbell sumo dead-lift	157	5 × 2–4	5 × 2–4	5 × 2–4
2b. Stability-ball pike rollout	206	4 × 8–12 with 2 min. rest between paired sets	4 × 8–12 with 2 min. rest between paired sets	4 × 8–12 with 2 min. rest between paired sets
SIZE				
3a. One-leg 45-degree cable Romanian deadlift	150	2 × 15–20 each side	4 × 6–8 each side	3 × 10–12 each side
3b. Stability-ball plate crunch	211	2 × 15–20 with 60 sec. rest between paired sets	4 × 6–8 with 60 sec. rest between paired sets	3 × 10–12 with 60 sec. rest between paired sets
4a. Dumbbell fighter's lunge	170	2 × 14 or 15 each side	4 × 6–8 each side	3 × 10–12 each side
4b. One-arm dumbbell farmer's walk	197	2 × 60 sec. each side with 60 sec. rest between paired sets	4 × 30 sec. each side with 60 sec. rest between paired sets	3 × 45 sec. each side with 60 sec. rest between paired sets
5a. Machine seated hamstring curl	186	2 × 15–20	4 × 6–8	3 × 10–12
5b. Machine leg exten-sion	187	2 × 15–20 with 60 sec. rest between paired sets	4 × 6–8 with 60 sec. rest between paired sets	3 × 10–12 with 60 sec. rest between paired sets

TABLE 12.13 **Performance and Muscle Program 4: Workout C—Pushing**

	Page	Days 1 and 4	Days 2 and 5	Days 3 and 6
SPEED				
1a. Medicine-ball horizontal punch throw (3–4 kg or 6.5–9 lbs.)	191	4 × 4 or 5 each side	4 × 4 or 5 each side	4 × 4 or 5 each side
1b. Lateral bound	148	4 × 3–5 each side with 90 sec. rest between paired sets	4 × 3–5 each side with 90 sec. rest between paired sets	4 × 3–5 each side with 90 sec. rest between paired sets
STRENGTH				
2. One-arm dumbbell rotational push press	80	4 × 2–4 each side with 90 sec. rest between sets	4 × 2–4 each side with 90 sec. rest between sets	4 × 2–4 each side with 90 sec. rest between sets
SIZE				
3. Angled barbell rotational push press	83	4 × 5 or 6 each side with 60–90 sec. rest between sets	3 × 8 or 9 each side with 60–90 sec. rest between sets	2 × 11 or 12 each side with 60–90 sec. rest between sets
4. Box crossover push-up	86	4 × max (–2)* with 60–90 sec. rest between sets	3 × max (–1)* with 60–90 sec. rest between sets	2 × max with 60–90 sec. rest between sets
5a. Dumbbell pec fly	98	4 × 6–8	3 × 10–12	2 × 15–20
5b. Dumbbell triceps skull crusher	100	4 × 6–8 with 60 sec. rest between paired sets	3 × 10–12 with 60 sec. rest between paired sets	2 × 15–20 with 60 sec. rest between paired sets
CARDIO CONDITIONING		SMIT**: gasser—1–3 with 3–4 min. rest between sets (page 26)	MCP***: 20-20-10-10 leg complex—2–3 sets with 2 min. rest between sets (page 37)	Steady-state cardio: brisk walking outside or on treadmill—25–35 min. (page 29)

*(–1) means to stop the set one rep before failure; (–2) means to stop two reps before failure.

**SMIT = supramaximal interval training.

***MCP = metabolic conditioning protocol.

TABLE 12.14 Performance and Muscle Program 5: Workout A—Pulling

	Page	Days 1 and 4	Days 2 and 5	Days 3 and 6
SPEED				
1a. Medicine-ball rainbow slam (3–4 kg or 6.5–9 lbs.)	105	5 × 3 or 4 each side	5 × 3 or 4 each side	5 × 3 or 4 each side
1b. Medicine-ball shot-put throw (3–4 kg)	192	4 × 3 or 4 each side with 90 sec. rest between paired sets	4 × 3 or 4 each side with 90 sec. rest between paired sets	4 × 3 or 4 each side with 90 sec. rest between paired sets
STRENGTH				
2. Angled barbell press	82	4 × 2–5 each side with 90 sec. rest between sets	4 × 2–5 each side with 90 sec. rest between sets	4 × 2–5 each side with 90 sec. rest between sets
SIZE				
3. Smith-bar underhand-grip row or suspension row	128, 127	3 × 10–12 with 60–90 sec. rest between sets	2 × 15–20 with 60–90 sec. rest between sets	4 × 6–8 with 60–90 sec. rest between sets
4. Cable compound straight-arm pulldown	135	3 × 10–12 with 60–90 sec. rest between sets	2 × 15–20 with 60–90 sec. rest between sets	4 × 6–8 with 60–90 sec. rest between sets
5a. EZ-Bar biceps curl	137	3 × 10–12 with 60–90 sec. rest between sets	2 × 15–20 with 60–90 sec. rest between sets	4 × 6–8 with 60–90 sec. rest between sets
5b. Bent-over dumbbell shoulder fly	130	3 × 10–12 with 60 sec. rest between paired sets	2 × 15–20 with 60 sec. rest between paired sets	4 × 6–8 with 60 sec. rest between paired sets
CARDIO CONDITIONING		MCP*: weight-plate push—4–6 sets 40–50 yd. with 90 sec. rest between sets (page 50)	Steady-state cardio: elliptical trainer or upright bike— 25–35 min. (page 29-30)	SMIT**: shuttle run—300 yd. × 2 or 3 with 3 min. rest between sets (page 25)

*MCP = metabolic conditioning protocol.

**SMIT = supramaximal interval training.

TABLE 12.15 Performance and Muscle Program 5: Workout B—Lower Body and Core

	Page	Days 1 and 4	Days 2 and 5	Days 3 and 6
SPEED				
1. Lateral power shuffle	143	4 × 5–8 in each direction with 60–90 sec. rest between sets	4 × 5–8 in each direction with 60–90 sec. rest between sets	4 × 5–8 in each direction with 60–90 sec. rest between sets
STRENGTH				
2a. Barbell hybrid deadlift	158	5 × 1–4	5 × 1–4	5 × 1–4
2b. Leg lowering with band	212	4 × 8–12 with 2 min. rest between paired sets	4 × 8–12 with 2 min. rest between paired sets	4 × 8–12 with 2 min. rest between paired sets
SIZE				
3a. One-leg offset traveling lunge	154	2 × 15–20 each side	4 × 6–8 each side	3 × 10–12 each side
3b. Rollout exercise variation indicated	204, 208, 208	Stability-ball rollout 2 × 15–20 with 60–90 sec. rest between paired sets	Medicine-ball walkout 4 × 6–8 with 60–90 sec. rest between paired sets	Arm walkout 3 × 10–12 with 60–90 sec. rest between paired sets
4a. Dumbbell anterior lunge	172	2 × 14 or 15 each side	4 × 6–8 each side	3 × 10–12 each side
4b. Low-to-high cable chop	198	2 × 14 or 15 each side with 60–90 sec. rest between paired sets	4 × 6–8 each side with 60–90 sec. rest between paired sets	3 × 10–12 each side with 60–90 sec. rest between paired sets
5. Leg-curl exercise variation indicated	184, 184, 178	Stability-ball leg curl 2 × 15–20 with 60 sec. rest between sets	One-leg stability-ball leg curl 4 × 6–8 with 60 sec. rest between sets	Hip thrust hamstring curl combo 3 × 10–12 with 60 sec. rest between sets
6. Barbell calf raise	188	2 × 15–20 with 60 sec. rest between sets	4 × 6–8 with 60 sec. rest between sets	3 × 10–12 with 60 sec. rest between sets

TABLE 12.16 **Performance and Muscle Program 5: Workout C—Pushing**

	Page	Days 1 and 4	Days 2 and 5	Days 3 and 6
SPEED				
1a. Medicine-ball horizontal punch throw (3–4 kg or 6.5–9 lbs.)	191	4 or 5 × 4 or 5 each side	4 or 5 × 4 or 5 each side	4 or 5 × 4 or 5 each side
1b. Power skip	142	4 or 5 × 8–10 each leg with 90 sec. rest between paired sets	4 or 5 × 8–10 each leg with 90 sec. rest between paired sets	4 or 5 × 8–10 each leg with 90 sec. rest between paired sets
STRENGTH				
3. Angled barbell press	82	4 × 2–5 each side with 90 sec. rest between sets	4 × 2–5 each side with 90 sec. rest between sets	4 × 2–5 each side with 90 sec. rest between sets
SIZE				
4. Dumbbell bench press	88	4 × 6–8 with 90 sec. rest between sets	3 × 10–12 with 90 sec. rest between sets	2 × 15–20 with 90 sec. rest between sets
5. Push-up lock-off	86	4 × max (–2)* each side with 60–90 sec. rest between sets	3 × max (–1)* each side with 60–90 sec. rest between sets	2 × max each side with 60–90 sec. rest between sets
6a. Dumbbell side shoulder raise	99	4 × 6–8	3 × 10–12	2 × 15–20
6b. Suspension triceps skull crusher	101	4 × 6–8 with 60 sec. rest between paired sets	3 × 10–12 with 60 sec. rest between paired sets	2 × 15–20 with 60 sec. rest between paired sets
CARDIO CONDITIONING		SMIT**: rower—4–6 sets of 45–60 secs. as fast as possible with 90 sec. to 2 min. rest between sets (page 28)	MCP***: boxing and kickboxing with heavy bag—3–5 3 min. rounds with 90 sec. rest between rounds (page 30)	Steady-state cardio: elliptical trainer or upright bike—25–35 min. (page 29-30)

*(–2) means to stop the set two reps before failure and (–1) means to stop the set one rep before failure.

**SMIT = supramaximal interval training.

***MCP = metabolic conditioning protocol.

Performance and Muscle Workout Programs (2 days per week)

Although I recommend training at least three times per week, you can still get positive results if your schedule allows only two training days per week. Designed to meet that need, the following programs are alternative versions of the programs provided in the preceding sections of the chapter.

Each of the following three programs consists of two workouts: workout A and workout B. Workout A focuses on pulling and pushing exercises, and workout B focuses on lower-body and core exercises. Perform the workouts in each program six times before moving on to a new program. In other words, if you're training twice per week, use the same program for six weeks before switching to the next program and performing that one for another six weeks and so on. In each of the following programs, workout B (lower body and core) is almost identical to the corresponding workout in the preceding sections, with the exception of an additional exercise application in the speed category. On the other hand, the version of workout A used in these programs is a combination of the corresponding workout A and workout C in the preceding sections. Therefore, although they feature exercises also found in the preceding sections, each workout A presented here involves performing several more exercises.

TABLE 12.17 Two-Day Performance and Muscle Program 1: Workout A—Pulling/Pushing

	Page	Days 1 and 4	Days 2 and 5	Days 3 and 6
SPEED				
1a. Medicine-ball step and overhead throw (3–4 kg or 6.5–9 lbs.)	104	4 or 5 × 6–8	4 or 5 × 6–8	4 or 5 × 6–8
1b. Medicine-ball front-scoop horizontal throw (3–5 kg or 6.5–11 lbs.)	195	4 or 5 × 5 or 6 each side	4 or 5 × 5 or 6 each side	4 or 5 × 5 or 6 each side
1c. Medicine-ball vertical squat push throw (3–5 kg)	73	4 or 5 × 4–6 with 90 sec. rest between tri-sets	4 or 5 × 4–6 with 90 sec. rest between tri-sets	4 or 5 × 4–6 with 90 sec. rest between tri-sets
STRENGTH				
2a. One-arm cable row	114	5 × 3–5 each side	5 × 3–5 each side	5 × 3–5 each side
2b. Angled barbell rotational push press	83	5 × 3–5 each side with 90 sec. rest between paired sets	5 × 3–5 each side with 90 sec. rest between paired sets	5 × 3–5 each side with 90 sec. rest between paired sets
SIZE				
3a. One-arm cable press	84	4 × 6–8 each side	3 × 10–12 each side	2 × 15–20 each side
3b. Bent-over dumbbell shoulder fly	130	4 × 6–8 with 60–90 sec. rest between paired sets	3 × 10–12 with 60–90 sec. rest between paired sets	2 × 15–20 with 60–90 sec. rest between paired sets
4a. Push-up lock-off	86	4 × max (–2)* each side	3 × max (–1)* each side	2 × max each side
4b. Wide-grip seated row	126	4 × 6–8 with 60–90 sec. rest between paired sets	3 × 10–12 with 60–90 sec. rest between paired sets	2 × 15–20 with 60–90 sec. rest between paired sets
5a. Dumbbell biceps curl	136	4 × 6–8	2 × 15–20	2 × 15–20
5b. Dumbbell triceps skull crusher	100	4 × 6–8 with 60 sec. rest between paired sets	3 × 10–12 with 60 sec. rest between paired sets	2 × 15–20 with 60 sec. rest between paired sets
6. Dumbbell side shoulder raise	99	4 × 6–8 with 60 sec. rest between sets	3 × 10–12 with 60 sec. rest between sets	2 × 15–20 with 60 sec. rest between sets
CARDIO CONDITIONING		SMIT**: shuttle run—250 yd. × 4 or 5 with 2.5 min. rest between sets (page 25)	MCP***: unilateral leg complex—1 or 2 sets with 2 min. rest between sets (page 34)	Steady-state cardio: elliptical trainer or upright bike—25–35 min. (page 29-30)

*(–1) means to stop the set one rep before failure; (–2) means to stop two reps before failure.

**SMIT = supramaximal interval training.

***MCP = metabolic conditioning protocol.

TABLE 12.18   Two-Day Performance and Muscle Program 1: Workout B—Lower Body and Core

	Page	Days 1 and 4	Days 2 and 5	Days 3 and 6
SPEED				
1a. 25-yard dash	141	5–8 sets	5–8 sets	5–8 sets
1b. Medicine-ball down-ward-chop throw (3–4 kg or 6.5–9 lbs.)	196	4 × 4–6 each side with 60 sec. rest between paired sets	4 × 4–6 each side with 60 sec. rest between paired sets	4 × 4–6 each side with 60 sec. rest between paired sets
STRENGTH				
2a. Trap-bar squat	164	5 × 1–5	5 × 1–5	5 × 1–5
2b. Ab snail	210	4 × 6–10 with 2 min. rest between paired sets	4 × 6–10 with 2 min. rest between paired sets	4 × 6–10 with 2 min. rest between paired sets
SIZE				
3a. One-leg one-arm dumbbell Romanian deadlift	149	2 × 15–20 each side	4 × 6–8 each side	3 × 10–12 each side
3b. Dumbbell plank row	197	2 × 14 or 15 each side with 60–90 sec. rest between paired sets	4 × 6–8 each side with 60–90 sec. rest between paired sets	3 × 10–12 each side with 60–90 sec. rest between paired sets
4a. Bench step-up	172	2 × 15–20 each side	4 × 6–8 each side	3 × 10–12 each side
4b. Leg lowering with band*	212	2 × 15–20 with 60–90 sec. rest between paired sets	4 × 6–8 with 60–90 sec. rest between paired sets	3 × 10–12 with 60–90 sec. rest between paired sets
5. 45-degree hip exten-sion	182	2 × 15–20 with 60 sec. rest between sets	4 × 6–8 with 60 sec. rest between sets	3 × 10–12 with 60 sec. rest between sets
6. Barbell calf raise	188	2 × 15–20 with 60 sec. rest between sets	4 × 6–8 with 60 sec. rest between sets	3 × 10–12 with 60 sec. rest between sets
CARDIO CONDITIONING		Steady-state cardio: brisk walking out-side or on tread-mill—25–35 min. (page 29)	SMIT**: rower—4–6 sets of 45–60 sec. as fast as possible with 90 sec. to 2 min. rest between sets (page 28)	MCP***: bilateral farmer's-walk com-plex—2 or 3 sets with 2 min. rest between sets (page 57)

*There is an inverse relation between the amount of reps indicated and the resistance load of band you use or how far you extend your legs. Extend your legs the farthest you can control on the days you perform 6 to 8 reps or use the heaviest band, and use the lightest band or don't extend your legs out as far on the days you perform 15 to 20 reps.

**SMIT = supramaximal interval training.

***MCP = metabolic conditioning protocol.

TABLE 12.19 Two-Day Performance and Muscle Program 2: Workout A—Pulling and Pushing

	Page	Days 1 and 4	Days 2 and 5	Days 3 and 6
SPEED				
1a. Medicine-ball rainbow slam (3–4 kg or 6.5–9 lbs.)	105	5 × 3 or 4 each side	5 × 3 or 4 each side	5 × 3 or 4 each side
1b. Medicine-ball side-scoop diagonal throw (3–5 kg or 6.5–11 lbs.)	194	4 × 4 or 5 each side with 90 sec. rest between paired sets	4 × 4 or 5 each side with 90 sec. rest between paired sets	4 × 4 or 5 each side with 90 sec. rest between paired sets
2. Lateral power shuffle	143	4 × 6–8 each direction with 90 sec. rest between sets	4 × 6–8 each direction with 90 sec. rest between sets	4 × 6–8 each direction with 90 sec. rest between sets
STRENGTH				
3a. One-arm freestanding dumbbell row	112	5 × 2–4 each side	5 × 2–4 each side	5 × 2–4 each side
3b. One-arm dumbbell rotational push press	80	4 × 2–4 each side with 90 sec. rest between paired sets	4 × 2–4 each side with 90 sec. rest between paired sets	4 × 2–4 each side with 90 sec. rest between paired sets
SIZE				
4a. Angled barbell rotational push press	83	3 × 7–9 each side	2 × 10–12 each side	4 × 5 or 6 each side
4b. Two-arm dumbbell bent-over row	124	3 × 10–12 with 90 sec. rest between paired sets	2 × 15–20 with 90 sec. rest between paired sets	4 × 6–8 with 90 sec. rest between paired sets
5a. Close-grip push-up	95	3 × max (–1)*	2 × max	4 × max (–2)*
5b. Pull-up or lat pull-down	120, 121	3 × 10–12 with 90 sec. rest between paired sets	2 × 15–20 with 90 sec. rest between paired sets	4 × 6–8 with 90 sec. rest between paired sets
6a. Cable biceps curl	137	3 × 10–12	2 × 15–20	4 × 6–8
6b. Rope Face Pull	134	3 × 10–12	2 × 15–20	4 × 6–8
6c. Cable triceps rope extension	101	3 × 10–12 with 60–90 sec. rest between tri-sets	2 × 15–20 with 60–90 sec. rest between tri-sets	4 × 6–8 with 60–90 sec. rest between tri-sets
CARDIO CONDITIONING		MCP**: Six-min. body-weight complex—2 or 3 sets with 2 min. rest between sets (page 32)	Steady-state cardio: brisk walking outside or on treadmill—25–35 min. (page 29)	SMIT***: gasser—1–3 with 3–4 min. rest between sets (page 26)

*(–1) means to stop the set one rep before failure; (–2) means to stop two reps before failure.

**MCP = metabolic conditioning protocol.

***SMIT = supramaximal interval training.

TABLE 12.20 **Two-Day Performance and Muscle Program 2:
Workout B—Lower Body and Core**

	Page	Days 1 and 4	Days 2 and 5	Days 3 and 6
SPEED				
1. 30-yard shuttle	142	4–8 with 60 sec. rest between sets	4–8 with 60 sec. rest between sets	4–8 with 60 sec. rest between sets
2. Deadlift jump with arm drive	145	4 or 5 × 5–7 with 90 sec. rest between sets	4 or 5 × 5–7 with 90 sec. rest between sets	4 or 5 × 5–7 with 90 sec. rest between sets
STRENGTH				
3a. Barbell hybrid dead-lift	158	5 × 2–5	5 × 2–5	5 × 2–5
3b. One-arm plank	201	4 × 10–20 sec. each arm with 2 min. rest between paired sets	4 × 10–20 sec. each arm with 2 min. rest between paired sets	4 × 10–20 sec. each arm with 2 min. rest between paired sets
SIZE				
4a. Lateral lunge with cross-body reach	152	2 × 14 or 15 each side	4 × 6–8 each side	3 × 10–12 each side
4b. Stability-ball plate crunch	211	2 × 15–20 with 60–90 sec. rest between paired sets	4 × 6–8 with 60–90 sec. rest between paired sets	3 × 10–12 with 60–90 sec. rest between paired sets
5a. Elevated barbell reverse lunge	163	2 × 14 or 15 each side	4 × 6–8 each side	3 × 10–12 each side
5b. Stability-ball abdominal exercise indicated	204, 206, 205	Stability-ball knee tuck 2 × 15–20 with 60–90 sec. rest between paired sets	Stability-ball pike roll-back 4 × 6–8 with 60–90 sec. rest between paired sets	Stability-ball pike 3 × 10–12 with 60–90 sec. rest between paired sets
6. Leg-curl exercise variation indicated	184, 184, 178	Stability-ball leg curl 2 × 15–20 with 60 sec. rest between sets	One-leg stability-ball leg curl 4 × 6–8 with 60 sec. rest between sets	Hip thrust hamstring curl combo 3 × 10–12 with 60 sec. rest between sets
7. Barbell calf raise	188	2 × 15–20 with 60 sec. rest between sets	4 × 6–8 with 60 sec. rest between sets	3 × 10–12 with 60 sec. rest between sets
CARDIO CONDITIONING		Steady-state cardio: elliptical trainer or upright bike—25–35 min. (page 29-30)	SMIT*: tread-mill—5–7 sets running at top speed for 15–30 sec. with 60 sec. rest between sets (page 28)	MCP**: boxing and kickboxing with heavy bag—4–6 2 min. rounds with 60 sec. rest between rounds (page 30)

*SMIT = supramaximal interval training.

**MCP = metabolic conditioning protocol.

TABLE 12.21   Two-Day Performance and Muscle Program 3: Workout A—Pulling and Pushing

	Page	Days 1 and 4	Days 2 and 5	Days 3 and 6
SPEED				
1a. Medicine-ball step and overhead throw (3–4 kg or 6.5–9 lbs.)	104	4 or 5 × 6–8	4 or 5 × 6–8	4 or 5 × 6–8
1b. Medicine-ball side-scoop horizontal throw (3–5 kg or 6.5–11 lbs.)	193	4 or 5 × 5 or 6 each side	4 or 5 × 5 or 6 each side	4 or 5 × 5 or 6 each side
1c. Medicine-ball step and push throw (3–4 kg)	77	4 or 5 × 4–6 with 2 min. rest between tri-sets	4 or 5 × 4–6 with 2 min. rest between tri-sets	4 or 5 × 4–6 with 2 min. rest between tri-sets
STRENGTH				
2a. One-arm compound cable row	116	4 or 5 × 3–5 each side	4 or 5 × 3–5 each side	4 or 5 × 3–5 each side
2b. One-arm push-up or one-arm cable press	85, 84	4 or 5 × 1–5 or 4 or 5 × 4–6 each side with 60–90 sec. rest between paired sets	4 or 5 × 1–5 or 4 or 5 × 4–6 each side with 60–90 sec. rest between paired sets	4 or 5 × 1–5 or 4 or 5 × 4–6 each side with 60–90 sec. rest between paired sets
SIZE				
3a. Angled barbell press	82	3 × 10–12 each side	2 × 15–20 each side	4 × 6–8 each side
3b. Fighter's cable lat pull-down	122	3 × 10–12 each side with 60–90 sec. rest between paired sets	2 × 14 or 15 each side with 60–90 sec. rest between paired sets	4 × 6–8 each side with 60–90 sec. rest between paired sets
4a. Dumbbell front-hold overhead press	90	3 × 10–12	2 × 15–20	4 × 6–8
4b. Cable compound straight-arm pull-down	135	3 × 10–12 with 60–90 sec. rest between paired sets	2 × 15–20 with 60–90 sec. rest between paired sets	4 × 6–8 with 60–90 sec. rest between paired sets
5a. Wide-elbow suspension row	128	3 × 10–12	2 × 15–20	4 × 6–8
5b. Suspension biceps curl	138	3 × 10–12	2 × 15–20	4 × 6–8
5c. Suspension triceps skull crusher	101	3 × 10–12 with 60–90 sec. rest between tri-sets	2 × 15–20 with 60–90 sec. rest between tri-sets	4 × 6–8 with 60–90 sec. rest between tri-sets
CARDIO CONDITIONING		MCP*: 20-20-10-10 leg complex—2 or 3 sets with 2 min. rest between sets (page 37)	Steady-state cardio: elliptical trainer or upright bike—25–35 min. (page 29-30)	SMIT**: shuttle run—300 yd. × 2 or 3 with 3 min. rest between sets (page 25)

*MCP = metabolic conditioning protocol.

**SMIT = supramaximal interval training.

TABLE 12.22 Two-Day Performance and Muscle Program 3: Workout B—Lower Body and Core

	Page	Days 1 and 4	Days 2 and 5	Days 3 and 6
SPEED				
1. Broad jump	146	4 or 5 × 3 or 4 with 90 sec. rest between sets	4 or 5 × 3 or 4 with 90 sec. rest between sets	4 or 5 × 3 or 4 with 90 sec. rest between sets
2. 180-degree squat jump with cross-arm drive	144	4 × 2 or 3 each direction with 90 sec. rest between sets	4 × 2 or 3 each direction with 90 sec. rest between sets	4 × 2 or 3 each direction with 90 sec. rest between sets
STRENGTH				
3a. Barbell Romanian deadlift	156	5 × 3–5	5 × 3–5	5 × 3–5
3b. Stability-ball stir-the-pot	207	4 × 4–8 in each direction with 90 sec. rest between paired sets	4 × 4–8 in each direction with 90 sec. rest between paired sets	4 × 4–8 in each direction with 90 sec. rest between paired sets
SIZE				
4a. Angled barbell cross-shoulder reverse lunge	155	2 × 14 or 15 each side	4 × 6–8 each side	3 × 10–12 each side
4b. Angled barbell tight rainbow	202	2 × 14 or 15 each side with 60–90 sec. rest between paired sets	4 × 6–8 each side with 60–90 sec. rest between paired sets	3 × 10–12 each side with 60–90 sec. rest between paired sets
5a. Bulgarian split squat and Romanian deadlift combination	168	2 × 14 or 15 each side	4 × 6–8 each side	3 × 10–12 each side
5b. Reverse crunch*	211	2 × 15–20 with 60–90 sec. rest between paired sets	4 × 6–8 with 60–90 sec. rest between paired sets	3 × 10–12 with 60–90 sec. rest between paired sets
6. One-leg dumbbell bench hip thrust	177	2 × 15–20 each side with 60 sec. rest between sets	4 × 6–8 each side with 60 sec. rest between sets	3 × 10–12 each side with 60 sec. rest between sets
7. Machine leg press	165	2 × 15–20 with 90 sec. rest between sets	4 × 6–8 with 90 sec. rest between sets	3 × 10–12 with 90 sec. rest between sets
CARDIO CONDITIONING		Steady-state cardio: brisk walking outside or on treadmill—25–35 min. (page 29)	SMIT**: rower—4–6 sets of 45–60 sec. as fast as possible with 90 sec. to 2 min. rest between sets (page 28)	MCP***: unilateral farmer's-walk complex—2 or 3 sets with 2 min. rest between sets (page 59)

*There is an inverse relation between the amount of reps indicated and the weight you'll use as an anchor, as the heavier the anchor the easier the exercise becomes. Use the lightest dumbbell, kettlebell, or medicine ball as an anchor on the days you perform 6 to 8 reps, and use the heaviest anchor on the days you perform 15 to 20 reps.

**SMIT = supramaximal interval training.

***MCP = metabolic conditioning protocol.

At this point in the book, you've been provided with a variety of functional-spectrum workout programs for emphasizing muscle, emphasizing performance, or pursuing a balanced mix of the two. And, you've also been provided with the simple rationale behind the organization of each workout program. As a result, you now know how to design your own, ongoing functional-spectrum programs for performance training, muscle training, and balanced training.

Your understanding of the concepts and techniques presented in this book shows you the power of the functional-spectrum training system. It is a programming model that enables great training and conditioning because it gives you a simple path for effectively and efficiently designing exercise programs to train both your hustle and your muscle. All that's left is to help you understand *how* to customize your functional-spectrum training workouts to best fit you so that the exercises you include hold up on the training floor. That's exactly what the next chapter does!

13

Customizing Programs for Personal Results

Whether you're using the workout programs provided in this book or designing your own workouts based on the training concepts and techniques you've learned here, it's crucial that you know how to personalize workouts to *best* fit you. Regardless of your training goal, the process of personalizing your workouts hinges on five key factors: your ability, your injuries and limitations, the two C's (comfort and control), your training environment, and the principle of specificity. To use these factors to your advantage, apply the following guidelines.

Adapt Exercises Based on Your Ability

One of the biggest training mistakes, made often by trainers and coaches, involves trying to fit the individual to the exercise instead of fitting the exercise to the individual. For example, many personal trainers and strength coaches attempt to fit everyone into the mold of performing deadlifts in the conventional style with a barbell. Though well intentioned, this approach is misguided. Given the natural variations between human beings, it doesn't make sense to lead people to believe that, just because some individuals can perform the conventional-style barbell deadlift, *everyone* should be able to perform that same movement in the same manner.

Indeed, taking a one-size-fits-all approach to deadlifting, or any other exercise, not only ignores the obvious physiological differences between humans, but also can be dangerous. Sure, we are all part of the human species, just like all makes and models of car, truck, and van are part of the category that we refer to as vehicles. But, as with vehicles, humans come in all shapes and sizes; your own size and shape are determined by your structure, which in turn determines function. For example, a Mini Cooper and a minivan are made up of the same basic parts (e.g., four wheels, two axles) and can perform the same basic driving functions (e.g., go forward and backward, turn right and left, stop and start). But you'd never expect a Mini Cooper to drive and handle in the same way as a minivan because of the different ways in which their (same) basic parts are put together.

This is exactly why it's unrealistic to expect a guy who's built like an American football running back to move in the same way as a guy built like a lineman. Granted, both can change levels, run, push, pull, twist, and so on; however, they perform the movements in different ways based on their differing structures. Because of these individual variations in the ways that humans move, no given exercise can exactly match everyone's movements. Therefore, each person must choose the particular exercise variations that best fit how he or she moves.

In the case of the deadlift exercise, because we all come in different shapes and sizes, it's smartest to choose a deadlift style and variation—and plenty are provided in chapter 6—that fits you, rather than trying to fit yourself to a specific type of deadlift. Depending on individual ability, some people can use several deadlift variations and styles, whereas other people are more limited in the options that they can use safely.

For example, some people—based on their unique structure, ability, or injury history—may be unable to maintain the back arch needed to optimize spinal stability when performing the Romanian deadlift with a barbell. Others may be able to maintain the arch but experience back issues when doing so. However, such individuals may be able to display better spinal control—or do so without experiencing back issues—when performing hybrid deadlifts or sumo deadlifts. These styles offer slightly different joint positioning, due to a wider stance and more upright torso position, that may be more conducive to a given person's unique structure, ability, or injury history.

This book provides a multitude of exercise variations not only to diversify your training but also to make note of the variations of "normal" in the way that humans move. Some exercises just don't fit well with certain bodies. We all move a bit differently, based on size and shape, which is dictated by each person's unique skeletal framework and body proportions. In addition, injury, loss of cartilage, and natural degenerative processes in joints (e.g., arthritis) can influence how we move. For these reasons, trying to fit every person to the same exercise movement is potentially dangerous. If doing so goes against an individual's movement capability, it could cause a new problem or exacerbate an existing one.

Work Around—Not Through—Injuries and Limitations

If an exercise hurts you—for whatever reason—find a modification or an alternative that doesn't hurt. Now, we're not talking here about the sensation associated with muscle fatigue. We're talking about aches and pains that exist outside the gym or flare up when you perform certain movements. Such problem areas may simply need time to heal through rest, or they may be injuries—compromised areas of your body that can no longer tolerate the same level of load and do not improve.

Either way, you're not helping the situation by training through pain. Although this fact should be obvious, many people are stubborn and use exercises that cause them pain—a practice that is often the product of having more ego than brains. Continuing to perform exercises that cause you pain could very well make things worse and lead to further damage, which could change a painful area from something you can easily train around to something that's more debilitating. In short, don't train through pain; train *around* it.

So, what if you can't squat because you have bum knees? What if you can't do bench presses or overhead lifts because of lingering shoulder injuries? What if your bad back makes barbell deadlifts a bad idea? Over the years, I've worked on these issues with lots of people at all fitness levels, and I've developed a list of alternative exercises that helped them get bigger and stronger. I do this with a concept that I refer to as *joint-friendly training*.

Drawing on that experience, I'm providing you here with a list of joint-friendly training exercises that you can use to work around sensitive spots and still make gains in muscle and performance! Before getting into specific exercises, however, it's time to wave the obligatory caution flag: Before switching out an exercise provided in the workout programs for one listed here, make sure that the aches and pains you have aren't caused by either suboptimal exercise techniques or too much training with too little recovery.

PROBLEM   Knee issues that are aggravated by traditional-style squats and lunges

SOLUTION   Try the following lower-body exercises to build stronger legs with bad knees.

One-leg one-arm dumbbell Romanian deadlift (page 149)

One-leg 45-degree cable Romanian deadlift (page 150)

One-leg one-arm angled barbell Romanian deadlift (page 151)

Lateral lunge with cross-body reach (page 152)

Barbell Romanian deadlift (page 156)

Barbell hybrid deadlift (page 158)

Barbell good morning (page 162)

Dumbbell anterior lunge (page 172)

Weight-sled push (page 173)

Weight-sled forward pull (page 174)

Weight-sled lateral pull (page 176)

One-leg dumbbell bench hip thrust (page 177)

Hip-thrust hamstring-curl combo (page 178)

One-leg hip-thrust hamstring curl combo (page 178)

One-leg hip lift (page 179)

Low lateral mini-band shuffle (page 180)

Lateral mini-band shuffle (page 180)

Supine hip-bridge march with mini band (page 181)

45-degree hip extension (page 182)

Nordic hamstring curl (page 183)

Stability-ball leg curl (page 184)

One-leg stability-ball leg curl (page 184)

Glute-ham roller leg curl (page 185)

Machine seated hamstring curl (page 186)

PROBLEM   Back issues that prevent you from loading your spine with a barbell or trap bar on squats and deadlifts

SOLUTION   Try the following lower-body exercises to build stronger legs despite a bad back.

One-leg 45-degree cable Romanian deadlift (page 150)

One-leg elevated offset reverse lunge (page 153)

One-leg offset traveling lunge (page 154)

Angled barbell cross-shoulder reverse lunge (page155)

Goblet squat (page 164)

Machine leg press (page 165)

One-leg knee-tap squat (page 166)

Bulgarian split squat (page 167)

Dumbbell reverse lunge (page 169)

Elevated dumbbell reverse lunge (page 169)

Dumbbell fighter's lunge (page 170)

Traveling lunge (page 171)

Bench step-up (page 172)

Weight-sled push (page 173)

Weight-sled forward pull (page 174)

Weight-sled backward pull (page 175)

Weight-sled lateral pull (page 176)

One-leg dumbbell bench hip thrust (page 177)

Hip thrust hamstring-curl combo (page 178)

One-leg hip thrust hamstring curl combo (page 178)

One-leg hip lift (page 179)

Lateral mini-band shuffle (page 180)

Low lateral mini-band shuffle (page 180)

Supine hip-bridge march with mini band (page 181)

Stability-ball leg curl (page 184)

Glute-ham roller leg curl (page 185)

Machine seated hamstring curl (page 186)

Machine leg extension (page 187)

PROBLEM   An injury or limitation that puts unwanted stress on the shoulder joint during traditional-style press-type movements (e.g., bench press, overhead press)

SOLUTION   Try the following pushing exercises to work around shoulder issues.

Angled barbell press (page 82)

Angled barbell rotational push press (page 83)

Heavy-band step and press (page 96)

One-arm cable press (page 84)

Remember, these are options to experiment with to see if you're able to perform them without pain. Certain injuries are more limiting than others, and there are no guarantees as to which, if any, of these exercises will work for you. Sometimes a joint has an issue that prevents a person from doing much of anything with it. That's okay, as long as you work around it and focus more on exercising the rest of your body.

If you are *not* limited by injury, aches, or pains, joint-friendly exercises can help you maintain that winning streak. Not only are they easier on your most vulnerable joints, but also they provide new and challenging ways to build muscle and improve your strength, athleticism, and work capacity. That's why they're included in the functional-spectrum training system and integrated into many of the workout programs provided in this book.

Use the Two C's When Selecting Exercises

You have a wide variety of exercise options to choose from in the pushing, pulling, lower-body, and core training chapters of this book. Therefore, if, say, a certain pulling exercise hurts you, simply experiment with other pulling options provided in the same exercise category until you find one that you can do without discomfort. When selecting exercises—whether you have limitations or not—use the following two simple criteria to make effective choices.

- Comfort—The movement is pain free, feels natural, works within your current physiology, and so on.
- Control—You can execute the movement technique and body positioning as indicated in the exercise description. For example, when squatting, you display good knee and spinal alignment throughout and use smooth, deliberate movement.

Again, when we talk about discomfort in this context, we are not talking about the sensation associated with muscle fatigue or "feeling the burn." Rather, we're talking about aches and pains that exist outside the gym or flare up when you perform certain movements.

To allow for comfort and control, you may need to modify (shorten) the range of motion or adjust the hand or foot placement of a particular exercise to fit your current ability to honor the joint alignment cues provided in the exercise description. In addition, in some cases, you may just have to avoid certain exercises and emphasize other options.

Work Within Your Training Environment

There's an old saying that a good craftsperson never blames the tools. This perspective applies perfectly to the training and conditioning arena because we're not always able to use all of the exercise equipment we'd like to. We may be limited, for example, due to being in a crowded gym or by training at home or in a small hotel gym with limited equipment and space.

The workout programs provided in the preceding chapters have been designed with the big-box gym member in mind. For instance, they group exercises requiring immobile equipment (e.g., squat rack or machine) with exercises using mobile equipment (e.g., dumbbells, resistance bands). This mixture enables you to bring the mobile equipment to the immobile equipment and remain there without having to walk all over the gym and lose the equipment you're using to another member. You can use this same strategy when designing your own functional-spectrum training workouts.

Of course, some training environments contain limited space or equipment and therefore are not conducive to performing certain exercises included in the programs provided in this book. In such cases, simply adjust the program by substituting another exercise option from the same category that better fits with your training environment. In most areas of life, success involves making good adjustments, and this book provides you with more than enough exercise options to adjust to any training environment.

Use the Principle of Specificity

If you want to become more explosive (i.e., improve movement speed), use explosive exercises (i.e., total-body power exercises). If you want to improve strength, incorpo-

A Word on Nutrition

It's no secret that what you eat affects not only your overall health but also your training results. Therefore, in order to help you achieve the best results from the training concepts and techniques provided in this book—and to help maximize your overall health—I offer the following simple nutritional guidelines: Eat mostly foods based on fruits and vegetables and on high-quality meats, eggs, and fish (or protein substitutes, for vegetarians and vegans). Limit your intake of refined foods, simple sugars, hydrogenated oil, and alcohol. And don't overeat.

If you start by focusing on the quality of the foods you eat—emphasizing fruits, vegetables, high-quality proteins—you'll likely end up taking in fewer calories without even counting them. Indeed, when it comes to calories, the easiest approach is to first emphasize the quality (i.e., nutrient density) of the foods you eat rather than the quantity (i.e., the number of calories) and see where that gets you. It spells success for most people because fruits, veggies, and lean proteins are generally lower in calories than are fast food and candy. You don't just want to be well fed; you want to be well nourished.

Sometimes it seems that contradictory scientific conclusions about nutrition appear almost daily. However, if you scrutinize them, remain skeptical of "magic" and "miracle" claims, and avoid being taken in by marketing hype, you will see that most legitimate studies amount to no more than tinkering with the basic nutritional principles and simple advice that I've provided here.

rate some training with heavier loads. This is specificity of adaptation. If you want to improve your rotational ability for a rotary-oriented sport, use a variety of rotational exercises at various speeds and loads. This is specificity of muscle action and movement. Put simply, your goals ultimately determine the exercises that need to be a part of your workout routine.

When designing your own functional-spectrum training programs, if you follow the principle of specificity—along with the other simple guidelines provided in this chapter—you won't go wrong with your exercise applications. In using your chosen exercises, look for improvements in the amount of weight lifted; your quality of movement and efficiency; your ability to go longer and harder; and your ability to recover between sets. In other words, if you're training, for example, to improve your strength, make sure that you're continually progressing by gradually working with heavier loads or performing more reps with the same load, during the duration of each workout program.

Along with good nutrition and good sleep, the other keys to successful training are continued intensity, variety, and specificity. The functional-spectrum training system enables you to apply these principles in a simple yet comprehensive, fully customizable programming framework in order to achieve better long-term training results.

In this book, I've given you everything you need to know—and nothing you don't—in order to safely and effectively build muscle, improve your performance, and get into record shape. Better still, you now have the tools to develop your own ongoing functional-spectrum training workouts that suit both your needs and the limitations of your gym.

My part has now come to an end, and the rest depends on you. It's your turn to put these great training methods and techniques into practice and get after it!

REFERENCES

Chapter 1

1. Harman, E. The biomechanics of resistance exercise. In: Baechle, ER, and Earle, RW (eds.), NSCA's Essentials of Strength Training and Conditioning. (3rd ed.) Champaign, IL: Human Kinetics; 25-55, 2000.

2. Otsuji, T., Abe, M., and H. Kinoshita. 2002. After-effects of using a weighted bat on subsequent swing velocity and batters' perceptions of swing velocity and heaviness. *Perceptual and Motor Skills* 94 (1):119-26.

3. Southard, D., and L. Groomer. 2003. Warm-up with baseball bats of varying moments of inertia: Effect on bat velocity and swing pattern. *Research Quarterly for Exercise and Sport* 74 (3): 270–76.

4. Brown, J.M., and W. Gilleard. 1991. Transition from slow to ballistic movement: development of triphasic electromyogram patterns. *European Journal of Applied Physiology and Occupational Physiology* 63 (5): 381–86.

5. Morrison, S., and J.G. Anson. 1999. Natural goal-directed movements and the triphasic EMG. *Motor Control* 3 (4): 346–71.

6. Brown, S.H., and J.D. Cooke. 1990. Movement-related phasic muscle activation. I. Relations with temporal profile of movement. *Journal of Neurophysiology* 63 (3): 455–64.

7. Meylan, C., T. McMaster, J. Cronin, N.I. Mohammad, C. Rogers, and M. Deklerk. 2009. Single-leg lateral, horizontal, and vertical jump assessment: Reliability, interrelationships, and ability to predict sprint and change-of-direction performance. *Journal of Strength and Conditioning Research* 23 (4): 1140–47.

8. Logan, G., and W. McKinney. 1970. The serape effect. In *Anatomic Kinesiology* (3rd ed.), ed. A. Lockhart, 287–302. Dubuque, IA: Brown.

9. Vleeming, A., A.L. Pool-Goudzwaard, R. Stoeckart, J.P. van Wingerden, and C.J. Snijders. 1995. The posterior layer of the thoracolumbar fascia. Its function in load transfer from spine to legs. *Spine* 20 (7): 753–58.

10. Santana, J.C., F.J. Vera-Garcia, and S.M. McGill. 2007. A kinetic and electromyographic comparison of the standing cable press and bench press. *Journal of Strength and Conditioning Research* 21 (4):1271–77.

Chapter 2

1. Schoenfeld, B.J. 2010. The mechanisms of muscle hypertrophy and their application to resistance training. *Journal of Strength and Conditioning Research* 24 (10): 2857–72.

2. Adam, A., and C.J. De Luca. 2003. Recruitment order of motor units in human vastus lateralis muscle is maintained during fatiguing contractions. *Journal of Neurophysiology* 90: 2919–27.

3. Cheung, K., P. Hume, and L. Maxwell. 2003. Delayed onset muscle soreness: Treatment strategies and performance factors. *Sports Medicine* 33 (2):145–64.

4. Grant, A.C., I.F. Gow, V.A. Zammit, and D.B. Shennan. 2000. Regulation of protein synthesis in lactating rat mammary tissue by cell volume. *Biochimica et Biophysica Acta* 1475 (1): 39–46

5. Stoll, B. 1992. Liver cell volume and protein synthesis. *Biochemical Journal* 287 (Pt. 1): 217–22.

6. Millar, I. D., M.C. Barber, M.A. Lomax, M.T. Travers, and D.B. Shennan. 1997. Mammary protein synthesis is acutely regulated by the cellular hydration state. *Biochemical and Biophysical Research Communications* 230 (2): 351–55.

7. Mitchell, C.J., et al. 2012. Resistance exercise load does not determine training-mediated hypertrophic gains in young men. *Journal of Applied Physiology* 113: 71–77.

8. Santana, J.C., F.J. Vera-Garcia, and S.M. McGill. 2007. A kinetic and electromyographic comparison of the standing cable press and bench press. *Journal of Strength and Conditioning Research* 21 (4): 1271–77.

9. Baechle, T.R., and R.W. Earle. 2008. *Essentials of Strength Training and Conditioning.* 3rd ed. Champaign, IL: Human Kinetics.

10. Werner, S.L., et al. 2008. Relationships between ball velocity and throwing mechanics in collegiate baseball pitchers. *Journal of Shoulder and Elbow Surgery* 17 (6): 905–8.

11. Rhea, M.R., et al. 2002. A comparison of linear and daily undulating periodized programs with equated volume and intensity for strength. *Journal of Strength and Conditioning Research* 16 (2): 250–55.

12. Prestes, J., et al. 2009. Comparison between linear and daily undulating periodized resistance training to increase strength. *Journal of Strength and Conditioning Research* 23 (9): 2437–42.

13. Miranda, F., et al. 2011. Effects of linear vs. daily undulatory periodized resistance training on maximal and submaximal strength gains. *Journal of Strength and Conditioning Research* 25 (7): 1824-30.

14. Simão, R., et al. 2012. Comparison between nonlinear and linear periodized resistance training: Hypertrophic and strength effects. *Journal of Strength and Conditioning Research* 26 (5): 1389–95.

Chapter 3

1. Neal, C.M., et al. 2013. Six weeks of a polarized training-intensity distribution leads to greater physiological and performance adaptations than a threshold model in trained cyclists. *Journal of Applied Physiology* 114 (4): 461–71.

2. Muñoz, I., et al. 2014. Does polarized training improve performance in recreational runners? *International Journal of Sports Physiology and Performance* 9 (2): 265–72.

3. Cicioni-Kolsky, D., C. Lorenzen, M.D. Williams, and J.G. Kemp. 2013. Endurance and sprint benefits of high-intensity and supra-maximal interval training. *Eur J Sport Sci* 13(3):304-11.

4. Zuhl, M. and L. Kravitz. Hiit Vs. Continuous Endurance Training: Battle Of The Aerobic Titans. *IDEA Fitness Journal* » February 2012. http://www.ideafit.com/fitness-library/hiit-vs-continuous-endurance-training-battle-of-the-aerobic-titans.

5. Mikkola, J., H. Rusko, et al. 2012. Neuromuscular and cardiovascular adaptations during concurrent strength and endurance training in untrained men. *Int J Sports Med.* 33(9):702-10.

6. Harber, M.P., et al. 2012. Aerobic exercise training induces skeletal muscle hypertrophy and age-dependent adaptations in myofiber function in young and older men. *J Appl Physiol.* 113(9):1495-504.

7. Konopka, A.R., M. Harber. 2014. Skeletal Muscle Hypertrophy after Aerobic Exercise Training. *Exerc Sport Sci Rev.* 42(2):53-61.

Chapter 7

1. Dominguez, R., and R. Gadja. 1982. *Total body training*. New York: Scribner's.

2. Nuzzo, J.L., et al. 2008. Trunk muscle activity during stability ball and free weight exercises. *Journal of Strength and Conditioning Research* 22 (1): 95–102.

3. Martuscello, J.M., et al. 2013. Systematic review of core muscle activity during physical fitness exercises. *J Strength Cond Res.* (6):1684-98.

4. Gottschall, J.S., J. Mills, and B. Hastings .2013. Integration core exercises elicit greater muscle activation than isolation exercises.. *J Strength Cond Res.* 27(3):590-6.

Chapter 9

1. DeFreitas, J.M., et al. 2011. An examination of the time course of training-induced skeletal muscle hypertrophy. *European Journal of Applied Physiology* 111 (11): 2785–90.

2. Seynnes, O.R., et al. 2007. Early skeletal muscle hypertrophy and architectural changes in response to high-intensity resistance training. *Journal of Applied Physiology* 102 (1): 368–73.

3. Horwath, R., and L. Kravitz. 2008. Postactivation potentiation: A brief review. *IDEA Fitness Journal* 5 (5): 21–23.

ABOUT THE AUTHOR

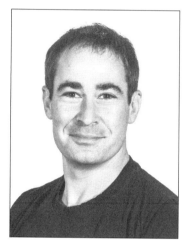

Nick Tumminello is the owner of Performance University International, which provides strength training and conditioning for athletes and educational programs for trainers and coaches all over the world.

As an educator, Tumminello has become known as the trainer of trainers. He has presented at international fitness conferences in Norway, Iceland, China, and Canada. He has been a featured presenter at conferences held by such organizations as the IDEA Health & Fitness Association, the National Strength and Conditioning Association, and DCAC Fitness Conventions, along with teaching staff trainings at fitness clubs throughout the United States. Tumminello holds workshops and mentorship programs in his hometown of Fort Lauderdale, Florida. He is the author of *Strength Training for Fat Loss* (Human Kinetics, 2014), has produced more than 20 instructional DVDs, and is the coauthor of the National Strength and Conditioning Association's *Program Design Essentials* and *Foundations of Fitness Programming*. Tumminello is also a continuing education course provider for the American Council on Exercise, the National Academy of Sports Medicine, and the National Strength and Conditioning Association.

Tumminello has been a fitness professional since 1998 and co-owned a private training center in Baltimore, Maryland, from 2001 to 2011. He has worked with a variety of exercise enthusiasts of all ages and fitness levels, including physique and performance athletes from the amateur to the professional ranks. From 2002 to 2011, Tumminello was the strength and conditioning coach for the Ground Control MMA fight team and is a consultant and expert for clothing and equipment companies such as Sorinex, Dynamax, Hylete, and Reebok.

Tumminello's articles have appeared in more than 50 major health and fitness magazines, including *Men's Health*, *Men's Fitness*, *Oxygen*, *Muscle Mag*, *Fitness Rx*, *Sweat Rx*, *Status*, *Train Hard Fight Easy*, *Fighters Only*, and *Fight!* Tumminello is also a featured contributor to several popular fitness training websites. He has been featured in two *New York Times* best-selling exercise books, on the front page of Yahoo and YouTube, and in the *ACE Personal Trainer Manual*. In 2015, Tumminello was inducted into the Personal Trainer Hall of Fame.

Tumminello writes a popular fitness training blog at PerformanceU.net.